D0948852

HEALTH AND SOCIETY IN REVOLUTIONARY RUSSIA

HEALTH AND SOCIETY
IN REVOLUTIONARY RUSSIA

EDITED BY

SUSAN GROSS SOLOMON

AND

JOHN F. HUTCHINSON

INDIANA UNIVERSITY PRESS
Bloomington and Indianapolis

This book was brought to publication with the assistance of a grant from the Andrew W. Mellon Foundation to the Russian and East European Institute, Indiana University, and the Center for Russian and East European Studies, University of Michigan.

The paper used in this publication meets the minimum requirements of American
National Standards for Information Sciences—Permanence of Paper for Printed
Library Materials, ANSI Z39.48-1984.
⊗™
Manufactured in the United States of America

Library of Congress Cataloging-in-Publication Data

Health and society in revolutionary Russia / edited by Susan Gross
Solomon and John F. Hutchinson.
    p. cm. — (Indiana-Michigan series in Russian and East
European studies)
    ''Published in cooperation with the Centre for Russian and East
European Studies, University of Toronto.''
    Includes bibliographical references.
    ISBN 0-253-35332-7 (alk. paper)
    1. Social medicine—Soviet Union—History. 2. Soviet Union—
History—Revolution, 1917–1921. I. Solomon, Susan Gross.
II. Hutchinson, John F. III. University of Toronto. Centre for
Russian and East European Studies. IV. Series.
RA18.3.S65S63 1990   89-45410
362.1'0947'09041—dc20   CIP
    1 2 3 4 5 94 93 92 91 90

CONTENTS

Acknowledgments

This book had its origins in a conference on the the the history of Russian and Soviet public health held May 7–10, 1986, at the University of Toronto. The conference brought together thirty scholars from Britain, Australia, the United States, and Canada. In planning and running the conference, we accumulated a number of institutional debts which we take pleasure in acknowledging. We are grateful to the National Council for Soviet and East European Research which generously both supported the conference and the editing of the volume and to Massey College (and its bursar, Colin Friesen) of the University of Toronto which so graciously hosted the conference. In a true spirit of international cooperation, the Centers for Russian and East European Studies of the University of Michigan (under the directorship of William G. Rosenberg) and the University of Toronto (under the directorship of Timothy Colton) jointly sponsored the conference. The Michigan center shouldered the job of administering the National Council grant; the Toronto center responded with sympathy to the periodic pleas of one of the editors for contingency funding.

The conference was greatly enriched by the presence of a *kollektiv* of outstanding commentators from the fields of Russian and Soviet history and the history of medicine and public health: the late Kendall Bailes, Mark Field, Loren Graham, David Joravsky, John Keep, Judith Leavitt, Russell Maulitz, Pauline Mazumdar, Peter Solomon, Barbara Rosenkrantz, Ronald Suny. Their combination of enthusiasm and high standards guided us as we edited the volume. To the authors of the essays, we express our special thanks for the good humor with which they endured the repeated queries we raised and the intellectual vigor with which they pursued the leads we suggested. To Edith S. Klein of the University of Toronto we are deeply indebted for the intelligence and care with which she undertook the tasks of editorial assistant and conference assistant. The staff of the Department of Political Science, University of Toronto, cheerfully executed a variety of technical tasks indispensable in bringing a volume such as this to fruition.

Introduction

The Problem of Health Reform in Russia

The Soviet health crisis of the 1980s has led the Soviet government to assign high priority to the reform of public health and medicine. This is not the first time that the reform of public health was high on the agenda of a Soviet leadership. Almost immediately after the Revolution, concerted attempts were made to transform the system of public health in order to deal with the devastating effects of war and revolution. Not surprisingly, the current commitment to health reform in the Soviet Union has directed the attention of Western observers to the earlier attempts at change. But those with an interest in history would do well to look back beyond 1917 for, as the essays in this book suggest, the problems encountered in reforming public health after the Revolution had important roots in the period before the Bolsheviks took power.

By the beginning of the twentieth century, thoughtful Russians had come to the conclusion that making their country healthy would require a struggle with the tsarist regime. In their view, it was the deadening hand of the St. Petersburg bureaucracy that was largely responsible for Russia's appallingly high morbidity and mortality rates. The country's most prestigious medical society, the Pirogov Society of Russian Physicians, propagated and perpetuated a credo according to which St. Petersburg bureaucrats were the embodiment of all evil whereas community physicians (those employed by zemstvos and municipalities) were the repository of all virtue. At the International Medical Congress in Moscow in 1899 and then at the International Hygiene Exhibition in Dresden in 1911, the community physicians successfully convinced their Western colleagues that they were the leading force for health reform in Russia and that the chief obstacle they faced was the tsarist regime itself.

The image of reform-minded community physicians standing firmly on the side of science and progress, battling a bumbling, recalcitrant, and obscurantist regime emerged in bold relief in Nancy Frieden's authoritative book, *Russian Physicians in an Era of Reform and Revolution, 1856–1905*.[1] However bold the relief, the image was tempered by Frieden's admission that community physicians strenuously resisted government attempts to raise the quality of local health programs even when those attempts "reflected current thinking among health planners and epidemiologists."[2] In the years since the publication of Frieden's book, the portrait of the "progressive" community physician has been called even more seriously into question. A study of the development of Russian psychiatry has shown that psychiatrists found community physicians aggressively hostile to both their scientific claims and their professional aspirations.[3] Moreover, according to research on the bacteriological revolution in Russia, community physicians initially opposed bacteriology on the grounds that it threatened the social and environmental orientation of their program of health reform. Only when they realized that the threat had been exaggerated did they come around to accepting the new field.[4]

Just as a review of the evidence suggests that the conventional portrait of community physicians bears revision, so too recent research points to the need for a more nuanced analysis of the attitudes of tsarist officials toward health reform and of the structural possibilities for bringing reform about. A full reassessment of these issues requires recognition that although the Russian empire was, by European standards, an unhealthy place to live, neither the tsar nor his ministers wished to keep Russians in an unhealthy state. Richard Robbins has drawn attention to the fact that the famine of 1891–92 was a considerable embarrassment to the regime, as was the cholera epidemic that followed it.[5] The government could only have welcomed the idea of making Russia healthier. A healthy people, as seventeenth-century mercantilists had argued, were likely to be industrious in their work, thrifty in their habits, stable in their moods, and valiant on the battlefield. The problem was not a lack of good intentions but, rather, that so many of the proposed avenues to better health conflicted with the traditions, ideology, and structure of the autocracy.

As an absolutist regime, tsarist Russia clung to a traditional medical police approach, in which state regulation of matters of health and disease was considered part of the "well-ordered police state."[6] (In this, the Russia of Nicholas II had more in common with the Prussia of Frederick the Great or the Austria of Joseph II than it had with the England of Joseph Chamberlain or the United States of Theodore Roosevelt.) This approach rested on two premises: the belief in the importance of centralized state direction and the conviction that health affairs constituted a branch of the general civil police. From the latter premise followed the belief that matters of public health could be best directed by a trained civil administrator and that the medical police administration properly belonged as a department within a ministry of the interior. Thus conceived, the medical police approach did not challenge monarchical authority, the estate structure of society, or the conservative teachings of the established church.

In contrast to the medical police approach, most proposals for health reform in tsarist Russia began from the assumption that matters of health ought to be the exclusive prerogative of physicians, to whose expert judgment lay persons—including, or course, civil administrators—ought to defer. For their part, officials of the enormously powerful Ministry of the Interior refused to defer to "expert medical opinion" even within the ministry and blocked any attempt to establish a separate ministry of health beyond their control. In this context, even the most conservative reformers found their proposals blocked. Little wonder then that the far more ambitious plans of the community physicians did not receive a positive hearing! It was not merely that the Pirogov physicians saw themselves as the representatives of a field which demanded expert knowledge, or even that they recited, like a litany, their opposition to centralized direction. It was that, at bottom, these reformers, with their insistence on the dictates of reason and science, appeared to threaten the monarchy, the social order, and the established church. Not surprisingly, health reform under the tsarist regime was severely limited.

Little changed when the tsarist regime was replaced by the Provisional Government in February 1917. Would-be reformers who were associated with the Pirogov Society hoped that a new day was dawning, but they were quickly disillusioned. The reform of public health took a back seat first to the imperatives of war and then to the social crisis which was intensifying throughout the late summer of 1917.

When the Bolsheviks seized power, the bureaucratic apparatus of the Ministry of the Interior disintegrated. With it died both the regulative approach of traditional medical police and the belief that matters of health were only a subordinate part of general civil police. The new regime professed dedication to the dictates of reason and science. Confident of its ability to discern, organize, and achieve a better society, it set about to overhaul medicine and public health. This was no easy task: the Bolsheviks had inherited from the tsarist regime a staggering variety of public health problems, most of which had been exacerbated by three years of war.

As early as June 1918 the outlines of Soviet public health policy began to emerge. In his report to the First All-Russian Congress of Soviet Medical-Sanitary Sections, N. A. Semashko, soon to become the RSFSR's first commissar of public health, declared that henceforth health care was to be free, accessible to all, and universal. This declaration promised a revolution in the delivery of health care. As part of that revolution, the Bolsheviks introduced a variety of progressive social programs that gave evidence of the high priority which the new regime placed on the prevention of disease. In July of the same year, the new approach to public health was given organizational form: the RSFSR Commissariat of Public Health (Narkomzdrav) was created for the express purpose of integrating, coordinating, and centralizing the delivery of health care.

The content and thrust of the policy reforms require interpretation. Were these reforms, like so many of the policy initiatives introduced in this period, primarily an ad hoc response to an urgent situation, or did they flow from a carefully thought out philosophy of health care?[7] And how should we understand the creation of the new Commissariat of Public Health? The founding of an agency for public health was a natural consequence of the collapse of the tsarist Ministry of the Interior, but the form of Narkomzdrav owed much to the determination of its Bolshevik architects to avoid the pitfalls of tsarist administration by unifying all medical affairs under one institution, thus providing themselves with a structure strong enough to shape the future direction of Soviet medicine.

The leading present-day Western studies of the development of Soviet public health do not address the historical questions posed here. In the main, they approach the postrevolutionary reforms largely in terms of their contribution to the contemporary Soviet health care system,[8] with the result that several major reforms which did not endure beyond the early 1930s are overlooked. More important, the current studies assume that the reforms that did survive carried the same meaning at the time they were adopted as they do now.

Nor can the writings of Western physicians who visited the Soviet Union in the 1920s and 1930s fill the void. With few exceptions, those physicians missed the real thrust of the health reform that followed the Revolution, not for lack of sympathy, but for want of an intellectual perspective in which to interpret Soviet developments. A telling illustration of the limits of cross-cultural understanding can be found in the evaluation by prominent American public health specialists of the Soviet approach to venereal disease. The Americans who visited Soviet venereal disease dispensaries in the 1920s spoke admiringly of the comprehensiveness of the Soviet approach to the disease: the facilities they visited treated the afflicted, taught prostitutes a trade, performed social work, and provided educational counseling.[9] What the American medical visitors failed to see was that the many-faceted approach they admired so much was a consequence of the fact that in the Soviet Union venereal disease was the province of the field of "social hygiene," which embraced all illnesses whose spread and incidence could be traced to societal factors. In the United States, social hygiene was much more narrowly conceived; its reach extended only to sexually related diseases.

For the historian, the subject of Soviet health reform poses numerous difficulties. The first problem is that of identifying the goals of the health reform. It is tempting to ascribe either a single goal or, at the very least, a clear rank-ordering of goals to those who made decisions about Soviet public health. Yet research reveals that Bolshevik specialists were almost always in pursuit of two goals, one practical, the other ideological: remedying appalling health conditions and differentiating themselves at any cost from the previous regime. In some instances, these two goals came into conflict. A striking example is Soviet insurance medicine of the twenties. In 1921, the Bolsheviks decided to dismember the workers' insurance movement they had inherited from the tsarist regime. Despite arguments that the prerevolutionary insurance movement had been effective in meeting the health needs of the workers, the new government refused to tolerate its existence because that movement was independent of the state-controlled trade unions which it had decreed to be the sole legitimate focus of workers' allegiance.[10]

Implementing goals proved even more difficult than formulating them. For between the design of a reform and its translation into practice there stood a formidable array of constraints—economic, geographical, and professional. These constraints had the effect of modifying, if not vitiating, goals. To be specific, notwithstanding the good intentions of those who made policy for health care, economic problems often torpedoed the aims of reform. An excellent illustration is the fate of the decree of 1920 legalizing abortion in the Soviet Union. As might have been predicted, the 1920 statute resulted in a deluge of women seeking abortions. In response to the inability of Soviet facilities to cope with the demand, the regime introduced a series of restrictions on eligibility and established commissions whose mandate was to assess whether the patient qualified for abortion under the new restrictions. At the same time, fees were introduced for those who could afford to pay. Regrettably, data were collected only on the patients who applied to the commissions for free abortions, but one Western physician who visited Soviet abortaria reported that requests from fee-paying patients were almost never refused.[11]

The sheer size of the Soviet Union made implementation of reform particularly difficult. In many instances reforms trumpeted at the center never penetrated the periphery. For example, in an effort to reform traditional medical education in line periphery. For example, in an effort to reform traditional medical education in line with the new philosophy of public health, the first *kafedra* of social hygiene was established in 1921 for the three medical faculties in Moscow. In keeping with the policy of standardizing medical education throughout the RSFSR, similar *kafedry* were mandated for all medical faculties. The transcript of a conference of medical teachers convened in 1928 revealed, however, that for many medical faculties on the periphery, the reform had remained a paper exercise. In outlying regions, new *kafedry* of social hygiene were often established without any staff; not infrequently, the head of such a *kafedra* occupied several other chairs simultaneously.[12] For all of its declared commitment to centralization, the Bolshevik regime had yet to conquer the periphery.

The entrenched interests of the medical profession constituted an obstacle of a different order. The medical profession had its traditions, its hallowed approaches, and its self-image, all of which affected its receptivity to reform. Despite the fact that the Soviet state served as the sole patron and client of all physicians, Soviet sources record instances of concerted resistance to change on the part of certain groups of medical specialists. For example, some prominent psychiatrists opposed the increasing tendency in the 1920s to funnel alcoholics into psychiatric hospitals. Decrying what they termed the "overpsychiatrization" of alcoholism, these psychiatrists argued that psychiatric facilities ought to be reserved for the most acutely mentally ill patients.[13] Likewise, a significant number of obstetricians and gynecologists voiced opposition to the 1920 decree legalizing abortion on the grounds that abortions adversely affected the childbearing capacity of women.[14] Finally, professors of clinical medicine resisted the new emphasis on prevention so widely touted in the medical schools.[15]

This book focuses on the dilemmas of reform in Russian and Soviet public health, but its essays also raise questions about the enterprise of health reform which cannot fail to intrigue both historians of the development of public health in other countries and historians of Russia after 1917. The Soviet reform effort began with all the propitious signs: a patron (the state) dedicated to rectifying longstanding inequities in health care delivery and to upgrading the health of the population as a whole, a willingness—even an eagerness—on the part of those who spoke for the field of public health to break with the past in their teaching and research, and a commitment by those who made policy for health to create new structures for the delivery of medical care. Even these advantages proved insufficient to ensure the viability of the reforms. This collection of essays documents in stunning detail the formidable array of obstacles, real and perceived, encountered by the Soviet reform effort. These findings force us to recognize that in some fields social change cannot be legislated from above. Change, like continuity, requires the support of those most affected—whether they be professionals administering medical care, clients receiving medical treatment, researchers who study the delivery of health care, or teachers of medicine. Without the support of at least some of these sectors, even the best-intentioned reforms will lack the legitimacy required for implementation and the staying power required to make a difference.

NOTES

1. Nancy M. Frieden, *Russian Physicians in an Era of Reform and Revolution, 1856–1905* (Princeton, N.J., 1981).

2. Ibid., p. 288.

3. Julie V. Brown, "The Professionalization of Russian Psychiatry, 1857–1911" (Ph.D. diss., University of Pennsylvania, 1981).

4. John F. Hutchinson, "Tsarist Russia and the Bacteriological Revolution," *Journal of the History of Medicine and Allied Sciences,* 40 (1985), pp. 420–39.

5. Richard G. Robbins, Jr., *Famine in Russia, 1891–1892* (New York, 1975); see also Nancy M. Frieden, "The Russian Cholera Epidemic, 1892–1893, and Medical Professionalization," *Journal of Social History,* 10 (1977), pp. 538–59.

6. See Marc Raeff, *The Well-Ordered Police State: Social and Institutional Change through Law in the Germanies and Russia, 1600–1800* (New Haven, Conn., 1983); George Rosen, "Cameralism and the Concept of Medical Police," *Bulletin of the History of Medicine,* 27 (1953), pp. 21–42; John T. Alexander, *Bubonic Plague in Early Modern Russia: Public Health and Urban Disaster* (Baltimore, 1980).

7. This debate has colored Western discussions of all Soviet social and economic policies put in place during the period of War Communism (1918–21).

8. For example, Michael Ryan, *The Organization of Soviet Medical Care* (Oxford, 1978); William A. Knaus, *Inside Russian Medicine* (New York, 1981); Michael Kaser, *Health Care in the Soviet Union and Eastern Europe* (London, 1976).

9. Rachelle S. Yarros, M.D., "Social Hygiene Observations in Soviet Russia," *Journal of Social Hygiene,* 16, no. 8 (1930), pp. 449–64; Ralph Reynolds, M.D., "Social Hygiene in Soviet Russia," ibid., pp. 465–82.

10. See Solomon Schwartz, *Sotsial'noe strakhovanie v Rossii v 1917–1919 godakh* (New York, 1968).

11. See Frederick J. Taussig, *Abortion: Spontaneous and Induced* (St. Louis, 1936). According to Taussig, the commissions which were originally charged with determining the medical eligibility of women for abortions came over time to be concerned primarily with the ability of the patient to pay. "Any pay case, with certain minor restrictions, was accepted, but in order to obtain free service the individual had to prove her inability to meet the charge, before the Commission." Ibid., p. 407.

12. The transcript of the entire conference was carried in "Trudy vtorogo soveshchaniia predstavitelei profilakticheskikh kafedr," *Sotsial'naia gigiena,* 13 (1928). For the assessment of developments on the periphery, see "Preniia," ibid., p. 235.

13. For a discussion of this attitude, see Susan Gross Solomon, "David and Goliath in Soviet Public Health: The Rivalry of Social Hygienists and Psychiatrists for Authority over the *Bytovoi* Alcoholic," *Soviet Studies,* XLI, no. 2 (April 1989), pp. 254–75.

14. For an unusually direct presentation of this case, see M. G. Serdukoff, "L'avortement artificiel en tant que traumatisme biologique et ses suites," *Gynécologie et Obstétrique,* 17, no. 3 (1928), pp. 196–208. Serdukoff was the director of the Grauermann Institute of Obstetrics and Gynecology in Moscow.

15. At the 1928 meeting of the representatives of prophylactic *kafedry* in Leningrad, two reliable speakers—Dr. Deichman, whose specialty was the study of alcoholism, and Dr. Gromashevskii, who was a leading authority on epidemiology—referred to a revolt among professors of clinical medicine against the new preventive emphasis in the medical schools. "Preniia," pp. 229, 232.

Part One

Public Health in Tsarist Russia

JOHN F. HUTCHINSON

"Who Killed Cock Robin?"

An Inquiry into the Death of Zemstvo Medicine

THE PROBLEM OF CONTINUITY AND CHANGE

In the summer of 1917, Charles-Edward Amory Winslow, professor of Public Health at Yale University and a leading figure in the public health movement, visited Russia with the American Red Cross mission.[1] On his return home, he lavished praise on Russian zemstvo medicine for its achievements in medical care and sanitary reform.[2] Like the European physicians who attended the Twelfth International Medical Congress in Moscow in 1899,[3] Winslow was impressed that zemstvo medicine provided the rural population with freely accessible scientific medical care, as well as with advice and education concerning hygiene and sanitation. Winslow was convinced that in the new democratic Russia which was being created by the Revolution much more could be expected from this vibrant force. As he said in his report to the American Public Health Association,

> The opportunity for developing preventive education work in connection with such a system is practically unlimited. . . . We may therefore look in the future, as zemstvo and municipal medicine develop and acquire the educational and preventive quality which is in accord with modern progress, for unprecedented successes in the control of preventable disease in the great sister Republic.[4]

Only one year after Winslow's visit to Russia, the monthly organ of the Pirogov Society of Russian Physicians, *The Community Physician [Obshchestvennyi vrach]*, published an article entitled "The Funeral of Zemstvo Medicine."[5] Written by K. G. Slavskii, a prominent Moscow zemstvo physician, the article predicted that the Bolshevik government's recent decision (July 1918) to establish a Commissariat of Public Health (Narkomzdrav) meant the death of zemstvo medicine. Bureaucratic controls reminiscent of the worst excesses of tsarism would, Slavskii predicted, choke the life out of zemstvo medicine; he concluded gloomily that "The old *prikaz* medicine is being reborn."[6] Many zemstvo physicians agreed; they saw the establishment of Narkomzdrav as proof that the Bolsheviks, like the tsarist government, would use bureaucratic centralization to destroy the zemstvo medical tradition.[7] In America, Winslow himself was soon singing a different tune, speaking and writing about the Bolshevik regime as if it had extinguished all hope that medicine and public health would benefit from the Russian Revolution.[8]

If Slavskii and Winslow were both correct, the conclusion to be drawn is that the Bolsheviks destroyed the zemstvo medical tradition and created an entirely new system of centralized state medicine. In broad outline, this was the picture painted by Mark Field some three decades ago when he argued that "the Bolshevik revolution profoundly affected the organization of medical services by bringing about their centralization and bureaucratization."[9] Relying on Barsukov's account of how the Bolsheviks had "silenced the most influential voice of the prerevolutionary medical profession,"[10] the Pirogov Society, Field pictured the Bolshevik Revolution as a radical break with prerevolutionary medicine. This view has been confirmed, from an entirely different viewpoint, by the Soviet historian I. D. Strashun, who argued that the failure of the 1905 revolution led the zemstvo medical tradition into a blind alley where its protagonists simply bickered and squabbled among themselves until the Bolshevik Revolution provided the impetus for the further development of Russian medicine.[11] Strashun understandably avoided any suggestion that Narkomzdrav might have had tsarist antecedents; indeed, he implied that its establishment was in fact a kind of funeral for zemstvo medicine. Yet, where Slavskii had protested against what he regarded as the stifling of a living organism, Strashun claimed that the Bolsheviks were simply burying a moldering corpse.

Not until 1979 was there a serious attempt to question this picture of the October Revolution as a decisive turning point in Russian medical history. Peter Krug's doctoral dissertation on the Pirogov Society in the years following the Revolution shattered existing assumptions—both Western and Soviet—by showing convincingly (1) that the Pirogov Society had not been suppressed in the months following the October Revolution but had remained in existence until 1922; (2) that, after a brief period of hostility and hesitation, many leading pirogovtsy worked with Bolshevik physicians and that some even joined the Communist party; and (3) that, far from engaging in the sabotage and political intrigue of which they had been accused in Stalin's day by M. I. Barsukov, Russia's former community physicians played a leading role in the building of Soviet medicine and public health.[12] To be sure, fifteen members of the Pirogov Society executive had hastily signed an anti-Bolshevik declaration on November 22, 1917; their action was soon approved by the community physicians of Moscow and later ratified by those attending the March 1918 Pirogov Congress. Nonetheless, Krug argued that too much had been made of these declarations, passed at a time when zemstvo physicians feared for their positions, salaries, and careers if the Bolsheviks destroyed the zemstvos and for their very lives if the new government incited or tolerated mob violence against the intelligentsia. Once they discovered that the commissars were largely interested in changing titles and that "local public health administration . . . remained the same as it had been for at least several decades,"[13] they began to sing a new tune. By May of 1919, Krug discovered, a meeting of leading *pirogovtsy* in Moscow resolved that " . . . the basic principles of public [community] medicine have remained vibrant, even in the new political and social conditions. As a matter of fact, the so-called Soviet medicine has assumed the same organizational forms and is seeking the same goals, which always constituted the essence of public medicine."[14] In Krug's opinion, the fertile zemstvo medicine that Winslow had observed not only survived October 1917 but used the Bolshevik Revolution to achieve many of its traditional goals. Reports of its death, like those concerning Mark Twain, were evidently an exaggeration.

Where do matters stand now? On the face of it, it would seem that Krug's work has revised all previous opinions: Winslow was wrong in thinking that zemstvo medicine failed to survive; Slavskii was clearly an alarmist; and Barsukov may be dismissed as a self-serving party hack. Instead of a sharp break with the past, 1917 was scarcely more than a ripple on the river of continuity which flows directly from the community medicine of prerevolutionary times to the so-called new Soviet medicine. Or was it? Can it be that Slavskii, a lifelong worker and publicist on behalf of zemstvo medicine, was so far off the mark that he mistook a helping hand for a mortal blow? If the "so-called Soviet medicine" was not essentially different from prerevolutionary zemstvo medicine, why did the former administrator of the Pirogov Society, D. N. Zhbankov—a man widely regarded as the very embodiment of the zemstvo medical tradition—refuse to have anything to do with Narkomzdrav and its agencies? And what of Strashun's claim that zemstvo medicine had burned itself out even before the outbreak of World War I: do we disregard his convincing evidence of factional strife because it does not fit the theme of continuity?[15]

The purpose of this paper is to reexamine the question of continuity and change during the Revolution through an inquest into the alleged death of zemstvo medicine. The term *zemstvo medicine* is used throughout this essay to mean not the day-to-day work of zemstvo physicians and sanitary doctors but, rather, the movement for medical, social, and political reform which was associated with the Pirogov Society. Precisely when this zemstvo medicine died is a matter of dispute. That something called zemstvo medicine was alive and flourishing at the turn of the century is contested by no one. That its "essence" was still alive in May 1919 is alleged by those who attended the meeting referred to above. There are no claims for its continued existence after May 1919 so this date may be taken as the last on which witnesses saw the victim alive. There is, however, a plethora of statements from credible witnesses who claim that zemstvo medicine was failing, dying, or even dead long before May 1919. Indeed, Slavskii's obituary notice was only the latest in a series of gloomy pronouncements, dating back to the 1905 revolution. Especially noteworthy is the fact that these statements originated not with the bureaucrats who often opposed zemstvo medicine, nor with uninformed bystanders, but with precisely those circles most closely identified with the advancement of medical science and the promotion of social progress: leading Russian specialists in public health, sanitation, bacteriology, epidemiology, and occupational hygiene. They disagreed about the date of death because there was no unanimity among them about the essence of zemstvo medicine. For some, the essence lay primarily in the apolitical humanitarian service ideal which received so much attention in the work of Nancy Frieden;[16] for others, it was active participation in radical, even revolutionary politics; for still others, it was found in local control over the type and extent of public medical services. As we shall see, the partisans of each of these viewpoints believed that "their" zemstvo medicine was dead or dying long before the Revolution of 1917.

The essential spirit of zemstvo medicine was defined by the leaders of the Pirogov Society, who planned the society's congresses, organized the work of its committees, and controlled its extensive program of publications. Between 1905 and 1917, there were significant changes in the composition of this leadership group, changes which resulted in the society's being identified with causes that it had in the past been loath to support. Indeed, it will be argued below that the substantive changes in the direction of public medical activity began to occur before and just after World War I, although their magnitude became apparent only in the course of the revolutionary year 1917. Slavskii may indeed have been correct in regarding the establishment of Narkomzdrav as the death knell of the zemstvo medicine so praised by the Pirogov Society before 1905, but he failed to acknowledge that the hands pulling the bell-rope in 1917 were not only those of Bolsheviks, but also those of his colleagues who had led the Pirogov Society during the war.

THE LEGACY OF 1905

Zemstvo physicians and the Pirogov Society shared in the bitter legacy which the Revolution of 1905 bequeathed to the Russian intelligentsia. The society's major contribution to the revolutionary upsurge had been the strongly worded political resolutions calling for a constituent assembly, universal suffrage, and basic civil liberties, which were passed at its extraordinary "Cholera" Congress, in March 1905. Although these resolutions have generally been treated within the context of the organizing campaign mounted by the political opposition to autocracy, Nancy Frieden has made a strong case for the importance of the underlying professional issues which impelled physicians to vote for an end to autocracy and the convocation of a constituent assembly.[17] It is, however, difficult to believe that anything other than left-wing political enthusiasm led participants to join the radical Union of All-Russian Medical Personnel which began to meet as soon as the formal proceedings of the congress were adjourned.[18] At its August congress, the medical union condemned the idea of a consultative assembly (the Bulygin duma proposal) and approved in principle the idea of a strike in order to achieve its political objectives. Such a strike never occurred because of the concessions granted in the tsar's Manifesto of October 17, 1905, but the resolution which approved the idea took the zemstvo physicians who voted for it closer to the revolutionary barricades than they had ever been before.

By no means all *pirogovtsy* approved of the stance taken at the 1905 "Cholera" Congress. The St. Petersburg Physicians' Mutual Assistance Society, itself an offshoot of the 1889 Pirogov Congress, included among its members most of the high-ranking bureaucrats and academics who composed the capital's medical establishment; its proceedings studiously avoided any mention of the resolutions passed at the "Cholera" Congress, and its members shunned participation in the medical union. When the next regular Pirogov Congress met in 1907, V. Ia. Kanel', himself a strong supporter of the medical union, noted the "conspicuous absence" of such Petersburg luminaries as Professor V. N. Sirotinin of the Military-Medical Academy, Professor S. M. Lukianov of the Imperial Institute of Experimental Medicine, and others who had "raised a friendly glass to the Russian physician" at the last regular Pirogov Congress in 1905.[19] Another noteworthy absentee was the leading hygienist, Professor M. Ia. Kapustin of the University of Kazan, who was one of the score of Octobrist deputies elected to the predominantly radical Second Duma. A lifelong supporter of the Pirogov Society, Kapustin had been honored by being elected president of its Eighth Congress in 1902, but, according to Kanel', the events of 1905 persuaded him that " . . . there is no longer any place for him at Pirogov Congresses."[20]

Also pointedly absent from the 1907 congress was the rising star of the St. Petersburg medical establishment, Professor G. E. Rein, who was soon to be named president of the Medical Council by Premier P. A. Stolypin. Rein had also been an active *pirogovets* in the past but, like Kapustin, he was now an Octobrist deputy in the Second Duma and thought it prudent to stay away from meetings of the "tainted" Pirogov Society. In his memoirs, Rein lamented that Pirogov Congresses

> strayed from the high ideals of their founder and were animated by narrowly understood political considerations. Scientific considerations were put in second place, and at the sections on community medicine, reports on tuberculosis, syphilis and alcoholism became the occasion for resolutions about the freedom of the person, assembly, speech and the press, for the "four-tailed" formula in elections to legislative institutions, and for the convocation of a constituent assembly to radically transform the life of our state and society.[21]

For conservatives such as Rein, zemstvo physicians who introduced politics into the Pirogov Society were guilty of betraying the ideals of zemstvo medicine itself. Yet it was not politics per se but opposition politics to which Rein objected; had the "Cholera" Congress sent a resolution of loyalty to the tsar, or hailed the Bulygin duma proposal, he would not then have objected that scientific considerations had been put in second place. Many of the distinguished figures who chose to keep their distance from the Pirogov Society after the events of 1905 later joined Rein in the work of the Interdepartmental Commission to Reform Medical-Sanitary Legislation which was established in March 1912. Not surprisingly, the work of this commission, especially its proposal for a ministry of public health, was later denounced by the Pirogov Society as a threat to the very existence of zemstvo medicine. We shall return to the work of the Rein Commission later in this essay.

Notwithstanding the attitudes of these conservative physicians, many *pirogovtsy* believed, with Kanel', that "real public health can only be achieved in an atmosphere of freedom and justice."[22] For them, the failure of the 1905 revolution and the reaction which followed it were devastating experiences. Throughout 1906 and early 1907, many physicians and other medical personnel who had openly supported the revolutionary cause found themselves dismissed, demoted, or otherwise harassed as a tide of reaction against the radicalism of professional employees swept through the zemstvos.[23] In Odessa, which had been the cradle of the bacteriological revolution in Russia, the city governor, General Tolmachev, carried out a purge which left several physician-radicals without employment.[24] The Pirogov Society's monthly *Journal* kept a careful record of all these arbitrary acts against physicians.[25] Of even greater significance was Stolypin's decision to backtrack in the face of gentry opposition to his proposed reform of local government.[26] Physician-radicals who had expected the establishment of democratically elected, all-class *volost'* zemstvo institutions to give them an opportunity to play a leading role in the renovation of Russian society now had to accept the bitter fact that Stolypin had caved into pressure from the United Nobility.[27] Morale among *pirogovtsy* who had sympathized with the Revolution of 1905, already sagging in the wake of these events, plummeted to a new low with the death of G. N. Gabrichevskii in 1907. Gabrichevskii had almost singlehandedly reversed the initial opposition of zemstvo physicians to the rise of bacteriology; as president of the "Cholera" Congress in 1905, he had come to symbolize the role which preventive medicine and social reform could play if only Russia's future could be wrested from the paralyzing hand of the tsarist regime. More than any other event during the months of reaction, Gabrichevskii's premature death (at age forty-seven) symbolized the extinction of that beacon of hope which the revolutionary movement had represented.

For the next several years, erstwhile physician-radicals spoke and wrote about finding themselves in a world where they had suddenly lost their bearings, where their pre-1905 assumptions were no longer relevant. The psychiatrist V. I. Iakovenko, whose career as a radical has been chronicled by Julie Brown,[28] tried to analyze the collective psyche of post-1905 Russia; his conclusion was that the healthy elements in Russian society had supported the revolutionary movement, whereas the morbid elements were responsible for government policy under Stolypin, a policy which he regarded as evidence of "moral insanity."[29] Faced with events which the positivism of nineteenth-century social thought had led him to believe could not happen, Iakovenko cloaked his shock and disapproval in the pejorative vocabulary of contemporary psychiatry. By contrast S. N. Igumnov, a well-known sanitary physician and pillar of the Pirogov Society, preferred honest confession to professional bluster. In a thoughtful essay which struck many responsive chords among Russian physicians, Igumnov openly admitted that the failure of the 1905 revolution had called into question the most cherished tenets of zemstvo medicine.[30] Like the populist movement which had provided its utilitarian direction, boundless optimism, and unquestioning self-assurance, zemstvo medicine now found itself adrift, unable even to analyze, let alone solve, the problems of contemporary society.

Marxist physicians, however, emerged from the 1905 revolution with their analytical tools not only intact but sharpened. Writing under his pen-name "E. M.," the Bolshevik physician E. G. Munblit argued that the so-called crisis of zemstvo medicine was only a part of the larger crisis of a Russia ruled by "black hundred" landlords.[31] Meanwhile, a Menshevik factory physician, L. B. Granovskii, went to great lengths to demonstrate that advancing capitalism was responsible for the prevalence of tuberculosis, alcoholism, and venereal disease in Russia.[32] If such arguments found an audience among community physicians, then zemstvo medicine might well be buried alongside the now discredited *narodnik* spirit of the 1870s.

The Revolution of 1905 and its aftermath left physicians convinced that zemstvo medicine was in a sorry state. Conservatives, posing as thoroughgoing professionals, took the position that the Pirogov Society had abused its proper role by permitting "politics" (read "opposition politics") to intervene in its deliberations. Radicals believed that the failure of the Revolution had shattered the ideological basis of zemstvo medicine; for populists like Igumnov, this realization provoked lamentation and confusion, while for Marxists like Granovskii it bred satisfaction that the weaknesses of populism had been demonstrated beyond dispute. No wonder that in a review of medical activities of zemstvos and the Pirogov Society for 1908, N. A. Vygdorchik described the past twelve months as "a dry and fruitless year."[33]

POPULIST IDEOLOGY AND RUSSIAN REALITY

The confusion on the part of the populist idealists of zemstvo medicine did not last long. Although Igumnov had confessed in 1908 that the "old house" in which zemstvo physicians had grown up no longer suited and that he had no idea what the "new house" should look like,[34] this indecision did not prevent him from speaking out over the next several years on any issue that seemed to threaten the kind of zemstvo medicine which had reached maturity in that "old house." Along with his friend and colleague D. N. Zhbankov, executive director of the Pirogov Society in fact if not in name, Igumnov occupied what might best be called the "moral high ground" in the many disputes which raged in the medical press and at medical congresses until the outbreak of war in 1914. In their crusades against private practice and the materialism of the younger generation, and in their hostility toward such innovations as zemstvo bacteriological clinics and sanitary engineering, there was one common theme: the need to rekindle the idealism and self-sacrifice of earlier generations. The names of Osipov, Molleson, Erismann, and of course the great Pirogov himself became a litany of saints to be called on whenever it was necessary to ward off evil. Yet for all their invocations, Igumnov and Zhbankov were unable to maintain the *narodnik* idealism of pre-1905 zemstvo medicine, not so much because of the changes wrought by the failure of the revolution as because they and their supporters failed to keep pace with the changing directions of medical and sanitary activity in the early twentieth century.

Nothing reveals more clearly the populist, even neo-Slavophile, elements in Zhbankov's conception of zemstvo medicine than the stance he took against zemstvo physicians who engaged in private practice on the side. Private medical practice in any form had always been anathema to the ideologists of zemstvo medicine; in their view, Russian medicine had to be saved from the contaminating entrepreneurship which, they claimed, characterized medical practice in Western Europe, England, and the United States. For any Russian physician to operate on a fee-for-service basis was, in their view, unfortunate; for a zemstvo physician to do so was despicable. The few instances of this practice which appeared before 1905 were quickly explained away by references to inadequate salaries and individual greed. In the aftermath of 1905, however, Zhbankov was able to take a new line: the growth of private practice was a symptom of the decline in idealism among zemstvo physicians,[35] a decline for which the new political situation was entirely responsible.

With the zemstvos now controlled by conservatives who cared nothing for social reforms, he claimed, morale among zemstvo employees had sunk to an all-time low. He was, however, aware that such lapses from grace could not continue, lest they "demoralize the whole family of zemstvo physicians and destroy their influence among the population."[36] Zhbankov went on to draw a revealing analogy between this "family" of zemstvo physicians and the peasant commune, arguing that both these quintessentially Russian institutions needed protection against harmful Western notions of individualism and financial gain.

A similar insistence on the primacy of the service ideal in zemstvo medicine ran through the campaigns which traditionalists waged during the prewar years against such "dangerous" innovations as clinical bacteriology and sanitary engineering. A fervent admirer of Erismann, Igumnov had built the zemstvo sanitary bureau of Kherson province on the environmental and ethical principles espoused by Erismann's mentor, Max von Pettenkofer. Convinced that the growing emphasis on laboratory work in bacteriology threatened to destroy the community direction (*obshchestvennost'*) of zemstvo medicine, Igumnov spoke out against this trend at the Pirogov Congress in 1910. Lamenting the current fad for bacteriology, he warned that "the old sociological emphasis" was in danger and called on his audience to reassert the "public tasks" of zemstvo sanitation.[37] This was a familiar theme: already in 1908, he had denounced another colleague (G. A. Berdichevskii) for trying to turn zemstvo physicians into clinicians.[38] Igumnov's reply struck the appropriate tone of moral indignation:

> He [the zemstvo physician] is a community physician who satisfies the needs of broad strata of the population and who studies its sanitary condition, and not a clinician who shuts himself away in his chamber or operating room; he is a physician-sociologist who has the broad masses of the population for the object of his study and activity, and not a physician-individualist who is interested only in a particular sick organism.[39]

In 1910 he grudgingly admitted that industrialization did demand some reconsideration of the qualifications necessary for zemstvo sanitary work, but adamantly maintained that any changes should only strengthen the principle of *obshchestvennost'*. Yet, since he made no proposals of his own, and condemned those of everyone else, his position appeared to be a wholly negative one.

Sanitary or hydrological engineering (usually called in Russian *sanitarnoe-tekhnicheskoe napravlenie*) found its greatest Russian exponent in A. N. Sysin, the dynamic young head first of the Nizhnii Novgorod (1911) and then of the Moscow (1913) province sanitary bureaus. Sysin had already departed from Pirogov orthodoxy by blaming zemstvo medicine rather than the government for the zemstvos' inadequate response to the 1910 cholera epidemic.[40] In an important 1912 report, Sysin explained his views on the role of sanitary engineering in zemstvo sanitary work.[41] The great challenge for sanitary physicians, he argued, was to provide communities with a dependable supply of pure water. To do this, they should work with other professional and technical zemstvo employees in a special hydro-technical bureau which would cooperate with the zemstvo sanitary bureau in carrying out sanitary reforms. The new bureau, headed by an engineer and employing geologists, hydrographers, and sanitary engineers, would carry out surveys, develop plans, budgets, and construction schedules for new schemes of piped water, sewage disposal, and sewerage.

Although Sysin tried to link his approach to the traditional responsibilities of the sanitary physician, his brand of sanitary engineering undoubtedly implied a fundamental transformation in zemstvo sanitary work. Sysin's ideal sanitary physician was neither the social researcher-statistician-topographer of Pirogov tradition nor the innovative hygienist at home in the laboratory; instead he was a new breed of technical specialist who was more likely to rub shoulders with engineers, architects, and town planners than with clinicians, *uchastok* physicians, or laboratory researchers. Moreover, his technical orientation meant that it was unnecessary for him to establish or maintain contacts with the common people, who became merely the passive beneficiaries of his work.

This professional, exclusive aspect of sanitary engineering was precisely what traditionalists feared most. Their ideal "physician-sociologist" was in constant contact with the people, meeting them as healer, teacher, adviser, and confidant. The Pirogov Society had worked hard for more than a decade to break down the barriers between physicians and ordinary people, to demystify medicine, and to simplify the principles of hygiene for popular educational work.[42] Sysin's sanitary engineering threatened to undermine all of these endeavors by turning sanitary improvement into a highly technical subject comprehensible only to a small group of experts. Even more ominous was the fact that improvements in water supply, sewage removal, and sewerage could be carried out, as it were, behind the scenes: there was no need, as there clearly was in hygiene education, to enlist the people as active participants in the struggle for better health.

Despite the threat it appeared to pose to the missionary role of the zemstvo physician, sanitary engineering was nevertheless difficult to oppose. For one thing, Sysin himself was no apolitical technician: he was every bit as radical in his social and political views as any of the *pirogovtsy* who had been on the revolutionary left in 1905. Moreover, supporters of sanitary engineering could argue that systems of water filtration and sewage treatment introduced elsewhere had led to reductions in mortality from cholera and typhoid fewer.[43] Finally, sanitary engineering was attractive: it offered tangible, measurable improvements within a relatively short period of time, whereas popular hygiene education was a neverending and always problematic enterprise. Nevertheless, the consequences of this new specialization aroused concern, and not only among traditionalists. E. G. Munblit blamed sanitary engineering for the collapse of what he called "broad *uchastok* activity" in Moscow province: zemstvo physicians were paying fewer home visits to the sick, and sanitary physicians preferred the new technology to their traditional role in combating epidemics, supervising schools, organizing creches, and stimulating public interest in sanitary issues.[44] For his part, Igumnov chose to behave as if Moscow province had been infected by a disease which had to be contained lest it destroy its neighbors. In a lengthy essay written in 1912, he argued that, while Moscow province was unique because of its industrial development and its emphasis on industrial hygiene and sanitary improvements, the rest of Russia did not need specialists in sanitary engineering and occupational hygiene but, rather, traditional "general tasks" sanitary physicians.[45] Behind this hostility to sanitary engineering was the preference of *narodniki* such as Igumnov for a Russia which was rural and agrarian rather than urban and industrial. From the point of view of traditionalists, the trouble with sanitary engineering was that by making large urban centers healthier, it would enable Russia to become more like the countries of Western Europe. The Russia which Igumnov wished to make healthier was the Russia of peasant villages.

From about 1910 onward, Zhbankov and Igumnov were fighting what was becoming a losing battle to maintain the traditional ideology of zemstvo medicine. Despite Igumnov's efforts to rally opinion against bacteriology, many of those who attended the 1910 Pirogov Congress were not persuaded that it was a menace and regarded its growth as both inevitable and desirable.[46] Sysin's rapid rise to a position of influence was itself evidence that Moscow province, tired of sermons and hand-wringing, was prepared to find its own way out of the post-1905 crisis. By 1912, two distinguished bacteriologists, P. N. Diatroptov and L. A. Tarasevich, were playing increasingly important roles in the Pirogov Society.[47] A new group of radical sanitary physicians, including Sysin, Tsvetaev, Kost', I. S. Veger, and Z. P. Solov'ev, threatened to push traditionalists such as Igumnov into obscurity.[48]

Ironically, the sagging fortunes of Pirogov traditionalists were suddenly bolstered by the tsarist regime itself. In March 1912, G. E. Rein, the energetic president of the Medical Council, was appointed to head an Interdepartmental Commission to Review Medical-Sanitary Legislation. A loyal monarchist and an avowed centralizer, Rein had formed an unflattering opinion of the capacities of zemstvo medicine while directing the battle against cholera in south Russia in 1910.[49] Since his return to the capital, he had lobbied both the tsar and the Council of Ministers on the necessity for Russia to create a separate, powerful ministry of health. The mandate given to him and his commission was broad: a complete revision of all medical, sanitary, and forensic medical legislation, antiepidemic measures, medical care, organized charities, medical education, and the rules governing the professional activity of physicians.[50] It was no secret in St. Petersburg that the commission would recommend the creation of a Main Administration for State Health Protection (*Glavnoe upravlenie gosudarstvennogo zdravookhraneniia*); Rein clearly saw himself being appointed its head and looked forward to taking a seat as a member of the Council of Ministers.

The Rein Commission was welcome grist for the mills of Zhbankov, Igumnov, and their adherents in the Pirogov Society. Just when it seemed that the old pre-1905 spirit of zemstvo medicine was becoming an anachronism, the specter of a ministry of health run by tsarist bureaucrats and headed by Rein enabled the traditionalists to regroup for battle against what was perceived to be the common enemy of all *pirogovtsy*. When Rein characteristically named all of the members of the commission without even a hint of consultation with the Pirogov Society, they were able to draw parallels with the earlier battles over the proposed Hospital Statute of 1894 and over the Sanitary-Executive Commissions in 1905.[51] A. S. Durnovo, himself a sanitary physician, used his regular column in *Obshchestvennyi vrach* for scathing attacks on the comission and all its works.[52] The Pirogov Society had opposed the establishment of a ministry of health when the idea had been advanced first by the Botkin Commission in 1889 and had continued to oppose similar proposals by V. K. von Anrep and S. E. Krizhanovskii.[53] At the Twelfth Pirogov Congress in 1913, Zhbankov easily persuaded participants to treat the work of the Rein Commission with disdain and to proclaim that only the Pirogov Society itself was capable of providing the appropriate leadership for medical and sanitary activity in Russia.[54]

The thrust of the Rein Commission's activity was by no means as reactionary as Zhbankov's rhetoric implied. To be sure, Rein was no advocate of unrestricted autonomy either for physicians or for zemstvos, but in some areas the work of his commission seemed to be more in tune with contemporary medical opinion than did the reflex responses of Pirogov traditionalists. For example, Rein's plans for medical research included the establishment of laboratory facilities for research in hygiene, bacteriology, and several other specialties, as well as a network of institutes for the study of sanitation. His views on the shortcomings of zemstvo antiepidemic measures, and on the type of improvements necessary, closely resembled those already articulated by Sysin himself. Most significant of all, the fact that Zhbankov had denounced Rein and all his works failed to carry weight with one of Russia's leading figures in bacteriology and hygiene, N. F. Gamaleia, who accepted Rein's invitation to participate in the work of the Interdepartmental Commission.

A former student of Mechnikov, Gamaleia was the director of the Odessa Bacteriological Station and a municipal physician in Odessa. As such he might have been expected to decline to work with someone who had as little time for zemstvo medicine and the Pirogov Society as did Rein.[55] Yet Gamaleia, while no aspiring medical *chinovnik*, held views on the future of public health in Russia which were far closer to those of Rein than to those of Zhbankov and Igumnov. In the spring of 1910, even before Rein set off for south Russia, Gamaleia published an essay in which he called for the establishment of a "supreme sanitary organ" in Russia to provide instruction, leadership, and control in matters of public health.[56] Thoroughly knowledgeable about developments abroad, Gamaleia was particularly impressed by the role played in Germany by the *Reichsgesundheitsamt* and in England by the Local Government Board in establishing the best methods of sanitary improvement and overseeing their implementation by local authorities.[57] In sharp contrast to the rhetoric emanating from the Pirogov Society, Gamaleia stressed the creative and positive role played by central government agencies and the debt owed to them by local government bodies. As a Russian counterpart to the Institute for Infectious Diseases in Berlin (the research arm of the *Reichsgesundheitsamt*), he proposed the formation of a State Institute for Social Hygiene under the aegis of the new ministry. Both the institute and the ministry would exercise control over the activities of zemstvos and municipalities, a development which, he claimed, would serve as "a corrective to their sometimes all too evident neglect of the interests of the poorest class."[58] It is hardly surprising, therefore, that Rein should have regarded Gamaleia as a kindred spirit in the field of medical and sanitary reform.

Gamaleia's support for central government direction was informed by his intimate knowledge of the administration of public health in Western Europe and Great Britain. Pirogov traditionalists were not ignorant of developments abroad, but they viewed them through the distorting prism of "zemstvo versus autocracy." A classic example of this tendency is the lengthy survey of British and European practices, written by G. I. Dembo, which appeared in serial form in *Obshchestvennyi vrach* during 1910.[59] On the one hand, Dembo hailed England as the ideal to be imitated because of its sanitary reforms, the success of which he ascribed entirely to the fact that parliament had left these matters to the jurisdiction of local government.[60] France, on the other hand, was denigrated for its backwardness in matters of public health, the blame for which Dembo (naturally) ascribed to the excessive centralization of its government.[61] In the same spirit, Ia. Iu. Kats attempted to rebut Gamaleia's argument for a ministry of public health: in doing so, he made the extraordinary claim that dirt could not be eliminated by police measures and predicted that all attempts to achieve sanitary reform through central government actions would result only in additional interference by bureaucrats in the work of physicians, hospitals, and local medical services.[62] According to Kats, all aspects of health reform in Russia—housing, water supply, hygiene, epidemic prevention—could be handled by zemstvos and municipalities if only they were given more powers, much more money, and complete autonomy to spend it as they saw fit.[63] The state apparently had no role except to dole out the money and ignore how it was spent.

The almost incredible naiveté of Kats's position serves as a reminder that the ideologists of zemstvo medicine—like the intelligentsia which had nurtured them—seemed unable to come to terms with the existence of the state. The "we-they" mentality of the *pirogovtsy,* forged in the decade before 1905, made it impossible for them to separate the idea of the state from the activities of the Petersburg bureaucrats, whom they saw as the enemy. When, at the Pirogov Congress in 1913, A. I. Shingarev attempted a less doctrinaire discussion of the roles of central and local governments in public health, he found himself confronting a hostile audience: most participants agreed with Kats that the state had no substantive role to play whatsoever.[64] Yet despite the unfriendly response, Shingarev was still the Pirogov traditionalist: he had, for example, argued that in Russia what the Germans called *soziale Medizin* would be the responsibility not of the state but of the zemstvos and municipalities, since they alone represented society (*obshchestvo*). He was subsequently criticized by one speaker who charged that Shingarev had confused essence with agency,[65] but the general silence that greeted his speech betrayed both his audience's ignorance of developments abroad and its blithe assumption that the future of zemstvo medicine was boundless.

In the years before 1914, Zhbankov and other Pirogov traditionalists found themselves unable either to prevent or to control the ferment which was taking place in zemstvo medical circles. While they continued to mourn the lost idealism of an earlier generation, others willingly discussed the shortcomings of zemstvo medicine, welcomed clinical bacteriology and sanitary engineering, and even began to question the traditionalists' negative attitude toward the role of the state. At the same time, the response of Russian physicians to the establishment of the Rein Commission was deeply unsettling: it was scarcely surprising that some of the conservatives who had deserted the Pirogov Society in 1905 were now working with Rein, but how was one to explain Gamaleia's willingness to participate? Even the well-known radical D. K. Zabolotnyi, Professor of Microbiology at the Imperial Institute for Experimental Medicine, accepted Rein's invitation to work with a subcommittee studying antiepidemic measures. Increasingly, those who clung to the pre-1905 *narodnik* ideology of zemstvo medicine appeared to be out of place in a world which was fast leaving them behind. The best minds in Russian medicine and public health no longer adhered to an outmoded ideology.

FROM 1914 TO 1917

The outbreak of war in the summer of 1914 immediately and decisively altered the terrain on which these conflicts were played out. The first to feel the war's effects was the ambitious *chinovnik* Rein, who was deeply disappointed when the Council of Ministers decided in September 1914 that his plans for the creation of a ministry of public health should be shelved until the end of the war. He tried to circumvent this decision by appealing directly to the tsar, but the latter had just appointed Prince A. P. Oldenburg to direct medical and sanitary assistance for the army and did not want to create a rival authority in the civil sector.[66] Those in the Pirogov Society who had opposed Rein's plans were delighted to learn that he had been thwarted; like Rein himself, they could not perceive how the war would alter their own fortunes.

To put matters succinctly, the circumstances of the war placed position, money, influence, and opportunity in the hands of those very individuals within zemstvo medicine and the Pirogov Society who had already parted company with the ideology of the *narodniki* and who had their own ideas on the course which medical reforms should take in Russia. The individuals in question were the score or so of physicians, bacteriologists, and sanitary engineers who staffed the medical bureaus established by the Union of Zemstvos and the Union of Towns in the autumn of 1914. These new job opportunities attracted a mixed bag of radical academics, planners, and would-be medical administrators, none of whom felt bound by the conventions of Pirogov traditionalism. They included the two leading exponents of clinical bacteriology, P. N. Diatroptov and L. A. Tarasevich; the apostle of sanitary engineering, A. N. Sysin, and his devotees N. F. Nikolaevskii and M. M. Kenigsberg; the leading Menshevik expert in industrial hygiene and occupational health, L. B. Granovskii; and the underground Bolshevik and secretary of the All-Russian League to Combat Tuberculosis, Z. P. Solov'ev. Many of these individuals had been elected to the Pirogov Society's board of directors during the prewar years, and four of them—Diatroptov, Tarasevich, Sysin, and Solov'ev—were also members of the editorial board of *Obshchestvennyi vrach*. Events, however, soon conspired to make their union positions more important than their Pirogov offices.

This is not the place to describe the phenomenal growth of the wartime unions between 1914 and 1916, a subject which has been ably treated elsewhere by William Gleason.[67] The medical bureaus of both unions grew rapidly and soon extended their activities far beyond the original aim of providing evacuation facilities and hospital beds for wounded and seriously ill soldiers. Because of their uniquely extralegal status—their only official standing derived from telegrams of thanks signed by the tsar—the unions and their medical bureaus were able to operate outside the constraints imposed by the Zemstvo and Municipal Statutes. This meant, for example, that they could organize their own local committees and could hold regional or national meetings without being obstructed at every step by the Ministry of the Interior. The money to support their operations came from credits approved by a special commission in Prince Oldenburg's office, credits that were eventually and grudgingly approved by the Council of Ministers, which resented the lack of accountability enjoyed by the unions.[68] Mindful of the dangers of epidemic disease both at the front and in the rear, Diatroptov and Tarasevich organized vaccination and disinfection programs, while Sysin and his colleagues planned vast schemes of urban sanitary improvements involving piped water supply, sewage removal, and sewerage. By late 1916, the Medical Bureau of the Union of Towns was planning a conference on urban sanitation in the postwar era.[69]

All of these wartime developments simply bypassed Zhbankov and the other Pirogov traditionalists. Although *Obshchestvennyi vrach* carried the occasional article lamenting the fact that the war was playing havoc with the provision of medical services on the home front, the *narodniki* had no weapons with which to combat the growing influence of bacteriologists and sanitary engineers—most of them Social Democrats or sympathizers—in the unions' medical bureaus. For their part, the union physicians made shrewd use of the scientific prestige which a Pirogov Society resolution could lend to a proposal: they arranged for all of their major proposals to be discussed first at hastily convened wartime conferences sponsored by the Pirogov Society so that each would be given the stamp of scientific legitimacy before becoming union policy. This enabled them to deny government claims that the unions were simply masks for covert political opposition to the regime.

Little by little, as the war dragged on, the physicians in the two medical bureaus began to behave as if they were the nucleus of a future ministry of public health. With plans to devise, budgets to prepare, funds to spend, and schemes to supervise, they were enjoying a taste of power and a sense of achievement greater than had been possible working in peacetime conditions at the level of a district, province, or city. They knew that their work counted because no matter how much Prince Oldenburg or the Council of Ministers tried to restrict their activities, the army commanders in the field always insisted that they play a greater role.[70] The plans which they had drawn up for urban sanitary improvements promised significant reductions in mortality from water-borne diseases, comparable to those which had occurred in Europe after the flowering of the "sanitary idea" in the third quarter of the nineteenth century. Indeed, by the end of 1916, the unions' medical bureaus were playing a role vis-à-vis local affairs which was similar to that played in England by the Local Government Board and in Germany by the *Reichsgesundheitsamt*. Recognizing what was afoot, the would-be minister of health, G. E. Rein, sidelined to the State Council for most of the war, finally persuaded the tsar in December 1916 to let him begin building his Main Administration for State Health Protection, but he had barely begun when revolution engulfed the tsarist regime.

In April 1917 the Pirogov Congress clearly demonstrated the extent to which the war had put the effective leadership of zemstvo medicine into the hands of the physicians employed by the unions. As soon as the tsarist regime collapsed, they forced themselves on the Provisional Government, insisting on taking over direction of both military and civil medical affairs. Two weeks before the Pirogov Congress opened, they met in Moscow to plan the composition and duties of a "Central Medical-Sanitary Council"—a body which they expected to dominate—that would advise the Provisional Government not only on immediate wartime needs, but also on the future direction of medical and sanitary reform in the new democratic Russia.[71] Several Union physicians were already regularly attending meetings in Petrograd of a temporary advisory committee formed by V. I. Almazov, the commissar who had been appointed to replace Prince Oldenburg. Their presence at these meetings appeared to lend the support of both the Pirogov Society and zemstvo physicians in general to these endeavors, although in reality the union physicians were acting almost entirely on their own initiative.[72] When the Pirogov Congress opened on April 4, they kept a low profile during its opening debates but were confident that the congress would endorse a carefully worded proposal for the establishment of a reforming body similar to the one envisioned at the Moscow meeting.

All of this stands in sharp contrast to the 1917 program of Zhbankov and his traditionalist supporters. The old *narodnik* mounted the rostrum soon after the congress convened to report with scarcely concealed joy that Rein and his hated ministry had been swept away by the "cleansing hurricane" of the February Revolution.[73] His vision of the future was contained in a speech entitled "Bases for the Reconstruction of Medical-Sanitary Affairs in Liberated Russia."[74] He began by asserting that any sort of central direction was "in complete contradiction to the local and community . . . sector"; central direction, he claimed, meant paralysis and inactivity, whereas local control meant growth and vitality. He called for the immediate abolition of all state medical-administrative agencies: the Medical Council, the medical departments and sections of all ministries, and the *guberniia* medical departments. Furthermore, he called for the abolition of all private medical institutions—schools, hospitals, sanatoria, pharmacies, and so on—and for the takeover by zemstvo and municipal institutions of all public medical work, including forensic medicine and the workers' hospital funds.[75] Zhbankov naturally looked to the people to provide future leadership: he expected that with reformed, democratic zemstvo and municipal institutions, the entire population would participate in creating a new order of "universally accessible and free medical assistance, and sanitary undertakings based on self-taxation and mutual assistance." To coordinate the activity of all these popular institutions Zhbankov proposed the creation of a council composed of representatives of medical faculties, of zemstvo and municipal physicians, and of local self-governing institutions, but the role of council was limited merely to ensuring that local initiatives not conflict with one another.

Zhbankov's program was as consistent with his lifelong struggle on behalf of *narodnichestvo* as it was out of touch with the political imperatives of the moment and with the current thrust of medical reform elsewhere. Whereas the union physicians had used the leverage which their wartime activities gave them to secure influence with the Provisional Government, Zhbankov completely ignored both the exigencies of the war and the constraints which the war might impose on the direction of future reforms. Whereas the union physicians were already thinking of a central state agency which would play an active part in directing medical reform and sanitary improvements throughout the country, Zhbankov wanted to put the future health of Russia into the hands of assemblies of peasants, trusting implicitly that they would look to local physicians for guidance as they embarked on this great endeavor. Both Zhbankov and the union physicians believed in the cause of making Russia healthy (*ozdorovlenie Rossii*), but they saw this goal in different terms: for Zhbankov, Russia would be made healthier when the peasants themselves took moral and civil responsibility for decisions about their environment and their medical needs; for the union physicians, Russia would be made healthier when undertakings planned and executed by professional experts yielded significant reductions in morbidity and mortality rates.

Participants at the 1917 Pirogov Congress turned away from Zhbankov's pleas for a peasant-led reform. Urged on by carefully worded speeches from Tarasevich, Diatroptov, and other union physicians, they reversed three decades of opposition to proposals for the centralized direction of medical affairs and endorsed a resolution which called for "the existing allied public organizations, both on the spot and in the center, to take into their hands the management of medical and sanitary affairs."[76] The same resolution called for the formation of a central council of representatives of the public organizations which would coordinate the activities of zemstvos, municipalities, and hospital funds, provide general leadership, deal with the financial matters, liquidate tsarist institutions, and " . . . elaborate questions concerning the reconstruction of the central medical organs of all-state significance."[77] To be sure, there was no intention here of turning the zemstvos into local agencies of a centralized bureaucracy; the whole thrust of the resolution was toward ensuring that local affairs would be locally controlled. The principle of central direction and coordination was, however, clearly accepted, and, as Tarasevich guardedly observed during a discussion of the war: "Together with collegiality and local activity, it is necessary to observe the principle of the correct arrangement and economy of medical labor; that is, in certain circumstances the centralization of technical and administrative forces—elected and responsible—may be necessary."[78] In fact, the union physicians had already discovered the virtues of centralized direction and were preparing to organize the transition from wartime to peacetime planning.

Zhbankov's virtual eclipse was underlined by the election of a new eighteen-member executive for the Pirogov Society: only he and one other *narodnik*, D. Ia. Dorf, could be put in the traditionalist camp; the other sixteen were primarily union physicians, many of them Menshevik or Bolshevik sympathizers. Needless to say, Tarasevich, Diatroptov, Sysin, and Solov'ev were all elected to the new executive.[79] In a stroke of bitter irony, Zhbankov was chosen one of ten representatives to the new council he had hoped would not be created, presumably a tactic to lend the council some semblance of Pirogov legitimacy. In fact, the quickening pace of social revolution during the summer of 1917 made the new council a poor instrument with which to carry on the fight for medical and sanitary reform. When it finally held its first plenary session in Petrograd in late August amid rumors of an impending military coup, Solov'ev, now the leader of the pro-Bolshevik cause among Pirogov physicians, denounced its ties to the now discredited Provisional Government and called on those who sincerely sought sweeping reforms in medicine and public health to work with the Soviets.[80] Perhaps not surprisingly, he and Sysin were among the first physicians with close ties to the Pirogov Society to support the Bolshevik regime.[81]

THE BOLSHEVIK REVOLUTION
AND RUSSIAN MEDICINE

What light does the foregoing analysis shed on the question of the role of the Bolshevik Revolution in the history of Russian medicine? Clearly the Bolsheviks did not begin the process of centralizing and bureaucratizing Russian medicine. That process was already under way even before Lenin seized power: had the war not intervened, it might well have been carried out by Rein and his planned Main Administration for Health Protection. Instead it was carried out by the bacteriologists, sanitary engineers, and planners who coalesced in the unions' medical bureaus, dominated the Central Medical Sanitary Council in 1917, and soon became leading figures in the Soviet public health apparatus. Slavskii's (and Zhbankov's) hopes for a locally controlled, "grass-roots" medical reform were dashed when the Pirogov Congress of 1917 lent its support to the plans of the union physicians who were already courting the Provisional Government. Nevertheless, it would be rash to minimize the significance of October: Lenin's victory undoubtedly accelerated the process of centralization and bureaucratization. If the Provisional Government had survived, the reformers most likely would not have created a body so reminiscent of Rein's proposed ministry as Narkomzdrav proved to be.[82]

It should also now be apparent that zemstvo medicine changed substantially after 1905. The zemstvo medicine that Winslow found flourishing in the Petrograd of 1917 had little in common with that of Pirogov traditionalists except for a commitment to medical care as a freely accessible public service. The reformers whom Winslow met were the union physicians who shared neither the antiurban, antiindustrial prejudices of the *narodniki* nor their resolute opposition to the centralized state as an instrument for social reform. The reformers' friendly attitude toward laboratory research and their enthusiasm for sanitary engineering stood in sharp contrast to the endless moralizing of the traditionalists. Indeed, it can be argued that the high moral tone adopted by Zhbankov and Igumnov doomed their conception of zemstvo medicine to extinction. In treating all criticism as heresy, they discouraged honest evaluations of the shortcomings of zemstvo medicine, especially in such areas as antiepidemic measures and patient care; it is not surprising, therefore, that reformers sought a new institutional base from which to transform Russian medicine.

The war provided the reformers with a temporary and uncertain base in the form of the unions' medical bureaus. At the outset the February Revolution seemed to promise them a more secure base: hence their support for the formation of the new Central Medical-Sanitary Council. When the Provisional Government proved to be a house built on sand, the reformers were forced to shift their hopes to Lenin's government and the new Commissariat for Public Health. Zhbankov and Igumnov inadvertently hastened this process: believing that only zemstvo medicine could meet the medical needs of all strata of the population, they had frowned on such "threatening" innovations as the workers' hospital funds; inevitably, the workers and their political leaders in 1917 came to regard zemstvo medicine as a tsarist legacy which should now be replaced by a new democratic social medicine. Even those reforming physicians who initially condemned the Bolshevik seizure of power soon recognized that they could no longer cling to the now discredited zemstvos.[83]

And condemn it they did: several union physicians were among the fifteen members of the Pirogov Society's executive board who, on November 22, 1917, issued a declaration condemning the Bolshevik seizure of power. The declaration denounced "those forces which are destroying the country" and called on physicians "to sharply and totally dissociate themselves from physicians, *operating in the camp of tyrants.*"[84] Ironically, this last group included Solov'ev and Sysin, two of the most important union physicians, as well as I. V. Rusakov who, like the other two, had been an active *pirogovets*. The impact of this declaration is difficult to measure. Presumably it influenced, at least in some measures, the actions of those physicians who participated in the strike of government employees in Petrograd and the strike of civic employees in Moscow. Yet as Peter Krug has convincingly argued, too much has been made of this piece of rhetoric by Western writers who have followed Barsukov (and, of course, Lenin) in claiming that the *pirogovtsy* led a campaign of sabotage against the new regime.[85] Not only was there no such campaign, but the seemingly intransigent tone of the declaration was soon belied by the actions of many of the signatories. A rapprochement was in the making: within months of the establishment of Narkomzdrav in July 1918, leading *pirogovtsy*, led by Sysin and Tarasevich, were working for the new regime.[86] Soon all of the leading medical reformers were playing important roles in Soviet public health institutions. Despite their initially hostile reaction to October (which was in any case not unanimous), the reformers found the new regime broadly sympathetic toward their own objectives: the formulation of health policy, the prevention of epidemic disease, the development of social hygiene, and the strengthening of sanitary education. As long as it was prepared to pursue actively such goals, the Soviet government could count on the support of the leaders of medical reform.

Why, then, was this support not forthcoming in November 1917? Many of those who signed the declaration did so because their radical and socialist sympathies impelled them to condemn Lenin's authoritarian behavior. In this, Menshevik sympathizers such as Granovskii and Diatroptov could join forces with a right Bolshevik such as Kanel' or even with SR sympathizers such as Zhbankov and Dorf. Moreover, in the absence of clearly articulated policies, it was easy to assume that the Bolsheviks both embodied and encouraged the worst elements of mob rule. One should recall that the escalating pace of social revolution during the summer months of

1917 jeopardized the future of any sort of zemstvo medical activity. For one thing, there was evidence that the peasants of rural Russia supported neither zemstvo institutions nor the work of zemstvo professionals such as physicians. It was, apparently, too late to democratize institutions which the peasants had come to regard as part of an obsolete prerevolutionary political structure. Yet the zemstvos were vitally important to community physicians both because they had provided employment and because they had helped increase the market for medical services in a still largely preindustrial society. Physicians could with good reason fear that both their jobs and this market would disappear if the Bolsheviks encouraged the peasants to destroy the zemstvos. Moreover, the crude egalitarianism which was rampant by the summer of 1917 threatened both the status of professional groups in general and the dominant position of physicians among medical personnel. Here again, physicians might reasonably fear that the Bolsheviks would encourage the assault on their privileged professional status by feldshers, nurses, and other lesser medical personnel. To be sure, fearful physicians vastly exaggerated Bolshevik responsibility for all of these developments, but railing against "the forces of destruction" was easier than facing up to the lack of popular support for the zemstvos or for privileged professional groups.

Medical reformers soon began to realize, however, that their long-term interests lay with the Bolsheviks. The rapprochement of autumn 1918 became possible as soon as they began to appreciate the extent of their misjudgment. Sysin and Tarasevich quickly found influential places for themselves and their colleagues within Narkomzdrav and its agencies. By the same token, Semashko, Solov'ev, and the other Bolshevik physicians who were running Narkomzdrav had no intention of compromising the professional status of physicians. Indeed, the physicians of Narkomzdrav would go on to save the medical elite from both the professional aspirations of feldshers and the syndicalist tendencies of Narkomtrud and its medical arm, Vsemediksantrud.[87] No wonder, then, that the November 1917 declaration was so soon forgotten: government support for public health programs directed by physicians had never been stronger than it was in the new Soviet Russia.

The analysis offered here may also add something to our knowledge of the development of sanitary science. In most of Western Europe, the great era of urban sanitary improvement occurred before the discoveries of the bacteriological revolution, at a time when improvements could be directed by social administrators such as Chadwick and by general hygienists such as Parent-Duchâtelet, Pettenkofer, and Virchow.[88] The situation was different in Russia, where as late as 1900 virtually all sanitary improvements had yet to be undertaken. One result was that old-fashioned believers in the civilizing mission of hygiene reform—among whom one must include Zhbankov and Igumnov—could no longer exert the degree of influence that, for example, Chadwick had in England: hence the bitterness with which Zhbankov and Igumnov condemned the emergence of specialists who seemed more interested in their own fields than in perpetuating the physician's role as teacher, advisor, and moral exemplar among the common people. The traditionalists looked back to Pirogov, Erismann, and their contemporaries and saw them as missionaries bearing the torch of enlightenment among the dark peasant masses. Although zemstvo medicine certainly played a role in transmitting medical ideas and scientific values to at least some of the inhabitants of rural Russia, there had always been more morality than medicine at the heart of the enterprise. By 1900, however, the situation had changed: although traditionalists might rail against bacteriology, sanitary engineering, and the transformation of the clinic, the day of the specialist had arrived. Both World War I and the Revolution of 1917 helped strengthen the role of specialists in the Russian public health movement. In Lenin's Russia, as many of the contributions to this volume demonstrate, specialists in social medicine, epidemiology, and various branches of hygiene enjoyed an unprecedented degree of patronage and encouragement.

NOTES

1. For an evaluation of Winslow, see Arthur J. Viseltear, "C.-E. A. Winslow: His Era and His Contribution to Medical Care," in Charles E. Rosenberg, ed., *Healing and History: Essays for George Rosen* (New York, 1979), pp. 205–28.

2. C.-E. A. Winslow, *Public Health Administration in Russia in 1917* (Washington, 1918; reprint no. 445 from *Public Health Reports*, December 28, 1917, pp. 2191–219).

3. It was for this congress that E. A. Osipov, I. V. Popov, and P. I. Kurkin produced their important work, *Russkaia zemskaia meditsina* (Moscow, 1899).

4. Winslow, *Public Health Administration,* p. 2219.

5. K. G. Slavskii, "Pokhorony zemskoi meditsiny," *Obshchestvennyi vrach,* nos. 13–14 (1918), pp. 116–17.

6. Ibid., p. 117.

7. For an analysis of these conflicts prior to 1905, see Nancy M. Frieden, *Russian Physicians in an Era of Reform and Revolution, 1856–1905* (Princeton, N.J., 1981), esp. pp. 135–99.

8. Viseltear, "C.-E. A. Winslow," p. 208.

9. Mark G. Field, "Medical Organization and the Medical Profession," in Cyril E. Black, ed., *The Transformation of Russian Society: Aspects of Social Change since 1861* (Cambridge, Mass., 1960), p. 541.

10. Ibid., p. 548. The classic Stalinist account of medicine and the Revolution is M. I. Barsukov, *Velikaia oktiabr'skaia sotsialisticheskaia revoliutsiia i organizatsiia sovetskogo zdravookhraneniia: X. 1917–VII 1918* (Moscow, 1951).

11. I. D. Strashun, *Russkaia obshchestvennaia meditsina v period mezhdu dvumia revoliutsiiami 1907–1917 gg.* (Moscow, 1964).

12. Peter F. Krug, "Russian Public Physicians and Revolution: The Pirogov Society, 1917–1920" (Ph.D. diss., University of Wisconsin, 1979), esp. pp. 128–267 and appendix, pp. 297–316.

13. Ibid., pp. 160–61.

14. As quoted in ibid., p. 219.

15. Strashun, *Russkaia obshchestvennaia meditsina,* esp. pp. 84–102, 125–35, 173–87.

16. Frieden, *Russian Physicians,* pp. 122–27.

17. Ibid., pp. 292–308.

18. For an assessment of the significance of the union, see J. F. Hutchinson, "Society, Corporation or Union? Russian Physicians and the Struggle for Professional Unity (1890–1913)," *Jahrbücher für Geschichte Osteuropas,* 30: 1 (1982), 45–47.

19. V. Ia. Kanel', "Soiuz vrachei," *Zhurnal Obshchestva russkikh vrachei im. N. I. Pirogova* [hereafter, *Zhurnal ORVP*], no. 2 (1908), p. 150.

20. Ibid.

21. G. E. Rein, *Iz perezhitogo* (Berlin, [1938?]), 1: 28.

22. Kanel', "Soiuz vrachei," p. 153. For a glowing but uncritical account of the activities of radical physicians in 1905, see S. I. Mitskevich, *Zapiski vracha-obshchestvennika (1888–1918)* (Moscow, 1941), pp. 133–40.

23. The definitive account of the gentry reaction after 1905 is Roberta Thompson Manning, *The Crisis of the Old Order in Russia: Gentry and Government* (Princeton, N.J., 1982).

24. On Tolmachev's purge, see John F. Hutchinson, "Tsarist Russia and the Bacteriological Revolution," *Journal of the History of Medicine and Allied Sciences*, 40 (1985), p. 438.

25. See, for example, the "Chronicle" section of *Zhurnal ORVP*, no. 7 (1906).

26. For a thorough analysis, see Neil B. Weissman, *Reform in Tsarist Russia: The State Bureaucracy and Local Government, 1900–1914* (New Brunswick, N.J., 1981), pp. 124–47.

27. The political repercussions are explored in detail in Ruth Delia MacNaughton and Roberta Thompson Manning, "The Crisis of the Third of June System and Political Trends in the Zemstvos, 1907–1914," in Leopold H. Haimson, ed., *The Politics of Rural Russia, 1905–1914* (Bloomington, Ind., 1979), pp. 184–218.

28. Julie V. Brown, "The Professionalization of Russian Psychiatry: 1857–1911" (Ph.D. diss., University of Pennsylvania, 1981).

29. V. I. Iakovenko, "Zdorovye i boleznennye proiavleniia v psikhike sovremennogo russkogo obshchestva," *Zhurnal ORVP*, no. 4 (1907), pp. 269–87.

30. S. N. Igumnov, "K voprosu o krizise v zemskoi meditsine," *Zhurnal ORVP*, no. 3 (1908), pp. 283–96.

31. E. M., "K voprosu o krizise zemskoi meditsiny," *Zhurnal ORVP*, no. 4, (1908), pp. 407–415.

32. L. B. Granovskii, "Obshchestvennoe zdravookhranenie i kapitalizm," *Zhurnal ORVP*, no. 5 (1907), pp. 371–405; and no. 6, pp. 539–64.

33. *Obshchestvennyi vrach*, no. 1 (1909), p. 11.

34. Igumnov, "K voprosu o krizise," pp. 293–95.

35. D. N. Zhbankov, "Zemskaia meditsina i chastnaia praktika," *Obshchestvennyi vrach*, no. 8 (1911), pp. 14–28. Other symptoms of the same phenomenon were the difficulties experienced by many zemstvos in trying to retain medical personnel and the almost chronic absenteeism of physicians from meetings of *guberniia* and *uezd* sanitary councils.

36. Ibid., p. 24.

37. As quoted in A. Amsterdamskii, "XI Pirogovskii S"ezd 21–28 apr. 1910 g. v Peterburge," *Vestnik Obshchestvennoi gigieny, sudebnoi i prakticheskoi meditsiny* [hereafter cited as *VOG*], t. 4 (1910), p. 1397. An abbreviated version of Igumnov's speech can be found in *Trudy XI Pirogovskogo s"ezda* (St. Petersburg, 1911), 1: 352–55.

38. G. A. Berdichevskii, "K otsenke polozheniia," *Zhurnal ORVP*, no. 1 (1908), pp. 5–27.

39. Igumnov, "K voprosu o krizise," p. 290.

40. Sysin blamed the poor performance of zemstvo medicine on its own organizational shortcomings and inappropriate measures, not on a shortage of funds or on administrative interference by the government. See *VOG*, t. 4 (1910), pp. 1681–83. Sysin's article first appeared in *Svedeniia san. biuro Nizheg. zemstva*, no. 7 (1910).

41. Strashun, *Russkaia obshchestvennaia meditsina*, pp. 91–92.

42. On the origins and work of the Commission for the Diffusion of Popular Hygiene Education, see Frieden, *Russian Physicians*, pp. 181–85.

43. Baldwin Latham's sanitary improvements in Croydon, England, would appear to have been particularly influential. For an appreciation of his work, see I. V. Poliak, "K voprosu ob ekonomicheskom znachenii narodnogo zdraviia," *Gigiena i sanitariia*, nos. 15–16 (1912),

pp. 137–40. For a full exposition of Latham's ideas and work, see Baldwin Latham, *Sanitary Engineering*, 2d ed., (London, 1878).

44. E. M., "Spetsializatsiia i obshchestvennost' v zemskoi meditsine," *Obshchestvennyi vrach*, no. 6 (1912), pp. 750–51.

45. S. Igumnov, "Kharakter i obshchie zadachi zemskoi sanitarii v eia proshlom i nastoiashchem," *Obshchestvennyi vrach*, no. 3 (1912), pp. 307–319.

46. Amsterdamskii, "XI Pirogovskii S"ezd," p. 1398.

47. Both were elected to the society's executive in 1910 and served on the editorial board of *Obshchestvennyi vrach*.

48. On the emergence of this group see Mitskevich, *Zapiski vracha-obshchestvennika*, pp. 158–59. Mitskevich also mentions N. A. Semashko, M. F. Vladimirskii, and Lenin's brother D. I. Ulianov, but all three were in exile after 1907.

49. Rein, *Iz perezhitogo*, 1: 65–73.

50. Rein's account of the establishment of the commission may be found in ibid., 1: 149–74.

51. On these battles, see Frieden, *Russian Physicians*, pp. 166–72, 292–304.

52. The column entitled "Sovremennaia zhizn' i narodnoe zdravie" appeared regularly from 1912 until the outbreak of World War I. See, for example, his comments on the composition of the Rein Commission, *Obshchestvennyi vrach*, no. 10 (1912), pp. 1218–24.

53. These events are discussed in Rein, *Iz perezhitogo*, 1: 91–103.

54. Hutchinson, "Russian Physicians," p. 51.

55. On Gamaleia's early career, see his *Vospominaniia* (Moscow, 1947); also Iu. I. Milenushkin, *N. F. Gamaleia, ocherk zhizni i deiatel'nosti* (Moscow, 1954).

56. N. F. Gamaleia, *K voprosu o ministerstve narodnogo zdraviia* (St. Petersburg, 1910), p. 29. The original version of this essay was published in *Gigiena i sanitariia*, vol. 2, nos. 20–21 (1910), pp. 398–428.

57. Ibid., pp. 16–18. For developments in Germany, see *Das Reichsgesundheitsamt 1876–1929*: Festschrift Herausgegeben vom Reichsgesundheitsamt aus Anlass seines funfzigjahrigen Bestehens (Berlin, 1926). For England, see W. M. Frazer, *The History of English Public Health 1834–1939* (London, 1950); and R. J. Lambert, *Sir John Simon* (London, 1964).

58. Gamaleia, *K voprosu*, p. 32.

59. G. I. Dembo, "V zakoldovannom kruge (k proektu o ministerstve narodnogo zdraviia)," *Vrachebnaia gazeta*, no. 43 (1910), pp. 1251–55; no. 44, pp. 1295–1301; no. 45, pp. 1338–1443; no. 46, pp. 1384–91.

60. For a recent evaluation of the English experience, see Anthony S. Wohl, *Endangered Lives: Public Health in Victorian Britain* (Cambridge, Mass., 1983), esp. pp. 142–65.

61. A recent work on public health reform in late nineteenth-century France concludes that private practitioners "successfully resisted the creation of a strong, centralized public health bureaucracy": Martha L. Hildreth, "Doctors, Bureaucrats and Public Health in France, 1888–1902" (Ph.D. diss., University of California–Riverside, 1983), p. 146. See also Anne-Louise Shapiro, "Private Rights, Public Interests and Professional Jurisdiction: The French Public Health Law of 1902," *Bulletin of the History of Medicine*, 54 (1980), pp. 4–22.

62. Ia. Iu. Kats, "O ministerstve narodnogo zdraviia," *Obshchestvennyi vrach*, no. 1 (1911), p. 46.

63. Ibid., p. 47.

64. *Dvenadtsatyi Pirogovskii s"ezd. Peterburg, 29 maia–5 iiunia 1913 g. Vypusk II* (St. Petersburg, 1913), pp. 150–52, 232–39; see also the comments of M. A. Neviadomskii in *Obshchestvennyi vrach*, no. 6 (1913), pp. 641–42.

65. V. Ia. Kanel' took Shingarev to task for his suggestion that in Russia the medical work of the public (zemstvo and municipal) institutions would constitute "social" medicine, whereas the work of government institutions would be "state" medicine: "Sotsial'naia meditsina, eia sushchnost' i znachenie," *Obshchestvennyi vrach*, no. 4 (1913), pp. 423–53.

66. This account of the war period is based on Rein's memoirs, *Iz perezhitogo*, 2: 49–

133, 190–221; see also his testimony in *Padenie tsarskogo rezhima,* P. E. Shchegolev, ed. (Moscow-Leningrad, 1926), 5: 1–31.

67. William E. Gleason, "The All-Russian Union of Towns and the All-Russian Union of Zemstvos in World War I: 1914–1917" (Ph.D. diss., Indiana University, 1971); idem, "The All-Russian Union of Zemstvos in World War I," in T. Emmons and W. S. Vucinich, ed., *The Zemstvo in Russia* (Cambridge, 1982).

68. See the frequent discussions of the unions in Yakhontov's notes of the meetings of the Council of Ministers during the summer of 1915: A. N. Yakhontov, "Tiazholyie dni," *Arkhiv russkoi revoliutsii,* 18 (Berlin, 1926), pp. 25–137.

69. The activities and plans of the two unions are described in N. F. Nikolaevskii, "Obzor organizatsii i deiatel'nosti Sanitarnogo Otdela Glavnogo Komiteta Soiuza Gorodov," *Vrachebno-sanitarnyi vestnik,* nos. 1–2 (1917), pp. 73–87; and Z. P. Solov'ev, "Itogi Vrachebno-sanitarnoi deiatel'nosti Zemskogo Soiuza i eia dal'neishie shagi," *Obshchest-vennyi vrach,* no. 7 (1916), pp. 363–73.

70. For a thorough evaluation of the work of the unions at the front, see Gleason, "All-Russian Union of Towns," chap. 4, pp. 56–85.

71. Minutes of this meeting were published in *Vrachebno-sanitarnyi vestnik,* nos. 1–2 (1917), pp. 101–3.

72. At the Moscow meeting referred to above, K. G. Slavskii, representing the Moscow *uezd* zemstvo organization, argued strongly that members of the unions did not represent either local zemstvos or municipalities. Although he received a handful of supporters, the union representatives dominated the meeting and overrode his objections. See ibid., pp. 102–3.

73. *Trudy chrezvychainogo pirogovskogo s"ezda (Moskva, 4–8 aprelia 1917 g.)* (Moscow, 1918), p. 55.

74. For a summary of this speech, see ibid., pp. 57–58.

75. The workers' hospital funds (*bolnichnye kassy*) were established in response to the 1912 sickness and accident legislation. For a description of the medical assistance scheme provided for, see B. G. D., *Strakhovanie rabochikh po zakonam 23 iiunia 1912 g.* (St. Petersburg, 1913), pp. 100–2.

76. *Trudy chrezvychainogo pirogovskogo s"ezda,* p. 75.

77. Ibid.

78. Ibid., p. 40.

79. The full list of eighteen members and six candidate members is printed in ibid., p. 80.

80. See his editorial in *Vrachebnaia zhizn',* no. 3 (September 1, 1917), pp. 3–5.

81. I. V. Rusakov also announced his adherence to the Bolshevik regime; these events are described in Krug, "Russian Public Physicians," p. 129.

82. When N. A. Semashko brought his proposal for the creation of Narkomzdrav to the Council of Peoples' Commissars on July 11, 1918, he was accused of "Rein-like belching" by three former Pirogov physicians who attended the meeting; Krug, "Russian Public Physicians," p. 187.

83. On popular opposition to the zemstvos in the summer of 1917, see William G. Rosenberg, "The Zemstvo in 1917 and Its Fate under Bolshevik Rule," in Emmons and Vucinich, eds., *The Zemstvo in Russia,* pp. 383–422.

84. *Obshchestvennyi vrach,* nos. 9–10 (1917), pp. 79–80 (emphasis in original).

85. Contrast Krug's description of the work of the Moscow zemstvo medical bureau in promoting the goals of the new regime ("Russian Public Physicians," pp. 152–75) with earlier accounts that emphasized the supposed incompatibility between the *pirogovtsy* and the Bolsheviks: Mark G. Field, *Soviet Socialized Medicine* (New York, 1968); Gordon Hyde, *The Soviet Health Service* (London, 1974); Vincente Navarro, *Social Security and Medicine in the USSR: A Marxist Critique* (Lexington, Mass., 1977). For Barsukov's account see note 10, above.

86. On the rapprochement, see Krug, "Russian Public Physicians," pp. 202–6. In his

view, it was well under way even before the typhus epidemic of 1918–19, which only accelerated it.

87. Krug, "Russian Public Physicians," pp. 229–67.

88. For a general discussion of sanitary reform in nineteenth-century Europe, see C.-E. A. Winslow, *The Conquest of Epidemic Disease: A Chapter in the History of Ideas* (Madison, Wisc., 1980).

JULIE V. BROWN

Social Influences on Psychiatric Theory and Practice in Late Imperial Russia

Psychiatry as a medical specialty first appeared in the Russian empire in the second quarter of the nineteenth century. The subsequent evolution of psychiatric theory and practice in Russia mirrored developments in those fields in the West. Russian psychiatrists advocated not only a new understanding of the phenomenon of insanity but also a markedly different societal response to it. Psychiatrists propagated the notion that insanity was an illness which, like others, could be understood scientifically and was amenable to treatment. Given proper care, they insisted, the mentally ill could be cured and the insane returned to productive roles in society.

This new approach required that large sums of money be spent on the construction and maintenance of asylums and that the responsibility of caring for the mentally disturbed be delegated to the new profession. Although there was an initial burst of activity along these lines, Russian psychiatrists soon encountered enormous obstacles, and for the next half century psychiatrists were forced to devote their best efforts to garnering support for the new asylums and to establishing an accepted role for themselves in the social and political order of late tsarist Russia. This essay focuses on their attempt to establish themselves as credible medical professionals while struggling against internal dissension and surrounded by the increasingly hostile opposition of other physicians and tsarist officials.

The first generation of Russian psychiatrists faced problems not dissimilar to those of their Western colleagues. Yet, the political and economic crises which enveloped the tsarist empire in the early years of the twentieth century significantly altered the context within which the profession functioned. The subsequent course of events revealed the extent to which "scientific" psychiatry can be influenced by its environment, while shedding new light on the policies and priorities of the tsarist empire during its final years.

THE ORIGINS OF PSYCHIATRY IN RUSSIA

The earliest institutions for the insane in Russia, like those in many other countries, predated the appearance of the profession of psychiatry. Madhouses, along with several other types of social welfare institutions, were established by Catherine II's enabling legislation of 1775 on provincial departments of public welfare (*Prikazy obshchestvennago prizreniia*). The concept of secular institutions for the insane was imported into Russia from the West, along with the basic design for the *prikaz* madhouses. Like their Western counterparts, these first madhouses were less institutions of healing than places of confinement. Reflecting the prevailing perception that the insane were insensitive to their environments, virtually all eighteenth-century madhouses were frightful places: inmates were routinely undernourished, underclothed, physically restrained, and subjected to abuse and ridicule.

The treatment of the insane in most Western societies underwent a significant transformation at the end of the eighteenth century. The dramatic removal of inmates' chains by Philippe Pinel and his assistant at the Bicêtre in Paris during the height of the French Revolution became a symbol of this "revolutionary" new approach. The nineteenth century ushered in an enormous expansion of organized care for the insane. Most of that care was given in "reformed" institutions administered by a new breed of physician, the psychiatrist, who claimed to be able to cure mental disorders using a combination of kindness and scientifically derived principles.[1]

Largely at the instigation of Tsar Nicholas I, in the 1820s and 1830s Russia too was overtaken by the spirit of psychiatric reform. Expressing shock at conditions in the *prikaz* madhouses, Russian reformers set out to build new institutions based on the latest Western principles. It was around these new "reformed" institutions that the nucleus of a psychiatric profession first appeared in Russia. This small group of specialists in the medical management of insanity added their voices to those of provincial governmental officials and bureaucrats in the Medical Department of the tsarist government's Ministry of Internal Affairs, who continued to press for additional reforms. The response to this sustained pressure was a plan to construct a series of regional (*okruzhnye*) asylums, which would replace the hated *prikaz* institutions. The first of these (in Kazan) was finally completed in 1869.

The Kazan Regional Asylum was a visible expression of many of the views of Russia's first psychiatrists, who played an active role in all stages of its planning and were particularly important in determining the architectural design of the structure. The man selected to be the institution's first director, A. Iu. Freze, was chosen in large part because he had written a monograph on asylum construction. Freze's writings and the construction of the Kazan asylum typified psychiatric thought at mid-century. Like their Western colleagues, Russia's first psychiatrists shared a strong belief in the curability of insanity and in the importance of the asylum in achieving that end. Successful treatment, according to this view, could be carried out only in a properly organized institution.

The therapeutic asylum as conceived by mid-nineteenth-century psychiatry abounded in paradoxes. It succeeded, so its advocates claimed, because it removed the mentally disturbed individual from his or her home environment. Thus, to effect a cure, the institution had to be different from the patient's home. Yet, if the milieu proved too foreign, the unbalanced mind would be unable to regain its moorings. Psychiatrists also acknowledged the carceral nature of the asylum, yet insisted that it could heal only if that coercive character was effectively concealed from its inhabitants.

Asylum management, in other words, was a delicate enterprise. The key to success, according to psychiatrists, was complete control over the institution. In their view, only properly trained experts could monitor all aspects of asylum management, and only medical experts possessed the knowledge necessary to ensure that patients were properly diagnosed and given the individualized attention that was the hallmark of enlightened psychiatric care.

Thus, the design of the mid-century asylum included a central role for specially trained medical professionals. Although the design was presumably derived from universal scientific principles, the therapeutic regimen, which the architecture was intended to facilitate, clearly reflected the values and the social hierarchy of the larger society. The most marked differences in treatment in the Kazan Regional Asylum were evident not as one moved from one category of pathology to another but as one crossed the boundaries which separated social classes. Virtually every aspect of a patient's experience in the asylum was determined by his or her social origins. The same was likely to be true of the psychiatric assessment of both the etiology of the individual's disorder and its probable outcome. In short, psychiatric theories at this time were clearly congruent with prevailing social values, and the asylum, in which the new profession placed so much confidence, fit easily into the existing order, reproducing the social structure within its thick and impenetrable walls.

PSYCHIATRY AND THE ZEMSTVOS

The important role played by psychiatric physicians in the construction of the Kazan Regional Asylum seemed to augur well for the future of the profession. The Kazan facility was to be only the first of a network of such institutions scattered across the vast empire. To ensure a domestic supply of experts to staff the new institutions, the tsarist government authorized the establishment of departments of psychiatry in Russian universities.[2] By the end of the nineteenth century the specialty of psychiatry had been introduced into the curricula of all Russian universities and the number of graduates of these programs had grown into the hundreds.

Its sponsorship of a psychiatric profession notwithstanding, the commitment of the tsarist government to providing institutional care for the insane began to waver almost as soon as the extraordinary costs of the endeavor became apparent. Indeed, even as the Kazan Regional Asylum was opening, the Ministry of Internal Affairs was in the process of transferring responsibility for mental institutions to the new organs of local self-government, the zemstvos, which had been created throughout European Russia after the abolition of serfdom to provide a number of services in their geographical areas. Members of the new zemstvo boards were unenthusiastic about the government's proposal to add the *prikaz* madhouses to their already numerous obligations.

The response of ministry officials in St. Petersburg to zemstvo protestations was a formal and unambiguous affirmation of zemstvo responsibility to provide institutional space for all the insane who needed it.[3] The ministry offered a modicum of financial assistance to local governments for additional asylum construction, but the bulk of the financial burden was shouldered by the zemstvos themselves. Many of the local governments devoted considerable resources to expanding and improving facilities for the mentally disturbed, but they naturally insisted on maintaining tight fiscal control over their operation. Indeed, most employed a nonphysician to manage the financial affairs of the asylum, a practice left over from the era of *prikaz* madhouses, when this official had been the sole administrator of the institution. Zemstvo psychiatrists sought to eliminate this post completely or, at the very least, to ensure that its occupant would be subordinate to the asylum's medical director. Few local governments were willing to delegate complete fiscal control to physicians, and the ones that did rarely hesitated to renege on their promises when it suited their purposes. Perhaps inevitably the result was repeated clashes between zemstvo officials and their psychiatric employees. Many of these clashes culminated in the resignation or firing of the latter.

One of the most widely publicized of these incidents occurred in the mid-1890s in the province of Tver, long regarded as a pioneer in its support for innovative programs for the insane. Tver's highly praised Burashevo Agricultural Colony for the Chronically Insane was directed by one of the early leaders of zemstvo psychiatry, M. P. Litvinov. For more than a decade the Tver provincial zemstvo's executive board supported Litvinov's efforts, approving a charter which gave the asylum director nearly autocratic control over the institution. Although the charter retained the position of manager of economic affairs in the institution, the individual occupying that post was clearly to be subordinate to the director. In the early 1890s the executive board suddenly revoked the charter and reclaimed for the lay manager (an individual appointed by the board) independent authority over the budget of the institution. The board then appointed to the post a man whom Litvinov had earlier denounced as incompetent. When the asylum director resigned in protest, it became apparent that the executive board had been anticipating his response and was ready to replace him with someone it regarded as more trustworthy.[4]

Outraged by the events at Burashevo, psychiatrists managed to mount a boycott of the institution. The Tver zemstvo was forced to appeal to the Ministry of Internal Affairs, which had to send three of its nonpsychiatric physicians to staff the facility. But even with this successful protest, the effect of the Tver incident and others like it added to the frustration and bitterness of Russian psychiatrists. V. P. Chizh, a professor of psychiatry, expressed the sentiments of many of his colleagues when he remarked in 1895, "How little respected are honest work and knowledge in our society. . . . Officials want neither knowledge nor honest labor but only deference and obedience."[5]

Russian psychiatrists were motivated in their dealings with their employers and with society at large by Western-inspired notions of professional autonomy and status. Their conviction that they deserved respect and authority was reinforced by their view that the therapeutic institution could cure only if at its helm it had an unfettered asylum director. Thus, their quest for control of their asylums was engendered not only by their sense of what was their due as professionals but also by their notions of what was necessary for therapeutic success with their patients.

Support for these demands proved difficult to attract. The fiscal conservatism of zemstvo assemblies was reinforced by widespread skepticism about the validity of the new expertise which the psychiatrists professed to possess. Popular notions regarding the nature of insanity continued to stress its supernatural character, and patterns of peasant use of asylums provided strong evidence that the masses used the institutions when they needed relief from life's burdens rather than because of any belief that the asylum doctors could help the disturbed.[6] The intelligentsia frequently idealized madness in such a way as to make psychiatric approaches largely irrelevant: the fictional heroic figure of the insightful fool was commonly portrayed as less in need of medical help than society itself was in need of his special—even divinely inspired—wisdom.

Even psychiatrists' colleagues within the medical profession remained skeptical of the legitimacy and the utility of psychiatric medicine. As one physician observed in the mid-1880s, "even a poorly trained feldsher could handle the insane and even without lectures on so-called theoretical psychiatry will know that they should be 'treated' and not subjected to torture. . . . In all probability these measures will not help, in which case a psychiatrist—albeit one sent from St. Petersburg—could do no more."[7]

To some degree the opposition of other physicians to psychiatrists was rooted in their perception that efforts by psychiatrists to establish an independent professional identity ran counter to the interests of the larger medical profession. Physicians' skepticism about the science of psychiatry was not without foundation. Psychiatrists were unable to demonstrate that they could cure many of the insane. Had they succeeded in returning a significant number of their charges to productive roles in society, greater support for their views might have been forthcoming. In the absence of such tangible indicators of effectiveness, the cynicism of other physicians and the reluctance of the zemstvos to give psychiatrists free rein over their costly asylums is hardly surprising.

PSYCHIATRISTS AND THE POLICE

Russian psychiatrists entered the twentieth century frustrated by their lack of success yet still dedicated to the therapeutic and professional goals articulated by early leaders of the profession. The next two decades, however, brought major changes. Russian psychiatrists set themselves a new and distinctive course which elaborated strategies for professional development and articulated goals for the organization of care for the insane. In these endeavors Russian psychiatrists differed markedly from both their predecessors and their counterparts in the contemporary Western world.

The Revolution of 1905 and the political reaction which followed altered the context within which Russian psychiatrists operated. These events shattered their confidence in their ability to direct the course of change, while the new political climate brought with it a host of fresh challenges to their authority. In response to these developments, they embarked on a largely uncharted course.

One immediate consequence of the political turmoil was a dramatic rise in the number of prisoners brought to psychiatric institutions by the tsarist police. The evaluation of mental competence had long been a responsibility of psychiatrists; many individuals who had run afoul of the law and whose mental status was in question had served out part or all of their sentences in psychiatric institutions. The profession had always insisted that such persons be treated as "patients" rather than as "prisoners." The asylum was a medical facility: the jurisdiction of the police ended at its doorway, and the methods of physical restraint utilized by police and prison guards were held to be unacceptable for a mental hospital. Prior to 1905 the profession had been reasonably successful in stopping the police at the gates of the asylum. After 1905, however, an increasing number of the prisoners brought to asylums were designated by the authorities as "political" prisoners who allegedly represented a serious threat to state security.

These new prisoners created difficult problems for psychiatrists. In August 1905, at the Second National Congress of Psychiatrists in Kiev, participants complained that prisoners were brought to them without any accompanying medical history, so that effective diagnosis and treatment became exceedingly difficult. Some psychiatrists added that they were compelled by the police to act as jail-keepers instead of healers: "we must conduct searches, provide extra supervision, and prevent escapes."[8] A most disturbing development was the unwillingness of tsarist prison administrators to entrust "dangerous" individuals to medical professionals; instead, hospitalized prisoners were shackled and surrounded with armed guards.

Psychiatrists protested against these measures on therapeutic grounds, although their notions of what was therapeutic remained inseparable from their notions of professional autonomy and respect. They protested the presence of chains and armed officials in the hospitals on the grounds that they were disturbing to all patients. Even the most passive patients became upset at the sight of physical restraints and armed strangers, they insisted, and those already in an agitated state grew even more difficult to control, much less to treat. More important, they protested, the presence of prison officials who paid no attention to the hospital regime undermined the authority of the psychiatric physician and seriously compromised his ability to retain the trust of patients. Without complete confidence of the patients in the asylum director, they stressed, the therapeutic mission of the institution was doomed to failure.

Russian psychiatrists' difficulties with the police were not without precedent. For decades the profession had been required by law to accept as patients individuals brought to them by the police. They had repeatedly protested this practice on the grounds that decisions about asylum admission were diagnostic in nature and as such should be made only by medical professionals. These protests led to naught. Instead, psychiatrists now found the police passing beyond the portals of their institutions and interfering in their internal operations. The profession's longstanding efforts to gain exclusive control over the right to diagnose insanity were now superseded by the more critical battle to eliminate a powerful competitor from their principal treatment setting.

The psychiatrists utilized every weapon at their disposal to remove the police from the asylum. They appealed to the Medical Council of the Ministry of Internal Affairs, a group which included among its members the influential professor of psychiatry V. M. Bekhterev. In 1907 the council issued a declaration condemning the use of manacles and leg-irons in mental institutions. Nevertheless the practice continued unabated. Many provincial officials simply ignored the recommendation of the Medical Council. Others protested it after local psychiatrists cited the council's statement as a pretext for refusing to admit individuals brought to the asylum in chains. The highly visible escapes of several political prisoners from mental institutions exacerbated the situation, prompting the Medical Council to create a special commission to explore the problem further.

The commission issued a ruling in 1909 which left no doubt as to who had the final authority. The commission concluded that shackles and manacles should not be used on insane prisoners, "as they are unequivocally injurious to the health not only of those madmen who wear them, but of others who are around them." Its decision was based, however, on a statute pertaining to political exiles which stipulated that shackles should be removed in the case of serious or debilitating illness, provided a physician certified that the patient's condition was such that fetters might prove dangerous or harmful and provided that the prison officials had given their consent.[9] In other words, final authority to remove the chains of prisoner-patients still rested with penal authorities and not with physicians.

Psychiatrists gradually reconciled themselves to the fact that they would not be able to compete successfully with the police for control over the asylum. Their response was to withdraw from the fray by advocating that responsibility for the "dangerous" insane be turned over entirely to penal authorities.

This represented a significant policy reversal for the profession. For the better part of a half century most Russian psychiatrists had argued that no clinical distinction could justifiably be made between insane criminals, prisoners, and other insane individuals and that there was no therapeutic rationale for the segregation of mental patients who were in trouble with the law. While the majority of psychiatrists continued to support this view, they also recognized the inevitability of police interference in the internal life of those institutions which counted among their residents individuals deemed dangerous by the state. Rather than risk losing control over all mental institutions, they reluctantly proposed that mentally disturbed prisoners be transferred to penal institutions. As the psychiatrists saw it, given the clearly stated priorities of the government, competition with the police was certain to end in their own defeat. Their only viable strategy was to distance themselves from responsibility for those whom the government regarded as dangerous. "That would remove from the physicians and other hospital personnel the painful role of jailkeeper and eliminate the basis for conflict with state organs."[10]

Discussion of this painful issue was characterized by a tone of bitter resignation. Psychiatrists in the West, some of whom also advocated the separation of insane prisoners, might have maintained the illusion that it was they who chose the path of separate facilities for criminals and subsequently directed the development of those institutions. For Russian psychiatrists, there was rather the sense that new arrangements were being thrust on them against their will. As longtime critics of tsarist prisons, many psychiatrists were greatly distressed by what they perceived as the unavoidable abandonment of a large group of their charges to settings which they had themselves repeatedly denounced as pathogenic.[11]

DECENTRALIZATION OF PSYCHIATRIC CARE

As the first decade of the twentieth century was drawing to a close, Russian psychiatrists had concluded that they could hope to establish professional dominance only over institutions which did not house patients regarded as dangerous. In practice there were no such institutions. The central government had indicated its intention to resurrect the regional asylums and to equip those institutions with security (*krepkie*) wards for mentally disturbed offenders, but progress in that direction had been exceedingly slow. In theory, institutions for the ''non-dangerous'' would be the responsibility of the local governments. Many psychiatrists therefore chose to dissociate themselves from the state and from what they disparagingly referred to as ''police'' psychiatry, casting their lot instead with other zemstvo medical practitioners.

By strengthening their ties to zemstvo medicine, psychiatrists clearly hoped to enhance their image as autonomous medical experts. That strategy proved to have far-reaching and largely unanticipated consequences. The return of psychiatry to the mainstream of Russian medicine was actively encouraged by the rest of the medical profession, but in the long run it worked to the disadvantage of psychiatrists. Given their inability to demonstrate their superiority as healers of the insane and the dominance of other medical practitioners over the structure of zemstvo medicine, psychiatric physicians were at a distinct disadvantage. In the attempt to establish a satisfactory relationship with zemstvo medical institutions, Russian psychiatrists began to advocate a radical reorganization of care for the ''nondangerous'' insane. As in the case of the ''dangerous'' insane, many psychiatrists were at best ambivalent about this new approach, perceiving it as a necessary compromise with the painful realities of Russian life.

Part of the reality was that zemstvo somatic physicians had advocated the decentralization of health care institutions throughout each province. In an effort to overcome the public distrust of medical institutions and practitioners which had been engendered by the *prikaz* facilities, zemstvo physicians strove to develop rural medical programs and to disperse medical personnel and institutions throughout the countryside. By the mid-1890s more than 60 percent of all zemstvo physicians lived in rural areas. They were justifiably proud of having made medical services available to many who had previously done completely without. Rural zemstvo medical service also provided physicians with a measure of corporate autonomy which they cherished and were willing to go to great lengths to protect.[12] Psychiatric care, focused as it was on the provincial mental hospital, became increasingly anomalous within the structure of zemstvo medicine.

Before the turn of the century, the overwhelming majority of psychiatrists opposed the decentralization of care for the insane. Since psychiatric care invariably meant institutional care, its decentralization would entail either the construction of still more mental institutions or the treatment of psychiatric patients in the small general hospitals scattered throughout each province. As the local governments were already staggering under the burden of one or two provincial asylums, they could scarcely be expected to respond favorably to the proposal that several more be constructed.[13] The profession's view was that there were not enough psychiatrists to staff dozens of small asylums. The alternative was to surrender control of the insane to the somatic physicians who staffed the general hospitals, thus denying the unique value of psychiatric expertise. This position was, for obvious reasons, untenable to the profession.

In short, the goals which psychiatrists and zemstvo somatic physicians set for themselves were strikingly at odds. Psychiatrists saw their professional future within the context of the large provincial hospital and naturally supported continued utilization—even expansion—of such institutions. Most zemstvo physicians, for their part, would have preferred to see those institutions eliminated and medical care decentralized throughout each province.

In the early years of the twentieth century, pressure for decentralization of psychiatric services began to mount. This pressure resulted from, on the one hand, the continually rising cost of maintaining provincial asylums and, on the other, the growing influence of certain groups of medical practitioners (especially sanitary physicians) with zemstvo assemblies in many areas of the country. The first psychiatric advocates of decentralization were two prominent psychiatrists, N. N. Bazhenov and V. I. Iakovenko, both of whom had exceptionally close ties to zemstvo medicine and had been active in the ongoing efforts to increase the autonomy and responsibilities of the local governments. They first presented their proposals to their colleagues at a meeting in 1902 of the Pirogov Society of Russian Physicians, an association dominated by zemstvo practitioners. Both Bazhenov and Iakovenko argued that, consistent with the organization of somatic medicine, the basic organizational unit for zemstvo psychiatry should be the smaller district (*uezd*) rather than the province. They based their arguments on data on asylum admissions which clearly indicated that the majority of patients in provincial asylums were residents of the immediate geographical area in which the institution was situated. Thus, in the words of Bazhenov, "the area of useful activity for the provincial psychiatric hospital is significantly smaller than the territory encompassed by the average province."[14] As it was, he continued, much of the population remained underserved. Large centralized institutions might be successful in the smaller and more densely populated countries in the West, he concluded, but they were totally inappropriate to Russia where distances were great and means of transportation poorly developed.

Iakovenko proposed the establishment in each district of a small psychiatric hospital with ten to twenty beds. Bazhenov went even further, urging the introduction of outpatient care programs for the insane who lived in areas remote from provincial hospitals.[15] Although Bazhenov and Iakovenko were both respected members of the profession, their views on this issue were shared by only a few psychiatrists, most of them staunch zemstvo partisans. While virtually all psychiatrists applauded the principle of making psychiatric services more accessible to the population, the proposals of Iakovenko and Bazhenov were denounced by the rest of their colleagues as "fantasies," "premature," and "unrealizeable."[16]

The issues were raised again at the next Pirogov Society meeting held in 1904. On that occasion the participants passed a resolution advocating the geographic dispersal of psychiatric services throughout each province. The resolution was not, as it might appear, a dramatic reversal in policy, but was in fact the result of increased efforts on the part of zemstvo somatic physicians to force on their psychiatric colleagues a new direction. It was indeed a sanitary physician who introduced the resolution on decentralization, and observers later reported that the room had been packed with nonpsychiatrists.[17]

Not surprisingly, there was much resentment at this intrusion by nonspecialists into psychiatric affairs. When psychiatrists held their own conference a year later in Kiev, a proposal to decentralize care was ignored by the conference participants. Only one discussant even responded to the proposal, and he did so with an offhand comment which suggested that there was virtually no concrete evidence to indicate the feasibility of such an idea.[18]

The position of the profession soon changed radically. Not only did many psychiatrists begin to advocate a reduced role for the provincial hospital, but their proposals for change began increasingly to include noninstitutional modes of treatment. This position distinguished Russian psychiatric policies from those of most of their Western counterparts.

Examination of the sequence of events suggests that the psychiatrists' about-face came largely in response to actions taken by their zemstvo employers rather than as a result of new research findings. The provincial zemstvos would not—at least some perhaps could not—support the further expansion of large psychiatric institutions. In increasing numbers, they simply ignored the recommendations of their psychiatrists and began to implement the proposal of somatic physicians that psychiatric care be provided at the district level. The knowledge that certain zemstvos had elected to send sanitary physicians rather than psychiatrists to the psychiatric section of that Pirogov Society meeting in 1904 was especially sobering to the psychiatric profession. In short, psychiatrists began to realize that the local governments intended to reorganize psychiatric care with or without their cooperation. Their new proposals appear to have been designed to reassert some control over the situation.

No one seriously believed that the district zemstvos would sanction the construction of dozens of small psychiatric hospitals. By the same token, they could scarcely be expected to employ enough psychiatrists to staff every district. In other words, it seemed clear that if psychiatric care were decentralized it would in the process be handed over to the somatic physicians who already staffed the small district hospitals. Psychiatrists' rejection of most of the proposals for decentralization was thus not surprising; virtually all of them would have given far greater responsibility for the insane to nonspecialist district physicians. Psychiatrists opposed this on therapeutic grounds. The district physicians were already overworked, they protested, and most had little interest in the insane. As one psychiatrist commented, "it is difficult to comprehend how one could turn over the responsibility for such an important matter to district physicians whose incompetence in psychiatric matters is all too well known to us."[19]

Psychiatrists also could not ignore the implications of decentralization both for their livelihood and for the role of their profession. To endorse decentralization was tantamount to admitting that their services were not essential. They could never hope to take the place of somatic physicians in the district hospitals, nor could they expect the zemstvos to employ a psychiatrist for each of the small district facilities. The possibility of unemployment was still too real for most physicians willingly to surrender salaried positions.

Support for noninstitutional alternatives thus emerged as an effort by the psychiatric profession to salvage for itself a role. The model most often proposed was a community-based program of foster care for chronic patients who were judged to pose little threat to the community. These extramural programs, which had been advocated since the 1880s by a small minority of Russian psychiatrists, were based on Western models (principally the Belgian village of Gheel and the Scottish home care system).[20] Most members of the Russian psychiatric profession, however, had remained avidly opposed to the idea that any mental patients could be successfully treated outside the confines of a psychiatric hospital. It was not good medicine, they argued, and it posed substantial risks to both the insane and their foster families. Before 1905 most psychiatrists denounced the idea at every opportunity. The few experiments attempted prior to this era were ridiculed and failures were held up to close public scrutiny in the professional media.[21]

By the outbreak of World War I more than half of all the provinces of European Russia had introduced foster care programs, and many of the rest had plans for them. In a number of provinces the initiative in this direction was not taken by psychiatrists, but most of them jumped quickly on the foster care bandwagon. From their standpoint, foster care for the insane was far from an ideal concept, but it was distinctly preferable to the decentralization of care for the insane in district hospitals. Extramural care could be organized, as Bazhenov had suggested, "at the hospital gates" or, after the fashion of Gheel, Belgium, in villages physically remote from the hospital. It could function either in conjunction with institutional care for the acutely ill, which would be provided in a centrally located facility, or on its own, independent of any institution. But the important point was that the foster care programs (generally referred to by the French term *patronage familial*) could, at least in theory, be under the direct supervision of a psychiatric specialist who worked closely with both the hospital and his professional colleagues. In other words, these programs were an opportunity for the zemstvos to reduce the cost of psychiatric care without depriving psychiatric practitioners of their independence and professional autonomy.

Psychiatrists' advocacy of the deinstitutionalization of much of Russia's insane population represented a desperate attempt by the profession to construct for itself a meaningful role. Although the alternatives may have been far worse, the position of psychiatrists within the *patronage familial* was hardly a firm foundation on which to build a professional identity. They certainly could not claim to play a major role in the "treatment" of those individuals boarded out to peasant families, nor could they claim to exercise much control over the conditions under which "care" was provided.

Psychiatrists represented the new idea of community treatment as a therapeutic advance: treating patients in more natural, homelike settings, they argued, in some cases improved their functional capacity. Nonetheless, close reading of their proclamations in support of foster care suggests strongly that most of those supposedly important therapeutic consequences were unanticipated. Psychiatrists introduced the programs with trepidation, discovering only after the fact that there were patients who benefited from them. Some members of the profession made no effort to hide the fact that they regarded the *patronage familial* as a painful compromise necessitated by the economic and political realities of Russian rural life. Although it might benefit a few patients, they feared that foster care held the potential for exploitation of both the helpless insane and Russia's destitute peasant population.

TURMOIL IN THE ASYLUMS

The local government assemblies had a number of reasons for wanting to divert resources away from the provincial asylums. Of greatest importance was the high cost of running these greedy institutions (not to mention the expense of new construction). But the facilities were also suspect in the minds of the increasingly conservative nobles who dominated many zemstvos after 1905, because some of the provincial asylums had been marked by unrest during the troubled months of Russia's first revolution. Like many other large institutions during that era, the mental hospitals of the empire at times were rocked by workers' demonstrations or strikes. Although most of these were relatively brief and insignificant incidents, on a few occasions the turmoil was prolonged and brought in its wake dramatic changes to the structure of authority in the institution.

These events not only stunned local authorities but shocked many members of the psychiatric profession as well. Although only a handful of psychiatrists had played an active role in the incidents, the effect of these disruptions on the profession was far-reaching. These attempts at "institutional revolution" became an additional basis for conflict between psychiatrists and their various employers. Even more significant, they led psychiatrists to reassess their role as a "professional" group within the larger hierarchy of workers, and ultimately to adopt a stand diametrically opposed to the ideals of autonomy and professional dominance which they had sought so ardently for more than a half century.

In some instances the demonstrations organized by workers had as their primary focus economic issues. The workers sought higher pay, shorter hours, and better working conditions. In at least two widely publicized incidents, however, workers in psychiatric institutions augmented their demands for economic change with an insistence on workplace democracy. In asylums in Khar'kov and St. Petersburg, medical directors were physically removed from the premises and the hospital "autocracy" was replaced with a "representative government" consisting of delegates selected by workers in the institution. Psychiatric physicians reluctantly participated in these new administrative organs but did not control them.[22] The workers professed to desire for the asylum the same form of governance which opposition groups (including many psychiatrists) were noisily demanding for society at large: a constituent assembly, selected on the basis of universal, direct, equal, and secret ballot.

These events created a moral and professional dilemma for Russia's psychiatrists. The problem of how to reconcile their commitment to equal representation in government with an insistence on professional privilege in the workplace was troubling for many. This was especially true for younger members of the profession, most of whom had already taken a stand against autocratic asylum directors.

The earliest generation of psychiatrists had unanimously endorsed the concentration of formal authority in mental institutions in the hands of one physician-director to whom all of the employees of the hospital were subordinate. The shared conviction about the central role of the asylum's medical director derived in large part from the concept of "moral treatment" which dominated the thinking of most nineteenth-century psychiatrists, in Russia as in other Western nations. "Moral treatment," according to a prominent historian of American psychiatry,

> meant kind individualized care in a small hospital; resort to occupational therapy, religious exercises, amusements and games. . . . Along with a rationale for care and treatment went a fairly elaborate vision of the structure of the ideal mental hospital. There was general agreement that hospitals should remain small (250 or less); that superintendents should have complete control of the medical, moral and dietetic treatment, and that all staff, professional and supporting, should remain under the unfettered control of the superintendent.[23]

The principles of "moral treatment" had inspired the architects of Russia's first asylums, and throughout the rest of the century the profession continued to rely on that model. They used it repeatedly in their efforts to wrest from nonspecialists control over asylums.

The argument that one individual should be in complete command of the asylum was relatively easy for psychiatrists to make when most asylums employed only one psychiatric physician. By the early twentieth century, however, many mental institutions were larger and had several psychiatrists on their payroll. Convinced of the superiority of their own credentials, most of the newer psychiatric physicians resented the bureaucratic organization of the asylum. They protested that it was incompatible with the ideals of collegiality and cooperation which they had been socialized to regard as inherent in the notion of "profession" and central to the medical practice of psychiatry. Increasingly, the result in a number of institutions was open conflict between asylum directors and this new generation of practitioners.

The younger psychiatrists urged that institutions introduce a form of "collective or collegial administration." In their view the posts of director, assistant director, senior and junior intern, and all other hierarchical designations should be eliminated. Each and every doctor should be responsible for the conditions in his department and answerable to the local governments, the central government, and society as a whole. Support for this concept grew rapidly in the first years of the twentieth century, a reflection both of the growth of this new generation of professionals and of the increasing politicization of the profession. In 1905, at their conference in Kiev, psychiatrists passed a resolution calling for the introduction into asylums of collective forms of administration which would include all physician specialists.[24]

While support for the idea was far from universal, those who did advocate collective administration couched the discussion in language which reflected their broader political concerns. In the eyes of this group, the asylum was the larger society in microcosm. Those values and organizational principles which dominated Russian society and against which they were raising their voices in protest were deeply embedded in the functioning of the empire's psychiatric institutions. The administrative structure of those institutions, they alleged, was rigidly hierarchical, exploitative, inefficient, and immoral.

Bolstered by the passing of the resolution at the Kiev gathering, most of these psychiatrists returned home ready to press for the introduction of collective administration in their own institutions. Within weeks, however, they found their position surpassed by the demands of nonprofessional workers to be included in this scheme for authority sharing. Though psychiatrists had acknowledged for years that the nonprofessional staff in the asylums played a vital role in its daily operation, all but the most radical were shocked by the workers' insistence that they be allowed to sit as equal partners on policymaking organs in the institutions.

The profession was at first deeply divided on this issue. There were those who insisted that no compromises be made with the workers. At the other extreme were a few psychiatrists who praised the workers' initiatives and encouraged their colleagues to support them. For most, however, the issues were not so clear cut. Having joined with the hospital proletariat in insisting that Russia be governed by a constituent assembly, physicians now found the workers demanding a similar government for their mutual workplace. The majority of physicians supported the principle of universal and equal suffrage for the empire as a whole; to support the workers' position within the confines of the hospital, however, was tantamount to the negation of their professional superiority, as that was presumably based on knowledge and capabilities possessed only by physicians.

In the years immediately after the Revolution of 1905 the majority of psychiatrists continued to insist on the inviolability of professional privilege. They were willing to admit nonprofessional workers to decision-making organs only when the interests of that group were directly involved. Only a few of the most radical members of the profession insisted on the full inclusion of nonprofessional workers in institutional administration. But by the eve of World War I, the profession's stand had changed. By 1910 the profession had twice unanimously endorsed resolutions calling for the introduction into *all* asylums of collective forms of administration which would include not only physicians but all other workers as well.

The first resolution was passed by the Pirogov Society's Section on Nervous and Mental Diseases at the society's tenth meeting in 1907. So strong were feelings on the subject by the end of 1909 that the topic headed the agenda of the Third Conference of Russian Psychiatrists which took place in St. Petersburg late that year.

With this new policy Russian psychiatrists had adopted a stand which seriously compromised their dominant position in the institutional division of labor. Their advocacy of such a policy was without precedent in the international psychiatric community. In espousing it they stressed the important role of nonprofessional workers in the asylum. They are our "coworkers and collaborators," argued one influential member of the profession in 1911, not "servants or assistants."[25]

As Elliot Freidson has pointed out, the central defining characteristic of a profession such as medicine or psychiatry is its autonomy, which "is sustained by the dominance of its expertise in the division of labor."[26] The adoption by an aspiring professional group of a stand which would undermine its autonomy seems puzzling. In the case of Russian psychiatrists, the sequence of events suggests that the profession adopted this position (as it did so many others) in reaction to external pressures rather than because of any independent assessment of its therapeutic worth. The years of reaction which followed 1905 had made it clear to psychiatrists that the profession would be allowed no say in how asylums were administered. Zemstvo assemblies across European Russia refused to work with the newly instituted councils of physicians and instead formally reinstated asylum directors and reaffirmed their dictatorial power over the institutions. These actions infuriated psychiatrists, and their anger grew even more intense as they witnessed those individuals who had been the most daring in their efforts to restructure the asylum being fired, imprisoned, and exiled.

Most of the leaders of the profession had been critical of attempts by the more radical of their younger colleagues in 1905 and 1906 to democratize the asylum. Nonetheless, when those individuals were made to suffer for their actions, their colleagues were quick to spring to their defense and to insist on the right of psychiatrists to determine how the asylum would be governed. At the heavily attended First Conference of the Russian Union of Psychiatrists and Neuropathologists in 1911, only one participant spoke out in strong opposition to the inclusion of support personnel in collective administration.[27] In short, the commitment of psychiatrists to asylum democracy grew in proportion to the insistence of their employers on maintaining a rigid hierarchy of authority in the institutions.

CONCLUSIONS

By the eve of the revolutions of 1917 the path taken by Russian psychiatrists had deviated in a number of significant ways from that followed by most of their Western counterparts. First, they had espoused an organizational scheme of care for the insane which involved abdicating responsibility for those insane persons judged dangerous by the government and returning many other patients to the peasant milieu from which they had come. While psychiatrists would retain nominal control over most of those patients, the conditions under which care would be provided were a far cry from those regarded as optimal. The need to develop an affordable system of care which would minimize competition and interference from both other physicians and the police had led them to embrace therapeutic concepts which they acknowledged to be inferior. Most were less than satisfied with this new direction and were deeply concerned about the future of the profession as well.

Second, mounting concern for their own welfare and that of their patients led many to elaborate a psychiatric critique of the society and politics of late tsarist Russia.[28] The tsarist regime itself was a direct threat to mental health, they maintained, and change was essential for the good of the entire population. A few senior members of the profession remained vocal supporters of the status quo (and of autocracy in particular), but their numbers were small. A somewhat greater range of opinion existed regarding appropriate strategies for change. Some psychiatrists actively participated in the revolutionary movement. Others opted for ''smaller deeds.'' The profession as a whole, however, spoke with an increasingly united voice on social and political issues. At the heart of their critique of Russian society was a firm conviction that ''prevention of the physical and psychological degeneration of the population was dependent upon fundamental political and economic reform of Russian life.''[29]

World War I diverted everyone's attention away from domestic concerns. The number of insane in the asylums plummeted, and much of the energy of psychiatrists was devoted to the treatment and evacuation of mentally disturbed soldiers. Even those individuals who remained at their institutional posts were similarly preoccupied. Asylums throughout the empire were reorganized during the war years to maximize the bed space available for the physically and mentally injured.

The events of early 1917 demonstrated that psychiatrists had not abandoned their earlier convictions. Their commitment to collective administration which five years earlier had seemed little more than a symbolic gesture of protest resurfaced after the abdication of Nicholas II in February of 1917. In April, Russian psychiatrists met to discuss their future. One after another, they described how they had welcomed the February Revolution by ousting the old hierarchy and introducing collective administration into their asylums.[30]

Understandably, many psychiatrists eagerly embraced the new regime which assumed power in October of 1917. With their commitment to workplace democracy and their conviction that fundamental change was essential to the construction of a mentally healthy society, psychiatrists shared a number of goals with the Bolsheviks. They also anticipated that the new regime would enhance the role of the profession, and a large number of them quickly assumed positions in the new government. The many consequences of that decision deserve to be chronicled in a separate essay.

NOTES

1. The literature on these developments in Western societies is quite extensive. See, for example, Norman Dain, *Concepts of Insanity in the United States, 1789–1865* (New Bruns-

wick, N. J., 1964); Klaus Doerner, *Madness and the Bourgeoisie: A Social History of Insanity and Psychiatry* (New York, 1981); Michel Foucault, *Madness and Civilization* (New York, 1965); Richard W. Fox, *So Far Disordered in Mind: Insanity in California, 1870–1930* (Berkeley, Calif., 1978); Jan Goldstein, *Console and Classify: The French Psychiatric Profession in the Nineteenth Century* (Cambridge, 1987); Gerald N. Grob, *Mental Institutions in America: Social Policy to 1875* (New York, 1973); David Rothman, *The Discovery of The Asylum* (Boston, 1971); Andrew T. Scull, *Museums of Madness: The Social Organization of Insanity in Nineteenth-Century England* (New York, 1979); and Nancy Tomes, *A Generous Confidence: Thomas Story Kirkbride and the Art of Asylum Keeping, 1840–1883* (New York, 1984).

2. S. Tekutev, *Istoricheskii ocherk kafedry i kliniki dushevnykh i nervnykh boleznei pri imperatorskoi voenno-meditsinskoi akademii* (St. Petersburg, 1898), p. 79.

3. J. V. Brown, "Psychiatrists and the State in Late Imperial Russia," in A. Scull and S. Cohen, eds., *Social Control and the State* (New York, 1983), pp. 267–87.

4. Indications are that politics played a significant role in this incident. The Tver zemstvo was known as a liberal stronghold and Litvinov was himself a member of the "liberal" nobility. His ouster came shortly after the newly crowned Nicholas II removed much of that liberal contingent from the local government assembly. This incident is discussed at length in Julie V. Brown, "The Professionalization of Russian Psychiatry, 1857–1911" (Ph.D. diss., University of Pennsylvania, 1981), pp. 141–45.

5. V. P. Chizh, "Letter to the Editor," *Nevrologicheskii Vestnik*, 3 (1895), p. 174.

6. J. V. Brown, "Peasant Survival Strategies in Late Imperial Russia: The Social Uses of the Mental Hospital," *Social Problems*, 34 (1987), pp. 311–29.

7. Cited in *Arkhiv psikhiatrii, nevrologii, i experimental'noi psikhologii*, 5 (1887), p. 154.

8. Excerpted from a discussion at the Second National Congress of Russian Psychiatrists: *Trudy vtorogo s"ezda otechestvennykh psikhiatrov proiskhodivshago v g. Kieve s 4-go po 11-go sentiabria 1905g* (Kiev, 1907), pp. 146–60.

9. V. M. Bekhterev and P. A. Ostankov, "O kandalakh u istpytuemykh i dushevno-bol'nykh arestantov," *Trudy pervago s"ezda russkago soiuza psikhiatrov i nevropatologov* (Moscow, 1914), p. 532; *Trudy tretiiago s"ezda otechestvennykh psikhiatrov* (St. Petersburg, 1911), p. 546.

10. N. N. Bazhenov, "Proekt zakonodatel'stva o dushevno-bol'nykh i ob'iasnitel'naia zapiska k nemu," *Trudy pervago s"ezda russkago soiuza*, p. 278.

11. J. V. Brown, "Revolution and Psychosis: The Mixing of Science and Politics in Russian Psychiatric Medicine, 1905–13," *The Russian Review*, 46 (1987), pp. 283–302.

12. Nancy M. Frieden, *Russian Physicians in an Era of Reform and Revolution* (Princeton, N. J., 1981).

13. In 1901 the zemstvos spent a total of 2,389,300 rubles on the operation and maintenance of psychiatric hospitals, an amount which represented nearly one-fourth of all zemstvo expenditures on hospitals and outpatient clinics. In several provinces (among them Tver and Riazan) the expenditures for psychiatric hospitals were greater than those for district and rural hospitals combined.

14. N. N. Bazhenov and V. I. Koliubakin, "V kakom napravlenii dolzhen byt' sdelan sleduiushchii shag v dele organizatsii prizreniia dushevno-bol'nykh," *Zhurnal nevropatologii i psikhiatrii im. S. S. Korsakov*, 2 (1902), pp. 145–55.

15. Ibid.

16. See Bazhenov, "Proekt." See also Obshchestvo Russkikh Vrachei v Pamiat' N. I. Pirogova, *S"ezd VIII: Vos'moi Pirogovskii S"ezd Moskva 3–10.I.1902* (Moscow, 1903).

17. N. V. Krainskii, "Vliianie 'nastroeniia' na evoliutsiiu psikhiatricheskago dela v Rossii," *Nauchnyi arkhiv vilenskoi okruzhnoi lechebnitsy*, nos. 1–2 (1904), 238.

18. P. P. Tutyshkin, "K voprosu o zakonodatel'stve o dushevno-bol'nykh i psikhiatricheskikh uchrezhdeniiakh," *Trudy tret'iago s"ezda*, pp. 403–4.

19. *Trudy tret'iago s"ezda*, p. 165.

20. These programs are discussed in William Ll. Parry-Jones, "The Model of the Gheel

Lunatic Colony and Its Influence on the Nineteenth-Century Asylum System in Britain,'' in Scull and Cohen, eds., *Social Control and the State*, pp. 201–217.

21. J. V. Brown, ''A Sociohistorical Perspective on Deinstitutionalization: The Case of Late Imperial Russia,'' *Research in Law, Deviance and Social Control*, 7 (1985), pp. 167–88.

22. These incidents are discussed thoroughly in Brown, ''Professionalization,'' pp. 352–61. See also J. V. Brown, ''The Deprofessionalization of Soviet Physicians: A Reconsideration,'' *International Journal of Health Services*, 17 (1987), pp. 65–76.

23. Grob, *Mental Institutions in America*, pp. 168–70.

24. *Trudy vtorogo s"ezda otechestvennykh psikhiatrov*, p. 106.

25. *Trudy pervago s"ezda rus_kago soiuza psikhiatrov*, p. 452.

26. Elliot Freidson, *Professional Dominance: The Social Structure of Medical Care* (New York, 1970), p. 136.

27. V. N. Ergol'skii, Director of the Voronezh Provincial Psychiatric Hospital, *Trudy pervago s"ezda russkago soiuza*, p. 743.

28. This critique is analyzed in Brown, ''Revolution and Psychosis.''

29. M. Ia. Droznes, *Zadachi meditsiny v bor'be s sovremennoi nervoznost'iu* (Odessa, 1907), p. 15.

30. L. A. Prozorov, *Trudy konferentsii vrachei psikhiatrov i nevropatologov sozvannoi pravleniem russkago soiuza psikhiatrov i nevropatologov v Moskve v 1917g 10–12 aprel'ia* (Moscow, 1917).

LAURIE BERNSTEIN

Yellow Tickets and
State-Licensed Brothels

The Tsarist Government and the Regulation of
Urban Prostitution

Like most European governments in the nineteenth century, the Russian government linked the control of venereal disease with the control of prostitution. Singled out as pernicious carriers of diseases, prostitutes were compelled to register with the local police, undergo regular physical examinations, and, if diagnosed as contagious, submit to hospitalization in locked wards. In most Russian cities government agencies known as medical-police committees issued prostitutes special licenses which identified their trade and certified their state of health. This combination of official toleration and tight control was also extended to brothels: medical-police committees permitted brothels to operate as long as they conformed to specific regulations.

Most European countries had experimented with the regulation of prostitution and, with a few exceptions, continued the practice into the beginning of the twentieth century.[1] Not surprisingly, Russia's medical-police committees suffered from many of the same problems which plagued other European regulatory agencies—quasi-legal status, corruption, arbitrary enforcement, and dubious, if not counterproductive, medical techniques. By the same token, after the turn of the century Russian educated society had begun to react against regulation; much of the same feminist critique and moral outrage that regulation had provoked among its European opponents (or "abolitionists") was beginning to be heard in Russia.

Because of the late emergence of a self-conscious and articulate civil society in Russia, the movement to end government regulation of prostitution took shape slowly. At first the most scathing denunciations of regulation came from the physicians and bureaucrats responsible for maintaining the system of regulation. Although few called for outright abolition, members of both these groups recognized that regulation simply did not work. Not until 1910 did educated society raise its collective voice against regulation. At the first All-Russian Congress for the Struggle against the Trade in Women it was resolved that "medical-police surveillance of prostitution does not attain its sanitary goals, enslaves women to prostitution, increases the number of prostitutes, acts in a fashion demoralizing to youth of both sexes, the whole population and agents of surveillance, and degrades and insults the dignity of women.''[2]

Reform lay within the purview of the Ministry of Internal Affairs (MVD). Fears about the spread of venereal disease in the late 1880s and in the early years of the twentieth century led the MVD to depart from its usually vigorous efforts to assert control over city councils and zemstvos and contemplate allowing local governments a measure of authority over regulation in certain circumstances.[3] This unusual concession on the part of the MVD was stimulated in this instance by the recognition that its task far exceeded its capabilities and by fears for public health should venereal disease be permitted to spread.

This essay traces the changing attitudes of the MVD toward prostitution and venereal disease in the early 1900s. Whereas throughout the nineteenth century the ministry had had full confidence in its regulatory operations, serious misgivings arose at the turn of the century because of growing evidence of shortcomings. MVD policies gradually acquired a more pragmatic edge, allowing for both local discretion and a more visible municipal role in the treatment of prostitutes and in the administration of regulation. Because the ministry was increasingly willing to accept whatever measures worked, it supported, paradoxically, some plans for local control that were intended to supplant its own medical-police committees. Moreover, when brothel prostitution became particularly controversial, the ministry went so far as to abdicate its authority over the granting of licenses to state brothels.

Despite the MVD's flexibility on this matter, most of the alternatives to regulation were also doomed to failure. Not only did most cities lack the financial means to realize reforms in the regulatory system, but reformers lacked muscle: a reluctant city governor or a slow-moving municipal bureaucracy could block any proposed improvements. Ministerial approval was obviously not enough; without active support from the MVD, the vast majority of municipal institutions could neither implement their own program nor make significant headway in the fight against venereal disease. At the same time, problems of funding, political rivalries, and a general unwillingness to be associated with a system that condoned prostitution made it unlikely that more than a handful of city councils and zemstvos would take advantage of the MVD's unexpected tolerance on this issue.

PROSTITUTION AND THE STATE

Prostitution had never received an official welcome in tsarist Russia. As early as the seventeenth century a law stipulated that "streets and alleys should be strictly patrolled day and night so that fighting, robbery, and whoring do not occur." In 1718, Peter the Great himself directed the police chief of St. Petersburg to stamp out "all suspicious houses, namely taverns, gambling parlors, and other obscene establishments." Under Catherine the Great it was forbidden by law "to open one's own home or to use a rented home day or night for indecency (*nepotrebstvo*); to enter a home by day or night for indecency; and to support oneself or another through indecency." Her son, Paul, went so far as to decree in 1800 that all "drunken and debauched women" should be exiled to forced labor in factories located in the remote Siberian city of Irkutsk.[4]

These repressive laws notwithstanding, prostitution thrived before the nineteenth century, sometimes with the tacit permission of the authorities. For example, in the mid-seventeenth century a German observer of Russian life commented on the tradeswomen near Moscow's Kremlin who, in addition to their wares, offered "something else for sale as well." In his *Journey from St. Petersburg to Moscow* (1790), Alexander Radishchev asserted that there were "painted harlots on every street in both the capitals" and went on to complain that the government allowed prostitution to flourish. Indeed, in the late eighteenth century certain sections of St. Petersburg were designated by the authorities for the operation of "free houses."[5]

In the 1840s the government decided to control prostitution according to a regulatory system modeled after the Parisian *régime des moeurs*.[6] Promoted by Count Lev A. Perovskii, Nicholas I's ambitious new minister of internal affairs, this new policy reflected the administration's acceptance of prostitution as a "necessary social evil" that, because of its public health implications, required government supervision. In the autumn of 1843 authorities in St. Petersburg organized a trial medical-police committee (*vrachebno-politseiskii komitet*) under the MVD, and in 1844 a similar committee was created in Moscow. Several other cities followed suit over the next few years. Nicholas accepted the necessity of regulating prostitution but, as he wrote in 1847, "by no means" did he wish to extend his "favor" to brothelkeepers. Perovskii swayed him, however, with a spirited defense of brothels: houses of prostitution, he argued, were controlled environments, "relatively useful for society," which would be administered by individuals functioning as "agents of the police."[7]

Initially, regulation was a relatively simple matter of identification, inspection, and incarceration. In the words of the 1844 rules: "When away from home, public women must always carry a medical ticket regarding the state of their health." This license (commonly known as a "yellow ticket") listed a prostitute's name, age, and address and left room for a physician to certify her as "healthy" or "menstruating." Prostitutes were to be examined on a weekly basis and were required to report immediately to a hospital if the examining physician discovered any sign of venereal disease.[8]

In 1861, amid Alexander II's Great Reforms, new rules added a different dimension to government regulation of prostitution: medical tickets were now to be issued in lieu of internal passports, thus depriving these women of the right to travel, find work, or move without official knowledge or permission. In addition to dooming thousands of women to full-time prostitution, this measure accelerated the professionalization of prostitution by removing the cloak of anonymity that women who turned to this trade on a casual or clandestine basis might have maintained. Deprived of their passports, women registered as prostitutes now had nothing to show prospective landlords or employers but their embarrassing yellow tickets.[9]

For several reasons regulation proved inadequate to the task of protecting public health. First and most obvious, regulation could hardly serve as an effective curb on venereal disease when only the prostitutes and not their clients were subject to medical scrutiny. Although the rules stipulated that prostitutes themselves examine their clients, this injunction was highly unrealistic in a world of drunken, dark, and hasty trysts. In 1851 the MVD prescribed medical examinations for "all persons of both sexes from the lower class who had been arrested by the police for deeds against public decency (*blagochinie*)"; it also directed provincial governors to compel factories and other institutions with large staffs to hire physicians to administer periodic examinations of male workers. Yet, these measures could affect only a fraction of the men who might patronize prostitutes, and there is good reason to doubt the effectiveness of the implementation of these directives.[10]

Second, although medical-police committees mandated regular and frequent examinations for prostitutes, the intervals between examinations left sufficient time for prostitutes to contract and transmit both syphilis and gonorrhea. Furthermore, examinations were far from foolproof because physicians knew so little about venereal disease. Until 1906, when the Wassermann test was invented, medical science was unable to differentiate syphilis from other venereal diseases with any degree of certainty.[11] Moreover, because microscopic examinations of women's vaginal secretions were rarely conducted, gonorrhea was frequently confused with simple vaginal infections and went undetected when not accompanied by severe discharge. Syphilis was also difficult to identify during its dormant, albeit still contagious, periods.

Third, if diagnosis was problematic, remedies were even less reliable. Penicillin was not developed as a cure until the 1940s; until 1910 the most common treatment for syphilis consisted of an ineffective series of painful injections of mercury.[12] Severe salivation (measured by the pint!) was only one of this drug's unpleasant side effects. Others included gastroenteritis, listlessness, anemia, liver and kidney diseases, loss of teeth, loss of hair, and even death. When a patient's gastrointestinal tract "could stand no more," inunctions made from mercury in a base of suet and lard replaced these injections. This ointment was gentler to the human organism, but it promoted skin diseases and condemned patients to walk around covered with a smelly blue-gray sheen.[13]

Finally, a lack of medical knowledge and expertise on venereal disease was compounded by the shortage of hospitals and qualified physicians. Venereal wards and venereal specialists outside the major cities were naturally even more scarce. Though syphilis was known to move in and out of its contagious phase over a period of years, prostitutes remained in the hospital for only three to six weeks. Lack of space compelled doctors to release their patients as soon as their sores, but not necessarily their contagion, disappeared.

Inadequacies of medical science and training were only a part of the problem. Funding also presented an enormous obstacle. Although the MVD had proclaimed in 1851 that every city should regulate prostitution, it failed to earmark funds for the implementation of this decree. At the very least, local agencies needed physicians, medical facilities, medical instruments, an administrative staff, and special hospital wards for housing diseased prostitutes. Only St. Petersburg received a stipend to operate its medical-police committee; other cities were expected to drain their already modest budgets.[14]

Further confusion was created by the fact that regulation policies violated the law that prohibited earning a living through "indecency." In 1845 the police were instructed to refrain from prosecuting prostitutes who were guilty of no other crimes, but later efforts by the ministries of internal affairs and justice to clarify the quasi-legal status of prostitutes suggest that provincial authorities remained bemused. Pointing to the paradox that was inherent in regulating an illegal trade, the State Council ruled in 1868 that, "without obviously contradicting itself," the law could not consider matters pertaining to the organization of prostitution.[15] Thus, prostitution in Russia, as in most European states, remained a part of the administrative realm, neither inside the law nor wholly outside it. Specific rules governing its regulation required approval from the Senate, but the MVD was responsible for their formulation and promulgation. Just as the state circumvented the courts by subjecting political prisoners to administrative prosecution, prostitutes were subject to rules rather than laws. Their fate was thus in the hands of the ministry's agents, namely, the police—and herein lay the source of most of the trouble.

Regulation gave the police effective power to monitor and pass judgment on the behavior of women in urban lower-class communities. Policemen in Russia's cities were empowered to identify those women who were practicing prostitution without a license by rounding up all "suspicious" women for medical examinations.[16] Regulation gave police the authority to determine what constituted unseemly female behavior, and thus encouraged an array of abuses. Not only did individual policemen harass, blackmail, and arrest innocent women, but local authorities also enjoyed carte blanche in supervising the activities of working-class and poor women. "Unseemly" behavior was a broad, arbitrary rubric that could include women who walked alone after dark and women whose conduct was not to the liking of the local police. Often, technical virginity was the sole evidence a woman could use to prove that she was not a prostitute, yet this "proof" was predicated on an intimate, mortifying examination in police headquarters and was of no help whatsoever to those with sexual experience.

By granting such broad powers to local police, the regulatory system could hardly be immune to corruption. Indeed, the press repeatedly mentioned incidents involving women who were unjustly apprehended during police round-ups. As the author of a 1906 pamphlet exclaimed, "Nobody knows how many girls have been ruined as a result of the coarse and hasty methods practiced by the medical-police committee!"[17] Simbirsk was the scene of a particularly scandalous episode. In 1889, distressed by reports about the prevalence of syphilis among the local military, the Simbirsk police subjected every female in one section of the city—including children, married women, and the old—to pelvic examinations.[18]

In 1892 the Senate moved to prevent further abuses of power by ruling that women could not be examined or registered as prostitutes against their will. Nonetheless, stories of mistaken arrests and police brutality attest to the likelihood that local authorities interpreted regulation to mean that all "suspicious" females were to be checked carefully and that every suspected prostitute was to be issued a yellow ticket, whether or not she agreed to accept one. Even the most ardent supporter of regulation, Dr. Veniamin M. Tarnovskii, head of dermatological and venereal medicine at the Academy of Military Medicine, estimated that one in every five women was registered without her permission.[19]

The efforts of the MVD to control prostitution provide an excellent example of the gulf between aspiration and reality in the tsarist administration. Given not only the limitations of contemporary medical knowledge, but also the difficulties of governing that vast empire, regulation could not by itself reduce the spread of venereal disease. By the end of the nineteenth century, Russia's medical professionals were acutely aware of this problem, just as they were convinced that syphilis was spreading inexorably.[20] Like their European colleagues, Russia's physicians tended to fall into one of two camps: those who believed that the regulatory system was in dire need of improvement and those who believed that regulation was, by its very nature, futile, if not counterproductive.

"PROSTITUTION IN THE CITIES"

Physicians and bureaucrats discussed the shortcomings of regulation in 1897 at the Congress on Measures against Syphilis. Although the express purpose of this congress was to discuss the control of syphilis, for many state officials prostitution and the spread of syphilis were almost synonymous, and thus prostitution became the implicit theme of the gathering. Sponsored by the Medical Department of the MVD, the 1897 congress was the regime's first attempt to address what was perceived to be a growing syphilis epidemic. More than 450 zemstvo, military, factory and private physicians, university professors, and state officials, a veritable "Who's Who" of Russia's administrative professional intelligentsia, participated in discussions of such issues as urban and rural prostitution, the proper nomenclature for venereal disease, and syphilis in the military and among industrial and commercial workers.

Tarnovskii, an adherent of the Italian school of criminal anthropology and the most renowned proponent of state regulation of prostitution, defined the problem for his colleagues: "Take any case of syphilis which apparently has nothing in common with prostitution and trace it back through several layers of individuals, sometimes through generations, to its original source. You will always find, in the long run, a prostitute who has spread the disease."[21] One faction of the congress echoed Tarnovskii's well-known theories about the nature of prostitution—that it was a pathological disease suffered by moral cripples and that prostitutes would wantonly spread syphilis and gonorrhea should the government abolish regulation.[22] In keeping with these notions, Tarnovskii and his partisans stressed the need for control and regulation.

Yet this view did not go unchallenged by other participants. Many zemstvo physicians and other professionals, representatives of Russia's "third element," were present, and they were critical of regulation itself, of the granting of licenses to brothels, indeed of repressive health policies in general. Their point of view had been summarized on an earlier occasion by Dmitrii N. Zhbankov, a physician and statistician for Smolensk's provincial zemstvo and an outspoken member of the Pirogov Society of Russian Physicians: the true culprits in the spread of syphilis were the "poverty, ignorance, and crowding" (*bednota, temnota, i tesnota*) of the Russian masses.[23] During the congress itself, Petr A. Gratsianov, a physician who headed Minsk's municipally run regulatory system, complained that government restrictions prevented him from speaking freely with workers about hygienic issues. Although the section chair attempted to deflect the political implication of these comments by steering the discussion in another direction, Gratsianov persisted, invoking the physician's "right to speak with those elements with whom he has business." A congress resolution criticizing the "difficult formalities" which prevented physicians from instructing workers about venereal diseases reflected strong support for Gratsianov's position.[24]

Despite vocal opposition to licensed brothels and efforts by several participants to debate the utility of regulation, the majority continued to support controls. Nonetheless, the congress proceedings forced physicians and MVD officials to take a more realistic look at regulation. Reports delivered at the congress made it clear that the empire's medical-police committees were in a sorry state. A paper by Konstantin L. Shtiurmer, "Prostitution in the Cities," inflicted the greatest damage on defenders of the regulatory system. Although Dr. Shtiurmer was associated with Petersburg's medical-police committee and considered himself a loyal supporter of regulation, he did not conceal the truth. His description of the actual workings of the regulatory agencies made it virtually impossible for anyone to defend their effectiveness.

In preparing his presentation for the congress, Shtiurmer had requested information from provincial governors on the operations of medical-police committees in their respective jurisdictions. The results were appalling. Few cities had even bothered to organize medical-police committees, and those that had were running them improperly. Outside of the nineteen cities with operating committees, the local police usually "controlled" prostitutes, albeit with little heed for safeguards and ministry regulations. Throughout the empire substandard medical practices with regard to examinations and hospitalization seemed to be the rule rather than the exception.

Although it is impossible to summarize all of Shtiurmer's information here, a few examples will demonstrate the extent of regulation's failure. Shtiurmer described the compulsory medical examinations in horrifying detail. Lacking the funding for medical facilities and equipment, local officials and doctors made do with what was already at hand when they carried out MVD instructions.[25] In Baku, for example, prostitutes were examined in the police station on a tattered couch or on a borrowed table. They awaited their turn with the usual "motley public" and were often too "ashamed" to arrive sober. From officials in Saratov, Shtiurmer learned that brothel prostitutes were examined on simple tables. They would undress, mount the table, and, because no speculum was available, spread their own vaginal lips (sometimes concealing venereal sores with their fingers). In Nikolaevsk and Tula police brought prostitutes into prison cells for their examinations. In Zamost' prostitutes were examined in a ground floor room that relied on windows facing the street for illumination; according to the district doctor, a crowd of spectators would stand outside on examination days to peek through the open windows and jeer.

Even Petersburg, though it had three special clinics, did not receive an exemplary report. The city's small medical staff often examined between two hundred and four hundred women in a single day. Clinics were so crowded and examinations so brief that prostitutes were not always required to undress fully. Under such harried conditions the physicians themselves admitted that it was impossible to diagnose disease accurately, let alone to observe the most rudimentary sanitary procedures.[26]

Shtiurmer also described the extreme inadequacy of hospital facilities.[27] With understaffing and overcrowding serious problems for all Russian hospitals, it is not surprising that special venereal wards for prostitutes were similarly affected. Shtiurmer reported that Nizhnii Novgorod's hospital regularly grew so crowded during the summer (when prostitutes would travel there from all over Russia to take advantage of the busy fair-time trade) that ailing prostitutes were turned away for want of space. In such cases the local medical-police committee would ask brothelkeepers to sign a paper "guaranteeing" that diseased prostitutes were abstaining from sex. Although Petersburg's Kalinkin Hospital was indisputably the best venereal facility in the empire, it too suffered from overcrowding; Shtiurmer reported that not only were prostitutes known to sleep two to a bed, but it was also not uncommon to place patients in corridors and dressing rooms.

Finally, Shtiurmer acknowledged that the phenomenon of clandestine (*tainaia*) prostitution posed a tremendous problem for medical-police committees. Extremely low numbers of registered prostitutes in most cities seemed to indicate that regulation had failed to encompass all women practicing prostitution rather than a decline in prostitution itself. For every woman who registered, Shtiurmer believed, many more engaged in prostitution clandestinely. He also noted prostitutes' great reluctance to appear for their examinations. While brothel prostitutes, whose examinations took place within the brothel, were relatively easy to monitor, streetwalkers (*odinochki*) were expected to appear at designated examination points. But few cities had special agents to pursue these women, and there was no way to compel them to appear. Shtiurmer suspected that the women who presented the greatest threat to public health —infected prostitutes who wished to avoid hospitalization—were precisely the ones who tried to circumvent the examination process. Without the personnel to compel the women to keep their appointments, the medical-police appeared virtually useless. Shtiurmer mentioned one city in which, within a five-year period, physicians had diagnosed 151 prostitutes as having venereal diseases; of this number, only 3 had admitted themselves to the local hospital.[28]

Shtiurmer's congress report graphically demonstrated how far existing practices deviated from ministry rules, whether the simple requirement that every city in the empire establish a medical-police committee or the more intricate instructions designed to ensure a prostitute's personal cleanliness. Nonetheless, like the majority of congress participants, Shtiurmer never wavered from his faith in the efficacy of regulation per se; he believed that the fault lay in the system's implementation, not its theoretical underpinnings. Confident that specific measures could be enacted to remedy these ills, Shtiurmer proposed some forty-nine resolutions addressing the most glaring shortcomings—slipshod sanitary procedures, hasty examinations, inadequate hospitalization, problems of clandestine prostitution, and violations of medical-police committee rules. He also recommended that no woman be issued a yellow ticket solely on one policeman's word and that police agents exercise "wariness" when rounding up women suspected of clandestine prostitution.[29]

The congress approved most of Shtiurmer's recommendations, but not before adding some additional resolutions which, if implemented, would have altered the regulatory system even more profoundly. Although none of the resolutions necessarily implied a complete loss of faith in the principle of regulation, many participants went much further than Shtiurmer in attempting to protect prostitutes and limit abuses within the system. For example, the congress voted to eliminate police round-ups completely. More significantly, whereas Shtiurmer had made no mention of abolishing brothels, the congress took a stand against these houses, calling them "undesirable in principle," tolerable "only until the improvement of surveillance of prostitution in general."[30]

Several measures promoted by Zhbankov and his supporters received favorable votes, indicating that many members of the congress shared the views of the zemstvo physicians who constituted nearly a third of its participants: the congress asserted the need for increased literacy, the broad dissemination of medical information, the publication of popular pamphlets on venereal disease, and a program of public lectures on these themes. But the participants' most radical recommendation was to shift the struggle against syphilis to the local level by placing control over regulation in the hands of city councils and zemstvos. In voting to establish "collegial institutions" as watchdogs over police activities, the congress held out a vision of regulation not only sharply at variance with Perovskii's original conception, but also more uncompromising than that of Shtiurmer. The congress resolved that: "Surveillance over prostitution must be placed in the hands of special collegial bodies which would manage both its medical and administrative aspects. Everywhere, management of this business must be transferred to city governments or institutions which substitute for them."[31] On the surface this change appeared to be purely administrative; by transferring responsibilities to municipal agencies, the necessary funding for examinations, physicians, and related expenses would have to come from city budgets. Moreover, municipal personnel could be required to fulfill managerial and medical duties. Yet such demands for authority over regulation implicitly challenged the central government and, set in the context of the more general struggle by zemstvo and municipal leaders for decentralization, had political implications.

Regulation served as a perfect political battleground because the local police were seen to operate as an arm of the autocracy. The free hand given the police in medical-police matters disturbed medical professionals, who increasingly regarded the control of venereal disease as properly their business. When individual policemen acted recklessly, they left the entire police department vulnerable to indignant complaints from physicians who resented such interference. Physicians demonstrated time and again at the 1897 congress how the police had foiled the regulatory process. By arresting innocent women, accepting bribes, and tainting the examination process with corruption and needless severity, the police were clearly responsible for many of the system's flaws.

THE GOVERNMENT RESPONSE

Regulation was indeed a thorn in the side of medical professionals and it is scarcely surprising to find them eager to assert their influence over it. That state officials joined progressive physicians in demanding local control over regulation is more noteworthy. After the 1897 congress, officials felt compelled to acknowledge that the struggle against syphilis and prostitution would lead nowhere without the support of zemstvos and municipal councils. Shtiurmer's "Prostitution in the Cities" had clearly demonstrated the need for a complete overhaul of the regulatory system; the MVD could therefore no longer ignore what might otherwise have been dismissed as the "senseless dream" of meddlesome physicians.

Fears about the rising rate of syphilis encouraged the ministry to heed the voices of Russia's doctors. According to one tally, there were 256,000 syphilitics in the Russian empire in 1880 and as many as 916,000 just ten years later.[32] Although the accuracy of these numbers is questionable, the crux of the matter is that officials and physicians *believed* that syphilis was spreading and that prostitution was a dire threat to public health. Haste in curbing syphilis was necessary, Tarnovskii warned his colleagues at the 1897 congress, or the Russian population could "so qualitatively deteriorate" that "biological evolution" would assume the direction it had for the vanishing natives of Siberia and North America.[33]

In 1903 the ministry issued a new set of regulations which reflected some of the concerns of the congress. These were embodied in "Circular 1611," the final product of lengthy deliberations by a commission of the Medical Council.[34] Though it began with the familiar claim that prostitution constituted "the chief source for the spread of syphilis and venereal disease," the circular contained new rules which suggested that the MVD had significantly altered its original vision of regulation. Most telling was the assertion that police measures associated with the regulatory process existed only to facilitate fundamental medical goals. Acknowledging that needless severity by policemen merely served to increase the number of prostitutes who sought to avoid regulation altogether, the circular warned that harsh treatment "can needlessly insult the honest woman and subject her to improper harm." On this basis, street round-ups and searches were expressly prohibited. In the words of the circular: "Humane attitudes toward prostitutes are obligatory for all ranks involved in medical-police surveillance because among prostitutes there are many unfortunate women who have fallen accidentally."[35]

The new rules clearly displayed a more humane attitude toward prostitutes. One provision, which echoed a similar resolution passed at the congress, required the use of special doctors and female assistants whenever a "significant" number of women fell under medical-police control. In no circumstances were police personnel permitted to be present during examinations. Medical-police committees were ordered to assume responsibility for a prostitute's possessions while she was in the hospital and to care for juvenile, pregnant, and sick prostitutes and for those women who wanted to return to an "honest life." In addition, the 1903 circular gave streetwalkers the freedom to retain their passports. No longer would the infamous yellow ticket replace their personal identification; now they could come and go as they pleased. (This ruling, however, did not extend to brothel prostitutes, who were still deprived of their passports.)

Circular 1611 reiterated previous calls for local control over the regulatory process. Yet, in keeping with the ministry's suspicion of local autonomy, it shied away from granting municipal governments complete administrative responsibility for medical-police surveillance. Instead, the circular gave local authorities the option to choose a form of regulation best suited for their area. According to its provisions, cities could choose either to leave their medical-police committees under police control or to split the functions of regulation into their component parts. In the latter case, city governments and zemstvos would take over medical matters, while the police would continue to be responsible for licensing and enforcement. To be sure, this option reflected neither the letter nor the spirit of the 1897 congress's recommendation to place both the medical and the administrative aspects of regulation exclusively in the hands of city councils and zemstvos.

Nonetheless, the ministry was not so inflexible as to prohibit local initiative completely. As early as 1891, the sanitary commission of Minsk, under the aggressive leadership of a new mayor, had received special permission from the Medical Council to assume responsibility for regulation, and Perm' had been granted similar discretionary powers three years later. In that spirit one remarkable clause in Circular 1611 contained the following intriguing sentence: "In cases where local conditions necessitate deviation from the present regulations, plans are to be presented to the Ministry of Internal Affairs for confirmation."[36] Thus, the MVD was not opposed unalterably to plans which eliminated the role of the police in the regulation of prostitution. Given the ministry's desire to combat venereal disease, alternative regulatory systems stood a chance of receiving ministry approval. Despite its usual desire to restrict the activity of town councils and zemstvos, the MVD left some room for lengthening its leash on this occasion.

EFFORTS AT REFORM

The new climate heralded by Circular 1611 sparked fresh efforts to put the medical aspects of regulation under city jurisdiction. Raised most often by zemstvo or municipal physicians, these alternative proposals usually attempted to introduce more humane policies toward prostitutes and other women of the urban lower classes. But despite good intentions, most municipalities failed to implement these plans. Funding was a major obstacle; because most city councils and zemstvos would not release funds for the establishment of clinics and the hiring of trained physicians, medical councils could do no more than invent ambitious designs which remained just that. At the same time, political struggles between provincial governors, municipal and zemstvo leaders, and professional employees also blocked the road to reform. No clear pattern emerges from the various struggles to shift authority over medical-police committees. In some instances a city council would promote reform while the city governor would block it, but the opposite scenario might hold as well.

In Kishinev it was the mayor who forestalled any significant reform. When, at the end of 1903, the city government of Kishinev decided to cooperate with the zemstvo administration of Bessarabia province to organize local regulation, the mayor stubbornly withheld his approval. Only in 1907, after the provincial governor had chided him for his refusal, did he assert that, although he supported the idea of municipal regulation, the city budget lacked the necessary funds. Consequently, a medical-police committee fully under the authority of the police was established. When this new committee asked for the relatively modest sum of 3,250 rubles annually to pay the wages of two police agents and a secretary and to fund and equip an examination facility, the mayor then claimed that the money was unavailable.[37]

In Odessa, where the city council proved to be a willing agent of change, resistance came from the city governor. Although prostitution and venereal disease were perceived as serious problems in Odessa, medical-police controls were extremely lax. According to reports submitted to the city council when Circular 1611 was disseminated, Odessa's medical-police committee had no facility in which to examine prostitutes and maintained no records of its meetings. It also appeared that the police still conducted street round-ups to root out unlicensed prostitutes and that examinations for prostitutes took place in local doctors' offices or in prostitutes' private residences. The fate of those diagnosed as contagious was uncertain because the city's venereal ward was grossly overcrowded. Meanwhile, a military physician in Odessa complained that more than half the men in some squadrons suffered from venereal disease.[38] Indeed, it appeared that the committee led a phantomlike existence. Not only did it fail to hold regular meetings, it did not even keep lists of women suspected of engaging in unlicensed prostitution. With only 500 women registered for the entire city, it was obvious that the vast majority of prostitutes conducted their business beyond official control.[39]

Surprisingly, the city council did not interpret these gloomy reports to mean that stricter controls were needed. On the contrary: in the spirit of Circular 1611 a commission consisting of local medical and administrative officials took a completely novel approach to the problem of public health by calling for the elimination of the term prostitute from the city's vocabulary. Instead of singling out prostitutes for compulsory inspections, the commission proposed that the city establish free medical clinics for all residents who suffered from any form of contagious disease. The commission's members evidently believed that prostitutes and nonprostitutes alike would be more inclined to seek treatment if shame and incarceration had no place in the process of medical treatment. If this plan succeeded, in Odessa at least, the yellow ticket and the state-licensed brothel would become relics of the past.[40]

Odessa was remarkable because it chose to take advantage of the clause in Circular 1611 which permitted alternative arrangements in cases ''where local conditions necessitate deviation from the present regulations.'' But elimination of the role of the police provoked strong opposition: the city governor flatly refused to sign a measure that so clearly undercut his authority and that of the police. He asked members of the council to reconsider, but they declined. Thus began a bureaucratic battle that would rage for the next several years: the city council would approve the commission's plan and submit it to the governor; he would return it, asking the council to discard the controversial provision which eliminated the police; the city council would read his letter at one of its sessions and then send back the proposal unchanged. Meanwhile, regulation remained under police control and continued to operate much as it had when the commission drew up its proposal. Finally, in 1913 a new city governor accepted the plan.[41] Ironically, his assent came too late; by the time the city was ready to act, the world war had begun, and more pressing problems came to the fore.

In several cities abolitionists blocked reform. As a matter of principle, some municipal governments and zemstvos categorically refused to participate in regulation. As the Chernigov city council ruled in 1904, only "the elimination of economic contradictions and ignorance, and the provision of medical aid to everyone, will help matters."[42] When the sanitary commission of Yalta met to discuss Circular 1611, it ruled simply that Yalta had no need for regulation. In the revolutionary year 1905, Kazan's council defiantly refused to participate in regulation because it was "immoral and useless," while the zemstvo in the district of Tiraspol rejected regulation because it "promotes debauchery, the degeneration of the population, and women's lack of rights."[43] Understandably, many zemstvo and city council representatives had no desire to sully their institutions by sanctioning prostitution. Yet their stand essentially freed the police to continue regulating prostitution according to the customary system.

Proposals to reform regulation met with failure throughout the empire. This is clear from a report published in 1910 by the MVD's Main Administration for Local Economic Affairs entitled "Medical-Police Surveillance of Urban Prostitution." It counted only nine cities which had succeeded in carrying out plans to transfer surveillance to municipal control.[44] Furthermore, this report made it plain that regulation still was not fulfilling its goals. Thirteen years after Shtiurmer had so carefully outlined its shortcomings, the new report read like a tragic sequel, full of familiar tales of violated rules, neglected duties, substandard examinations, and inadequate hospital facilities, all made worse by a chronic paucity of funds. The 1910 report recommended measures that harked back both to the 1897 congress and Circular 1611. Rather than concluding (as had many physicians and members of the intelligentsia) that regulation should be rapidly dismantled, this report reaffirmed the necessity for medical-police operations. Echoing their many predecessors, the authors advocated increased funding and sounded the old call for municipal control over regulation.

"Medical-Police Surveillance of Urban Prostitution" is a sterling example of the ministry's willingness to engage in self-criticism. Although the MVD had proved adept at issuing orders to provincial authorities, it had not yet found a way to ensure that they were carried out. Good intentions could not provide funding or training of medical facilities where none had existed before, nor could they force local bodies to make these reforms a high priority. Moreover, as Shtiurmer had observed in 1897, most bureaucrats and police officials preferred to regulate prostitution as they saw fit, without any interference whatsoever. More often than not this meant the continuation of abuses and arbitrary behavior during inscription, inspection, and incarceration. As long as there were no decisive efforts to enforce the new rules, regulation would ultimately depend on the will of local authorities. As the old saying went, "God and the tsar were very far away."

REGULATING RUSSIA'S BROTHELS

Like regulation, the control of brothels was subject to local medical-police committees. Although the MVD in principle continued to endorse brothel prostitution, its enthusiasm for licensing brothels began to falter at the beginning of the twentieth century. Whenever it encountered resistance of any sort on the local level, its policy at once became vague and ambivalent.

State-licensed brothels served as an uncomfortable reminder of what was wrong with the system of regulation. By granting licenses to brothels the medical-police system left itself wide open to criticism; far from serving as the useful police agents whom Perovskii had described to Nicholas I, brothelkeepers were generally regarded as unscrupulous exploiters with criminal connections. The sources are full of descriptions of the terrible suffering of brothel prostitutes at the hands of madams and clients, the prostitutes' chronic indebtedness, and the frequent scandals involving corrupt policemen and mercenary madams.[45]

Opposition to brothels was not confined to feminists and other members of the liberal intelligentsia. Sympathetic reformers and staunch regulationists alike complained of the inordinately high rates of venereal disease and alcoholism found in state-licensed brothels.[46] At the 1897 congress fully a third of the participants objected so strongly to their colleagues' tacit approval of licensing that they issued a dissenting opinion which called for the immediate abolition of all brothels. In their words, brothels were "immoral in their very essence" and did not "attain their goals in the struggle against syphilis."[47]

After the turn of the century the mounting dissatisfaction with government sponsorship of brothels blossomed into a broad movement which spanned Russia's entire political and social spectrum. Increased awareness of the trade in women and of the ways in which brothelkeepers and their associates exploited brothel prostitutes played a major role in shaping public and professional opinion about the licensing of brothels. Russia's daily newspapers helped propel the movement against brothels with their lurid stories of rape, torture, and secret dens stocked with child-virgins. In 1900 the *Volga Herald* reported how a brothelkeeper had tried to force a consumptive sixteen-year-old prostitute to drink alcohol and take customers. When the girl refused, the madam beat her and tossed her into the snow-covered street, where she remained until members of the Kazan Society for the Defense of Unfortunate Women came to her rescue. One of them melodramatically described how the girl had died before their eyes, muttering how glad she was finally to be rid of the terrible yellow ticket.[48]

In the medical community statistics attesting to the epidemic proportions of syphilis and gonorrhea among brothel prostitutes added scientific arguments to the emotional ones. Although in the nineteenth century brothels had been seen as more amenable to controls than street prostitution, new studies undermined this view by showing that brothel prostitutes would inevitably contract syphilis and that their clients would likely contract some form of venereal disease.[49] Even Tarnovskii, once a strong advocate of brothel prostitution, came full circle on this issue. When the Medical Council in its commission report failed to propose compulsory examinations of male guests, he protested, arguing that brothel prostitution was much more harmful to public health than prostitution in the streets.[50]

Once educated society began to regard brothels as "citadels of syphilis and venereal disease" and centers of white slavery, the clamor grew louder and louder.[51] In 1910 the First All-Russian Congress against the Trade in Women called for the elimination of state-licensed brothels.[52] The existence of brothels also stimulated various forms of grass roots, collective protest from small-town residents, home-owners, and housewives, who petitioned city officials and telegraphed the Minister of Internal Affairs to complain of the demoralizing effects of brothels on their neighborhoods and of the hardship caused by living so close to them.

Although the ministry never changed its policy on licensed brothels, there is evidence that officials in its Chief Medical Inspectorate listened carefully to both the criticisms of the medical profession and the indignant public outcry. When city councils and zemstvos throughout the empire disregarded ministerial directives and shut down brothels, the MVD generally did not interfere with such decisions. It was likely to intervene only when it became obvious that corruption was involved and that there were flagrant violations of the rules. More often than not, the MVD was willing to let local priorities prevail.

From ministerial documents it is possible to trace the fate of brothel licensing in several cities. In the military island-city of Kronstadt, despite evidence of serious breaches in medical-police committee rules and numerous complaints from residents about a nearby brothel, the Chief Medical Inspectorate permitted the military governor to make the final decision. Kronstadt's governor, not surprisingly, turned out to be a strong defender of brothels. He claimed that a committee of military personnel had identified five categories of local citizens as patrons of prostitutes and had accordingly made appropriate arrangements for brothels; to move the brothel in question would disrupt the overall plan.[53]

In the city of Dvinsk the MVD responded twice to charges of corruption by sending an investigator. In 1899, Dvinsk residents had petitioned the provincial governor to move the city's brothels to a more remote area. Although the governor recommended this to the city council in 1901 and the council assented in 1902, the brothels remained. In 1906 another governor asked the city council what had happened, only to hear the brothels defended as establishments which permitted "better and more suitable control of prostitutes." Frustrated homeowners soon began to complain to the MVD, expressing their "outraged moral sensibility" and pointing to the depreciation of property values. In 1908 an investigation revealed numerous violations of the rules. Not only were prostitutes as young as sixteen living in these brothels, but the doors were also frequently kept open to the street so that the revelries might attract customers. It emerged as well that the chief of police had been accepting bribes from Dvinsk brothelkeepers.[54]

Even this damaging report did not succeed in shutting down the city's brothels. The city council held its ground, claiming that "despite some discomfort for residents resulting from the existence of state-licensed brothels . . . , the houses will remain there in light of the impossibility of finding another, more suitable area.'' When the ministry and local residents pressured the medical-police committee to find a more ''suitable'' location for these brothels, the first site proposed turned out to be too close to a school and synagogue. A second site was designated in 1911, but it housed the Twenty-Fifth Russian Infantry Division, as well as the military high command. In the meantime, much to the chagrin of local residents, the brothels remained in place. In 1913, prompted by a telegram from a doctor's wife alleging that seventeen new brothels had sprung up to replace the five original ones, yet another MVD official traveled to Dvinsk. Only with his arrival did the city council finally force the brothels to relocate. In spite of the evidence of corruption and violations of rules, it had taken fourteen years for the ministry to bring the city council into line.[55]

Ministerial inactivity worked both ways. When several cities voted to eliminate brothels completely, the MVD made no attempt to reinstate the licensing procedure. In 1908, as part of a campaign to reform the regulatory system, officials in Moscow ruled that brothels could no longer be tolerated in their present form. A specially appointed commission which included the city governor, police officials, physicians, and a member of the municipal government dubbed them ''open dens of depravity'' whose existence ''could be justified neither from a medical, hygienic, nor moral point of view.'' Tashkent, Omsk, Irkutsk, and Rostov-on-the-Don also chose to close down the brothels in their cities.[56]

The city of Kharkov shut down local brothels in 1915 at the behest of residents who claimed that brothels in their neighborhood were ''tremendously uncomfortable for everyone living there,'' had a ''ruinous influence on our children,'' and had ''deprived us of the possibility to rent apartments to our own people.'' Thirty-eight petitioners convinced the city council ''to free us from a horrible nightmare.''[57] In its ruling against brothels the Kharkov Medical Department proclaimed: ''Public brothels are official employment agencies of women for the purpose of prostitution, arenas of criminality and open provocation to debauchery. [Brothels] are schools in which our youth loses its health, its honesty, and its respect for women and the family hearth. [Brothels] are sources of venereal disease and alcoholism.''[58]

What is especially interesting here is that the ministry did not interfere with any of these decisions. In fact, when the city of Iaroslavl reopened its brothels in 1908 after seven years, the MVD demanded an explanation from the provincial governor for this about-face.[59] Kiev also succeeded in closing its brothels. In November 1916 the Chief Medical Inspectorate readily acceded to the governor's request for official permission, asking only whether the city had developed concrete plans to combat venereal disease.[60]

As evidence proving that brothels served no medical purpose accumulated and as public sentiment grew more hostile toward them, the ministry seems to have implicitly withdrawn its support from Russia's bawdy houses. Although the MVD would not abolish brothels completely, it would no longer actively defend them. For example, when the local authorities in Tomsk attempted to close the brothels in 1913, no action was taken. Only in January 1917 did the State Senate enter the fray, ruling that city councils did not have the right to prohibit the opening and maintenance of state-licensed brothels.[61] It must be pointed out that even after such a long hiatus it was not the MVD that had forced the issue; rather, Tomsk's governing bodies had solicited legislative guidance from St. Petersburg in order to resolve their particular political struggle. The ministry, for its part, seemed content to leave decisions concerning licensing to local authorities.

CONCLUSION

Like so many of its European counterparts, the Russian government chose to tie the prevention of venereal disease to the control of prostitution, and, as so many European states discovered, the regulatory system often turned out to be more trouble than it was worth: regulation was embarrassing, cumbersome, expensive, and of uncertain value in protecting public health. Every European state wrestled with the question of regulation and faced opposition to whatever decision it made. Both the increased visibility of prostitution and the seemingly exponential rise in the rates of venereal disease had appeared to make regulation a logical choice, but with mounting evidence of its shortcomings and its failure to stem the number of syphilis cases and prostitutes, regulation appeared less and less tenable.

In Russia the contradiction between the ideals of public health and the reality of medical-police administration loomed particularly large. Police control over regulation served as a perfect example of the obstacles which physicians faced as healers. Opposition to the system of regulation gave them an indisputably noble cause that transcended other differences. Clearly, the battle against venereal disease could not be won by licensing brothels that housed large numbers of syphilitic women, nor could it be won by singling out only prostitutes for medical surveillance.

What is noteworthy is that Russia's physicians did not encounter much official resistance to their protests against medical-police surveillance. Within the government there was a bona fide desire to protect public health. Despite the MVD's reluctance to follow medical recommendations to the letter, Circular 1611 demonstrated that the ministry was willing to listen to the suggestions of the medical world. Nonetheless, good intentions on both sides were not enough to solve problems at the provincial level: one obdurate provincial or city governor could obstruct reforms, as could a city official or a municipal council or zemstvo that refused to participate in the licensing of prostitution. Nor did the ministry ever act decisively enough to guarantee that its careful instructions would, in fact, be implemented. Confusion and ambivalence about its role and the very provisions of its reforms assured the failure of regulation in any guise.

The MVD would only carry its recommendations to a certain point, particularly in regard to jurisdiction over regulation, for true municipal control represented a threat to bureaucratic control. Although the ministry was sufficiently concerned over venereal disease to loosen the reins in regard to regulation, ministerial flexibility went only so far. This is understandable: at the very moment the ministry was distributing Circular 1611, it was involved in the parallel process of attempting to restructure local administration in such a way as to increase its responsibilities, even while subjugating it to additional ministerial authority. Because a clear change of course for regulation was necessarily tied to the fate of local government, regulation suffered from the same problems that hindered general municipal reforms.[62]

Although the ministry appeared willing to let Odessa experiment in voluntarism, it did not intervene energetically enough to force the city governor's hand. Just as the ministry did not actively compel cities throughout the empire to obey the instructions for regulation, it did not assist Odessa's council with its radical program. The ministry was serious about halting the spread of venereal disease, but not serious enough to push its mandate through in Russia's hundreds of cities. It was prepared to back almost any policy on paper, but its support would go no further than that.

Of course, even if regulation had worked according to the letter of Circular 1611, it remained flawed in essence: it singled out only women for medical-police controls, and its organizing principles made little sense in light of recent discoveries about the nature of venereal disease. Indeed, had Russia's cities actually succeeded in operating their regulatory committees in keeping with ministry rules, neither syphilis nor gonorrhea would have abated. Only Odessa's city council had the foresight to outline a program of broad public health measures that removed elements of stigmatization, punishment, and coercion from the treatment of venereal disease, and eliminated gender-based examinations.

The regulation of prostitution was no way to control venereal disease. Increasingly aware of the shortcomings of regulation, the Russian intelligentsia joined European society in calling for its abolition. The MVD clung to regulation only as a means of controlling prostitution, but with slackening confidence and in the face of strong social opposition.

NOTES

I would like to thank John Hutchinson, Robert Weinberg, and Reginald Zelnik for their careful and attentive readings. I am also grateful to Laura Engelstein for her comments on an early draft. This paper is taken from chapters 1, 2, and 6 of "Sonia's Daughters: Prostitution and Society in Russia" (Ph.D. diss., University of California, Berkeley, 1987).

1. For recent treatments of the regulation of prostitution in other European states, see Richard Evans, "Prostitution, State, and Society in Imperial Germany," *Past and Present*, 70 (1976), pp. 106–129; Mary Gibson, *Prostitution and the State in Italy, 1860–1915* (New Brunswick, N.J., 1986); Jill Harsin, *Policing Prostitution in Nineteenth-Century Paris* (Princeton, N.J., 1985); Judith R. Walkowitz, *Prostitution and Victorian Society: Women, Class, and the State* (Cambridge, 1980). Richard Stites discusses Russian prostitution in "Prostitute and Society in Pre-Revolutionary Russia," *Jahrbücher für Geschichte Osteuropas* 31 (1983), 348-64.

2. *Trudy pervago vserossiiskago s"ezda po bor'be s torgom zhenshchinami i ego prichinami* (St. Petersburg, 1911–12), 2: 539.

3. See Edward H. Judge, *Plehve: Repression and Reform in Imperial Russia, 1902–1904* (Syracuse, N.Y., 1985); Neil B. Weissman, *Reform in Tsarist Russia: The State Bureaucracy and Local Government, 1900–1914* (New Brunswick, N.J., 1981), for useful

treatments of the MVD's efforts to decentralize local government while strengthening ministerial control.

4. The seventeenth-century law is quoted by Veniamin M. Tarnovskii, *Prostitutsiia i abolitsionizm* (St. Petersburg, 1888), pp. 98–99. Mikhail M. Borovitinov described Peter's decree during a speech on the history of regulation of the 1910 All-Russian Congress against the Trade in Women. See *Trudy pervago vserossiiskago s"ezda*, 2: 337–38. The Catherinian law was published in *Polnoe sobranie zakonov Rossiiskoi Imperii*, vol. 21, nos. 15106–15901, 1781–83 (St. Petersburg, 1830), p. 480. Paul's ruling is mentioned in *Belyia rabyni. V kogtiakh pozora* (Moscow, 1912), p. 48, and quoted in full by N. I. Solov'ev, "Presledovanie prostitutok v tsarstvovanii Imperatora Pavla Pervago," *Russkaia starina* (February 1916), pp. 363–64.

5. *The Travels of Olearius in Seventeenth-Century Russia*, trans. and ed. by Samuel H. Baron (Stanford, Calif., 1968), pp. 114, 241; Alexander Radishchev, *A Journey from St. Petersburg to Moscow* (Cambridge, Mass., 1958), p. 170. See also S. Bogrov, "Prostitutsiia," in *Entsiklopedicheskii slovar' t-va F. Granat i K.*, 33: 582.

6. See Harsin, *Policing Prostitution*, pp. 72–95, for a discussion of Paris regulation.

7. Quoted in *Trudy pervago vserossiiskago s"ezda*, 2: 349–50.

8. A complete set of the 1844 rules for "public women" is printed in *Sbornik pravitel'stvennykh rasporiazhenii kasaiushchikhsia mer preduprezhdeniia rasprostraneniia liubostrastnoi bolezni* (St. Petersburg, 1887), pp. 49–51.

9. For the 1861 rules, see ibid., pp. 52–55. Walkowitz describes, in her *Prostitution and Victorian Society*, pp. 201–13, how the promulgation of regulation in Great Britain accelerated the creation of a professional class of prostitutes.

10. The ministry's 1851 instructions can be found in Konstantin L. Shtiurmer, "Prostitutsiia v gorodakh," *Trudy Vysochaishe razreshennago s"ezda po obsuzhdeniiu mer protiv sifilisa v Rossii* (St. Petersburg, 1897), pp. 13–14; *Vrachebno-politseiskii nadzor za gorodskoi prostitutsiei* (St. Petersburg, 1910), p. 11.

11. For an excellent general history of syphilology, see John T. Crissey and Lawrence C. Parish, *The Dermatology and Syphilology of the Nineteenth Century* (New York, 1981). My description derives from this work.

12. It was not until 1910 that Paul Ehrlich developed salvarsan as a more effective treatment for syphilis. M. A. Waugh, "Venereology," *The Oxford Companion to Medicine* (Oxford, 1986), 2:1429.

13. Crissey and Parish, *Dermatology and Syphilology*, pp. 360–62.

14. The 1851 MVD circular mandating regulation for the entire empire is described by Shtiurmer, "Prostitutsiia v gorodakh," pp. 13–14; *Vrachebno-politseiskii nadzor*, p. 11. For a discussion of funding, see A. I. Smirnov, "Ob uchrezhdenii vrachebno-politseiskikh komitetov," *Trudy Vysochaishe razreshennago s"ezda*, p. 2.

15. The State Council's ruling is in "Ob"iasnitel'naia zapiska," *Izvestiia s-peterburgskoi gorodskoi dumy*, 21 (May 1914), p. 2085. The best descriptions of the legal muddle created by regulation can be found in *Trudy pervago vserossiiskago s"ezda*, 2: 336–51; "Zakonodatel'noe predpolozhenie ob otmene reglamentatsii prostitutsii," *Izvestiia s-peterburgskoi gorodskoi dumy*, 21 (May 1914), pp. 2072–77.

16. The rules regarding police round-ups are in *Sbornik*, pp. 61–69; Arkadii I. Elistratov, *O prikreplenii zhenshchiny k prostitutsii* (Kazan, 1903), p. 27.

17. Ape, *Prostitutsiia* (St. Petersburg, 1906), pp. 4–5.

18. This incident was described by Elistratov, *O prikreplenii zhenshchiny*, pp. 44–45; Boris I. Bentovin, "Torguiushchiia telom," *Russkoe bogatstvo*, 11–12 (1904), p. 150; D. L. Muratov, "Vrachebno-politseiskii nadzor," *Zhizn'*, 10 (October 1899), p. 408.

19. Tarnovskii, *Prostitutsiia i abolitsionizm*, p. 229. Senate ruling in A. L. Rubinovskii, "Povinnost' razvrata," *Vestnik prava*, 8 (October 1905), p. 171; Shtiurmer, "Prostitutsiia," *Real'naia entsiklopediia meditsinskikh nauk* (St. Petersburg, 1897), 16: 478.

20. Figures on the number of syphilitics believed to be in Russia are in *Otchet o sostoianii*

narodnago zdraviia i organizatsii vrachebnoi pomoshchi naseleniiu v Rossii za 1902 g. (St. Petersburg, 1904), pp. 18–19; *Otchet . . . za 1896–1901 gg.* (St. Petersburg, 1905), p. 18.

21. "Protokoly obshchikh zasedanii s"ezda," p. 10.

22. Tarnovskii's speech to the 1897 congress is in ibid., pp. 5–21, but see his *Prostitutsiia i abolitsionizm* for a full statement of his view that prostitutes were irrevocably depraved.

23. Zhbankov, quoted in Lazar Granovskii, *Obshchestvennoe zdravookhranenie i kapitalizm* (Moscow, 1908), p. 39.

24. "Protokoly obshchikh zasedanii," pp. viii, 27–28.

25. This description derives from Shtiurmer, "Prostitutsiia v gorodakh," pp. 44–46.

26. Ibid., p. 40; Shtiurmer, "Prostitutsiia," *Real'naia entsiklopediia meditsinskikh nauk,* p. 471.

27. The following paragraph is based on Shtiurmer, "Prostitutsiia v gorodakh," pp. 52–57.

28. Ibid., pp. 47–51, 59.

29. Shtiurmer's medical recommendations were published in ibid., pp. 77–81.

30. The resolutions approved by the congress are in "Protokoly obshchikh zasedanii," pp. xvi–xxi; for the specific comment on brothels, see p. xxi.

31. Ibid., p. xx.

32. From a July 15, 1910, report by Privy Councilor Mollerius to the Minister of Internal Affairs: Tsentral'nyi Gosudarstvennyi Istoricheskii Arkhiv SSSR (TsGIA), Upravlenie glavnago vrachebnago inspektora (UGVI), fond 1298, delo 1730, opis' 1, "O nadzore za prostitutsiei," June 1910–December 1911.

33. "Protokoly obshchikh zasedanii," p. 18.

34. The commission's decision are in "Svod postanovlenii komissii po razsmotreniiu dela o vrachebno-politseiskom komitete v Moskve, v sviazi s proektom obshchei organizatsii nadzora za prostitutsiei v Imperii," *Vestnik obshchestvennoi gigieny, sudebnoi i prakticheskoi meditsiny,* 3 (March 1901), pp. 41–55.

35. I saw a copy of the actual circular in the files of St. Petersburg province's Medical Division. Leningradskii Gosudarstvennyi Istoricheskii Arkhiv (LGIA), fond 255, delo 852, opis' 1, entitled "Po tsirkuliarnomu predlozheniiu Meditsinskago Departamenta ob organizatsii nadzora za prostitutsiei." The rest of this section derives from Circular 1611.

36. LGIA, fond 255, delo 852, opis' 1, "Po tsirkuliarnomu predlozheniiu Meditsinskago Departamenta."

37. Kishinev's problems with regulation were described in a March 31, 1912, report to the Chief Medical Inspectorate from a local clerk. TsGIA, UGVI, fond 1298, delo 2332, opis' 1, "O nadzore za prostitutsiei," January 1912–March 1913. Also see *Vedomosti kishinevskoi gorodskoi dumy,* 119 (December 4, 1907), p. 2; 21 (February 19, 1908), p. 2.

38. "Svedeniia o vrachebno-sanitarnoi organizatsii i epidemicheskikh zabolevaniiakh g. Odessy," *Izvestiia odesskoi gorodskoi dumy,* 17 (October 1904), p. 560.

39. Ibid., pp. 555–607.

40. Meeting of January 25, 1906, *Izvestiia odesskoi gorodskoi dumy,* 6 (March 1906), pp. 802–4. Odessa's radicalism must be seen in the context of growing disillusionment throughout Russia with regulation and the concomitant rise of an abolitionist movement. I discuss these issues in "Sonia's Daughters," pp. 317–95.

41. Something of the conflict between the city governor and the Odessa city council is revealed in "Doklad po predlozheniiu g. odesskago gradonachal'nika ob iskliuchenii iz proekta organizatsii nadzora za prostitutsiei v g. Odesse primechaniia k p. 3, st. 11, postanovleniia gorodskoi dumy," *Izvestiia odesskoi gorodskoi dumy,* 13–14 (July 1912), pp. 2101–8, as well as in a February 13, 1913, letter from Odessa's city governor to the Ministry of Internal Affairs: TsGIA, UGVI, fond 1298, delo 2400, opis' 1, "O nadzore za prostitutsiei," January 5, 1915–February 27, 1917.

42. G. A. Kovalenko, "Reglamentatsiia prostitutsii," *Fel'dsher,* 19 (October 1, 1904), p. 585.

43. Developments in Yalta, Kazan, and Tiraspol reported in *Russkii vrach,* 50 (1903), p. 1810; 5 (1905), p. 175; 19 (1905), p. 644.

44. *Vrachebno-politseiskii nadzor,* p. 3.

45. For a more detailed discussion of brothel prostitution, see "Sonia's Daughters," pp. 254–316.

46. See, for example, Nikolai P. Fiveiskii, "K statistike sifilisa sredi prostitutok domov terpimosti g. Moskvy," *Protokoly moskovskago venerologicheskago i dermatologicheskago obshchestva za 1892–93 gg.,* (Moscow, 1894), 2.

47. "Protokoly obshchikh zasedanii," pp. 159–60.

48. *Volzhskii vestnik,* 45 (February 23, 1900), p. 3; Aleksandr N. Baranov, *V zashchitu neschastnykh zhenshchin* (Moxcow, 1902), pp. 119–20.

49. Figures which supported the argument that brothel prostitution was more dangerous to clients than street prostitution can be found in *Conference Internationale pour la Prophylaxie de la Syphilis et des Maladies Veneriennes* (Brussels, 1899), pp. 227–30. See also K. M. Grechishchev, *Pritony razvrata* (Tomsk, 1913), pp. 4–7; A. L. Rubinovskii, *Kontsentratsiia prostitutok* (Kamenets-Podol'sk, 1905), pp. 9–12.

50. Tarnovskii's objections to the proposals of the Medical Council commission are in "Svod postanovlenii komissii," pp. 56–58.

51. A Siberian physician used this expression in "Protokoly zasedanii vrachebno-sanitarnago soveta," *Vrachebno-sanitarnaia khronika g. Tomska,* 9 (September 1912), p. 403.

52. For the congress vote, see *Trudy pervago vserossiiskago s"ezda,* 2: 575.

53. TsGIA, UGVI, fond 1298, delo 1730, opis' 1, "O nadzore za prostitutsiei," June 1910–December 1911.

54. The description of Dvinsk's struggle to relocate its brothels is from TsGIA, UGVI, fond 1298, delo 2332, opis' 1, "O nadzore za prostitutsiei," January 1912–March 1913.

55. Ibid.

56. Moscow's new plan for regulation is in "Vrachebno-politseiskii nadzor za prostitutsiei v gorodakh v Rossii," *Izvestiia s-peterburgskoi gorodskoi dumy,* 21 (May 1914), pp. 2050–53, 2067–71. *Gorodskoe delo,* 10 (1914), p. 650, mentions several cities which successfully shut down local brothels.

57. "Doklad o zakrytii domov terpimosti v gorode Khar'kove," *Izvestiia khar'kovskoi gorodskoi dumy,* 9–10 (September-October 1915), p. 133. Interestingly, brothel owners in Kharkov counter-petitioned to save their property.

58. Ibid., p. 138.

59. TsGIA, UGVI, fond 1298, delo 2332, opis' 1, "O nadzore za prostitutsiei," January 1912–March 1913.

60. TsGIA, UGVI, fond 1298, delo 2400, opis' 1, "O nadzore za prostitutsiei," January 5, 1915–February 27, 1917.

61. For the arguments in favor of shutting down Tomsk brothels, see Grechishchev, "K voprosu o tom, v prave li gorodskoi dumy vospretit' otkrytie i soderzhanie pritonov razvrata," *Vrachebno-sanitarnaia khronika g. Tomska,* 4 (April 1913), pp. 259–61; Grechishchev, *Pritony razvrata,* p. 13. The Senate's decision is in TsGIA, UGVI, fond 1298, delo 2400, opis' 1, "O nadzore za prostitutsiei," January 5, 1915–February 27, 1917.

62. See Judge, *Plehve,* pp. 53–69, 90–92; and Weissman, *Reform in Tsarist Russia, passim.*

Part Two

Building the New Soviet Medicine

SALLY EWING

The Science and Politics of Soviet Insurance Medicine

For at least a century, the "social dimension" has figured prominently in our understanding of medical practices, so much so that today few scholars would attempt to account for developments in medicine by reference to biology alone. There are, however, differing approaches to the "social dimension" of medicine. Some writers use the term to evoke the physician's responsibility to the community. For example, Richard Titmuss emphasizes the redistributive potential of a medical system grounded not in the possessive individualism of the marketplace but in the notion of man as a social being.[1] Other writers are less sanguine about the social dimension of modern medicine. According to Michel Foucault, medical knowledge is a principal mechanism for exercising power in modern society, a way of imposing order through "disciplinary normalization." Indeed, he warns of the dramatic consequences that follow from what he calls the "medicalization of behaviors, conducts, discourses, desires, etc."[2] These contrasting perspectives suggest that when we attempt to move beyond the biological we give up the seemingly unambiguous terminology of textbook medicine for the politically volatile and conceptually fluid categories of the human sciences.

If sociological categories have gradually, and often inadvertently, transformed medical practices in the West, in revolutionary Russia the transformation was sudden and deliberate. From the first days of the October Revolution, the Bolsheviks declared that theirs would be a social medicine, a medicine that rejected the individualistic, patient-centered practices of the capitalist West and responded instead to the medical needs of a class—the proletariat.[3] This decision was no doubt facilitated by the fact that an extensive public medical system had already been established in tsarist Russia under the jurisdiction of the zemstvo and private physicians serving individual, paying patients remained the exception. But the Bolsheviks' goal was not simply to create a public medical system. They planned to tailor that system to meet the specific medical needs of the working class, something that zemstvo medicine had never attempted. This, along with the Bolsheviks' ardent commitment to social science as the way to achieve that goal, was bound to place a distinctive stamp on Soviet medical practices. Perhaps this was already apparent in 1923 when E. Iakovenko, who had been a leading sanitary physician during the zemstvo era, made the following observation about Soviet medicine: "Medicine more and more approaches sociology, and, not renouncing its methods from the biological sciences, it blends its formal conclusions into sociological sciences, sciences of society.''[4]

This essay focuses on insurance medicine as it evolved from the prerevolutionary workers' insurance movement until the late 1920s. Scholars have largely ignored the insurance dimension of the Soviet medical system, thus obscuring the fact that a principal Bolshevik objective after the Revolution—to provide the working class with adequate medical care—was undertaken within the context of a comprehensive state insurance system.[5] In fact, the prerevolutionary insurance movement provides the immediate institutional and ideological background against which the Soviet system of class medicine gradually evolved. In 1912 the Social Democrats organized a workers' insurance movement to mobilize workers to demand medical coverage as well as sickness and disability benefits. Adequate medical care was a major goal of this movement, but workers also demanded the right to administer their own hospitals and medical centers.

Although the Bolsheviks themselves had articulated the most radical variant of this demand for working-class self-administration in the prerevolutionary movement, they quickly maneuvered to withdraw their support from workers who persisted in this demand after the October Revolution. In the evolving political discourse of many leading Bolsheviks, the Soviet state had been transformed into a workers' state, and the goal of self-administration was technically fulfilled. According to this logic, workers' organs that continued to expect autonomy from the workers' state became highly suspect.

Thus, if during the workers' insurance movement it had seemed that the working class was the revolutionary subject, destined to administer its own insurance organs according to varying local conditions, by the 1920s that same class had been transformed from the revolutionary subject into the privileged object of various benefits administered by a vast state insurance system. From now on, the working class would be studied and categorized and assigned benefits according to abstract sociological criteria. With this transformation, one begins to see how the infiltration of the medical by the sociological changed medical practice in ways and to an extent that even the most insightful participants did not anticipate at the time.

The determination of the criteria for entitlement became a central political task in the administration of a class-oriented medicine. Although these criteria were supposed to derive from the objective findings of a sociological medicine, entitlement decisions were in fact profoundly, and inevitably, political.[6] Two commissariats, the Commissariat of Labor (Narkomtrud) and the Commissariat of Public Health (Narkomzdrav), emerged as the agents of the Bolshevik effort to provide medical care to the working class. It was obvious from the outset that each commissariat approached the task with a different set of priorities, and those priorities determined how each viewed what all agreed was a revolution in medical practice. As we shall see, the outcome of that revolution would depend directly on whether Narkomtrud or Narkomzdrav managed to gain jurisdiction over working-class medical care.

Two controversies in particular drove the competing commissariats in ever more antagonistic directions. First of all, they argued over the merits of providing specialized, and privileged, medical services for the insured. Narkomtrud favored this policy, whereas Narkomzdrav, with its slogan of unified Soviet medicine, argued for a centralized medical system which would provide relatively uniform care for all citizens under the auspices of a single commissariat, namely, Narkomzdrav. Second, in the interests of fiscal efficiency, Narkomtrud sought to institutionalize strict control over the physicians who served the insured and over the experts who studied their illnesses, whereas Narkomzdrav fought to maintain the professional autonomy of its physicians and the scientific integrity of its experts. These were some of the dilemmas that surfaced when the medical system shifted its focus from the individual to the working class. As this account will show, there were no obvious solutions, especially to the question that dominated the entire period: which commissariat best represented the interests of workers? The most that can be said is that Narkomtrud articulated the exigencies of a class medicine, even if individual workers might have preferred the patient-oriented perspective of Narkomzdrav. Narkomtrud, which was given jurisdiction over the insurance system, viewed medical care as an insurance matter, with funding, entitlement, control, and administration the main concerns, whereas Narkomzdrav subscribed to a more traditional, patient-oriented practice with a long-term, theoretical approach to medical science. By the 1930s, during the most radical phase of this working-class revolution, the insurance perspective of Narkomtrud prevailed.

WORKERS' INSURANCE MEDICINE

The working-class demand for adequate medical care, provided at the owners' expense but administered by workers, was controversial, even before the Revolution. Ironically, the tsarist government itself set this controversy in motion when it decided, in response to working-class unrest in 1904, that a state-sponsored social insurance system could effectively coopt the working class and undermine the influence of the Social Democrats. From 1904 until 1912 the government prepared the way for insurance legislation which would placate workers without unduly antagonizing owners, but the resulting 1912 social insurance law managed instead to alienate the workers further. The provision for medical care was particularly inadequate, with the result that the demand for self-administered medical care became one of the rallying slogans of a workers' insurance movement. Instead of coopting workers, the government had helped them articulate a set of grievances that the Social Democrats could then exploit to further their revolutionary cause.

The debates leading up to the 1912 law centered on who should pay for medical care and who should administer it. Since 1866, the owners had borne the legal responsibility for both, but their performance was notoriously inadequate.[7] As early as 1903 the government had proposed that owners, while continuing to pay for medical care, should transfer the burdensome administrative functions to civil authorities. An official report stated that the 1866 law "forces upon the employer a function utterly foreign to him, which in the very nature of things cannot be satisfactorily fulfilled."[8] The 1903 plan was shelved because the impending insurance law was supposed to resolve the problem by incorporating medical care into an obligatory insurance system.

In spite of the intentions of reformers, a significant restructuring of factory medicine proved extremely controversial. The insurance legislation presented to the Duma in 1911 included a plan to introduce factory-based sickness kassy for administering sickness benefits and some types of medical care. Workers and owners would make obligatory financial contributions to these organizations, and they would jointly administer them with their respective vote being proportional to their contribution—the workers would pay for three-fifths of the kassa budget and control three-fifths of the vote in the general meeting.[9] When the Duma Commission on Worker Questions, dominated by owner representatives, tried to turn this kassa system to the owners' advantage by transferring to the kassa some of the medical costs for which owners were legally responsible, an unusually heated debate ensued in the Duma.[10] Government spokesmen found themselves siding with the Social Democrats against the commission's proposal on medical care.[11] Pravda sarcastically reported that the finance minister, V. N. Kokovtsev, and the minister of commerce and industry, S. I. Timashev, "gave socialist speeches in the Duma. . . ."[12] Kokovtsev, who had always considered medical care to be the responsibility of the owners, complained that the proposal "would give the owners 9,500,000 rubles profit (the amount paid in 1907 for medical care),"[13] while Timashev objected to the commission's revision of the insurance project on the grounds that it had "destroyed the interests of the workers."[14]

In spite of the government's strenuous objections that the commission's proposal would so weaken the insurance law as to completely undercut and alienate the working class, the final legislation transferred much of the financial burden for medical care to the kassa.[15] At the same time, it effectively rejected the demand that workers be allowed to administer their own medical facilities through the kassy. The law stipulated that a kassa, with the owners' consent, could take over medical services and collect a fixed yearly fee from the owners to cover the resulting expenses, but the designated fee was far less than a kassa would require for such an undertaking. Only by pooling the resources of several kassy could the workers hope to establish their own hospitals, but the legislation made such joint ventures difficult if not impossible. On the whole, the provisions for medical care were blatantly retrogressive, more likely to inspire cynicism among the workers than to pacify them. It is not surprising that the demand for comprehensive medical care funded by owners and administered by workers became a major slogan of the workers' insurance movement which the Social Democrats organized in the wake of the disappointing insurance legislation. To overcome the barrier to working-class self-administration, the movement demanded that factory sickness kassy unite into general kassy, either territorial or professional, pooling their resources and appropriating existing medical facilities or building their own. All this was to be paid for with substantial contributions by owners.[16] Owners resisted all such efforts at unification, but some joint facilities did surface, especially during the war.[17]

The impact of the insurance campaign on the organization of medical care for the working class lay not so much in concrete accomplishments, which were few, as in the fact that during these early years the issue of workers' insurance medicine became highly politicized. After the February Revolution the demand for self-administered medical care became even more insistent,[18] and by the time of the October Revolution no one involved in organizing the new Soviet medical system could afford to ignore the history of workers' insurance medicine. As N. A. Vigdorchik, a prominent physician and left Menshevik who had been active in this early campaign, wrote in 1923: "This period left a deep impression on the Russian workers' movement, and that impression is still felt to this day."[19] Two issues in particular carried over from the workers' insurance movement and figured centrally after the Revolution: first, the notion that insured workers should be provided with special medical facilities and receive better medical care than that available to the general public and, second, that insured workers should administer these medical facilities. What appeared during the revolutionary upheaval as two inseparable aspects of a system of working-class medicine proved instead to be not only separable but also (at least according to Lenin) the product of two distinct and profoundly contradictory political perspectives.

FROM WORKERS' INSURANCE MEDICINE TO UNIFIED SOVIET MEDICINE

After the October Revolution, the Bolsheviks had to contend with a network of sickness kassy that had in many cases become effective in providing sickness benefits and medical care to their members. As early as October 30, 1917, the new Commissariat of Labor published an official communication that promised to extend social insurance to all hired labor and to cover all incapacities at full wage.[20] This ambitious promise proved unrealistic, but even the modest coverage that was eventually provided forced the Bolsheviks to make difficult choices about the institutions that would distribute those benefits. The existing factory-based sickness kassa was an obvious choice, and Mensheviks like Solomon Schwarz, who had already worked extensively with the kassy before the Revolution, insisted that these democratic working-class organs should continue to operate, at least until the revolutionary upheaval had settled. The Mensheviks argued that an abrupt shift from the sickness kassa system would lead to a general deterioration in existing services rather than the extension of those services to all workers as the Bolsheviks envisioned.[21]

The Bolsheviks, however, were suspicious of these self-administered workers' organs from the outset, on the assumption that a well-funded factory-based kassa would inevitably concentrate on providing the best possible services to its own members, and thus undermine the government's plan to distribute insurance benefits to all insured workers according to uniform entitlement criteria based on labor.[22] The Bolsheviks were haunted by the specter of such trade unionist tendencies and thus decreed in December 1917 that existing factory-based sickness kassy be replaced by territorial kassy.[23] By early 1918 these territorial kassy came under the jurisdiction of the department of social insurance and labor protection of Narkomtrud. The avowed aim was to discontinue the autonomous sickness kassy while preserving the connection between the working class and social insurance and to

coordinate social insurance with other Narkomtrud labor policies.[24] Already the
two-fold legacy of the workers' insurance movement—working-class self-administration and autonomy from the state, and the provision of special insurance benefits
for the working class—was revealing its internal contradictions. Narkomtrud would
remain committed to the principle of working-class privilege, but it had participated
in delivering the decisive blow against working-class self-administration.[25]

However premature this Bolshevik attack on the sickness kassa may have been—
for Schwarz was right that a factory-based kassa was better than nothing at all—
the policy at least inaugurated the task of providing medical care to insured workers
through the territorial kassa. A principal objection to the factory-based sickness
kassa had always been, as we have seen, that an individual kassa could not afford
to maintain its own medical facility. After the February Revolution factory-based
kassy had begun to unite into territorial kassy in order to appropriate the owners'
facilities. In December the Bolsheviks formalized this process, first by requiring
that the territorial kassa provide its members with medical care and then by em-
powering kassy to requisition all factory treatment facilities. They also increased
the insurance tax paid by owners to help the kassa cover its medical expenses.[26]

All this suggests that the push for kassa-based insurance medicine had begun
in earnest in those first months after the Revolution. The kassy moved to confiscate
not only factory medical facilities, but also those run by private charities. The
Petrograd all-city kassa even contemplated requisitioning Red Cross facilities on
the grounds that, "with all their resources, if we don't take them now, someone
else will later."[27] According to Vigdorchik, who continued throughout the twenties
to advocate kassa medicine as the most progressive choice for Soviet medicine, the
kassa medical stations began to enlist their own "service" physicians and these
stations were, on average, better than the public hospitals.[28]

If Vigdorchik and the Bolshevik insurance activists associated with Narkomtrud
were committed to the concept of working-class social insurance and to kassa
medicine as an integral part of that system, the civil war introduced new constraints
which undermined their plans and efforts. An acute food crisis, combined with the
escalating civil war during the second half of 1918, changed working-class politics
dramatically, introducing organizational imperatives that had not figured in early
Bolshevik conceptions of socialist administration. Under the rubric of War Communism there was a radical shift toward extreme egalitarianism, a shift that undermined the original Bolshevik commitment to providing special insurance benefits
and medical services for the working class. Increasingly one heard that all citizens,
from peasants to ex-landlords to workers, should be compensated according to need
rather than labor performed, and all should have free and equal access to medical
care.

The administrative consequence of this brand of communism in social insurance
as in other realms was extreme centralization through the incorporation of all local
organs into the state apparatus. During 1918 two new state commissariats, the
Commissariat of Social Welfare (Narkomsobes) and the Commissariat of Public
Health (Narkomzdrav), were created, and their respective commissars, A. N. Vinokurov and N. A. Semashko, campaigned to incorporate social insurance functions

into their state organs. The idea was to separate insurance benefits such as sick pay and pensions from medical services, with the former going to Narkomsobes and the latter to Narkomzdrav. Bolsheviks in Narkomtrud and the unions defended the existing territorial kassy and vehemently resisted what they perceived as an attack on working-class privilege. (Some union representatives were still defending self-administration and autonomy from all state organs, including Narkomtrud, but by now that issue was more or less settled.) A jurisdictional struggle ensued, with some Bolsheviks defending the importance of retaining the link between insurance benefits and the working class and others demanding the elimination of class privilege so that scarce resources could be spread evenly over the population as a whole.

The radical climate of War Communism insured that the extreme central control and egalitarianism espoused by these two new commissariats would eventually overpower social insurance principles, despite the considerable revolutionary tradition of the latter. Already in April 1918 at the Insurance Council meeting, the social welfare commissar Vinokurov suggested replacing the concept of social insurance, which included a tax on owners and distributed benefits proportional to wage, with principles of universal social welfare. A. N. Paderin, the head of the department of social insurance of Narkomtrud, managed to pass a resolution rejecting Vinokurov's proposal and defending the class character of social insurance.[29] But Vinokurov was determined to expand his commissariat's domain, and he proposed again at the June session of the All-Union Central Council of Trade Unions (VTsSPS) that the department of social insurance be absorbed by his commissariat. Labor representatives were still in a position to resist this attempt to blur the distinction between workers and the general population, and therefore Vinokurov's proposal was rejected in favor of a resolution submitted by the head of VTsSPS, M. P. Tomsky, which underlined "that the question of social insurance was inextricably linked with general workers' politics."[30] Yet, notwithstanding this firm stand by Tomsky and others in Narkomtrud, and in the face of warnings that Narkomtrud would become "a piece of sugar" if the professional conditions of the working class were equated with the conditions of peasants and invalids,[31] Vinokurov's proposal to replace social insurance with social welfare was officially sanctioned on October 31, 1918, by the "Decree on the Social Welfare of Workers."[32] This decree signaled a fundamental break with the workers' insurance movement which had begun in 1912: by extending coverage to virtually everyone in need, it severed the link between a specific incapacity and the social right of a worker to receive compensation relative to his or her wage. In the months that followed, Vinokurov's commissariat managed to appropriate virtually all insurance functions from Narkomtrud, and social insurance itself was condemned as a bourgeois institution.[33]

In his campaign against social insurance principles, Vinokurov had a powerful ally in Semashko, the head of the newly created Narkomzdrav. While Vinokurov was campaigning to replace the territorial kassa with Narkomsobes organs, Semashko was demanding that kassa medical services be transferred to the health departments of Narkomzdrav. Thus, Vinokurov's advocacy of social welfare had its counterpart in Semashko's strident campaign for unified Soviet medicine. At a time when the kassy were scrambling to seize control of factory medical facilities, Semashko denounced this trend toward local consolidation as a wasteful dispersal of scarce medical resources.

The labor representatives who had opposed Vinokurov were equally insistent that working-class medicine remain under kassa jurisdiction, and for a time they managed to postpone the full-scale implementation of Semashko's plan for unified Soviet medicine. A July 1918 law placed Narkomzdrav in charge of all aspects of Soviet medicine, but as a concession to the insurance activists this legislation nevertheless acknowledged the "distinctiveness and particular features of insurance medicine," so that "in the unification of insurance medicine with general state medicine, the particular features of insurance medicine should be preserved."[34] In practical terms this meant that a special department for insurance medicine would be established within Narkomzdrav and that the territorial insurance kassy would continue to administer medical facilities for the insured. At the beginning of 1919, B. I. Faingold, a leading insurance activist from Narkomtrud who would be locked in a continuing confrontation with Semashko throughout the twenties over the issue of insurance medicine, declared that the call for the proletarianization of medicine and its administration by the insurance organs was becoming "louder and louder."[35] Yet that call, however loud, was destined to go unheeded. Since the kassy themselves were on the verge of extinction, it was only a matter of time before their medical facilities were transferred to Narkomzdrav and workers' insurance medicine was officially liquidated in favor of unified Soviet medicine.[36] In February 1919 a decree to this effect was issued and workers' insurance medicine seemed to come to an end. The newly declared goal of unified Soviet medicine was to raise all medicine to the level already attained in some areas by local insurance medicine, but inevitably the reverse occurred—the successful kassa medical stations were simply absorbed into a rudimentary public health system.[37]

WORKING-CLASS PRIVILEGE

The Civil War had barely ended when the debate over social insurance, like so much else that had been rendered irrelevant by War Communism, was cautiously but urgently renewed. Insurance activists who had been overruled by proponents of egalitarianism and extreme centralization now claimed that social insurance was not the bourgeois institution Vinokurov and others made it out to be but was, rather, a progressive socialist principle forced on bourgeois governments by the working class.[38] In the atmosphere created by the "trade-union debate" in the winter of 1920–21, these activists once again proposed that special working-class organs, specifically the territorial kassy, be reestablished to administer an insurance system geared to the specific needs of the working class.[39]

In their efforts to rebuild the insurance system, insurance advocates in Narkomtrud and the unions moved to regain the ground lost to Vinokurov and Semashko in 1918. Their attack on Vinokurov and his social welfare principles was well organized and highly successful. N. A. Miliutin, who occupied the post of assistant director under Vinokurov in Narkomsobes, had already admitted in an article in

1920 that Narkomsobes had failed the workers completely. He boldly proposed that it was time to draw on the experience of "the world's largest workers' insurance organization [the Petersburg workers' kassa of social insurance]" in order to re-structure the hopelessly bureaucratic social welfare system.[40] This article was the first indication that the territorial insurance kassa, the principal goal of the pre-revolutionary movement and the short-lived organizational form for the postrevolutionary insurance system, would once again become the foundation for Soviet social insurance.

Vinokurov and his Narkomsobes employees correctly interpreted this new talk of insurance kassy as a direct threat to their turf and a violation of the statist principles to which they subscribed. Times were changing, and their commissariat, buried as it was in bureaucratic red tape, was rapidly losing its credibility. Miliutin himself played a key role in the demise of his commissariat. It appears that Miliutin, unbeknownst to Vinokurov or his staff, worked with a small group of Narkomsobes employees to determine the tariffs and organizational reforms that would make it possible to replace the social welfare system with a kassa system.[41] This secret project culminated in the Sovnarkom (SNK) decree "On the Social Insurance of Persons Engaged in Labor for Hire" issued on November 15, 1921. After that, it was only a matter of time before Narkomsobes completely lost its jurisdiction over workers. In January 1922, VTsSPS formed a commission to draw up a plan for local workers' insurance organs, and its members included Narkomtrud head N. P. Shmidt, the long-time insurance advocates Paderin and Faingold, and Miliutin as the Narkomsobes representative. The commission predictably endorsed the re-crea-tion of workers' territorial insurance kassy.[42] In December 1922 these kassy were officially transferred from Narkomsobes to Narkomtrud, and the former, left to preside over war invalids, peasants, and the indigent, suffered a dramatic loss of prestige and all but disappeared in the mid-twenties because of a complete lack of funds.[43]

With the kassa back in place, preparing to distribute generous sickness benefits and rather meager labor invalid pensions, long-time insurance activists like Faingold and Vigdorchik turned their attention to the medical front. If events had demon-strated that workers would be served best by a social insurance system organized around territorial kassy, it seemed equally obvious, at least to many insurance activists, that another revolutionary tradition, that of insurance medicine, should also be revived. Vigdorchik, who firmly believed that insurance medicine was a necessary stage in the evolution of a modern medical system, wrote an impressive history of kassa medicine in 1923 in which he accused unified Soviet medicine of parading as socialist medicine when in fact it was no more than public medicine born of catastrophic civil war conditions, a step backward from kassa medicine.[44] He explained its survival beyond the war in purely negative terms: "In mid-1922 sickness kassy began to appear, providing the conditions for kassa medicine. But then there came a completely unexpected phenomenon: it turns out that [unified] Soviet medicine acquired such a power of inertia over the preceding years that it begins to oppose any attempt to reduce its significance."[45]

A. I. Vishnevetskii, another staunch kassa enthusiast, similarly traced unified

Soviet medicine to War Communism, noting that "this principle in the present, after the transition to the new economic policy and to a fundamental restructuring in all spheres, still rules in the organization of medical aid. Whether this is simply from inertia, or has serious objective foundations, is not something we will decide here."[46] Although Vishnevetskii was hesitant to express his opinion, the implication was obvious. According to Vishnevetskii and to those associated with Narkomtrud and the unions, it was essential that the kassy regain their control over medical care for insured workers.

Whereas the defeat of Vinokurov and Narkomsobes had been swift and complete, Semashko and his unified Soviet medicine proved to be a far more formidable and resilient opponent. Apart from the important element of inertia referred to by both Vigdorchik and Vishnevetskii, Semashko had on his side the fact that, for physicians and patients alike, kassa or insurance medicine, organized to serve a specific class rather than individual patients irrespective of their social location, not only disturbed traditional physician-patient relations, but also introduced blatant inequalities in a domain that seemed, perhaps more than any other, to call for egalitarianism in a country aspiring to socialism. Even more important, in spite of the possible advantages of kassa medicine, the government was reluctant to hand over to relatively autonomous workers' organs an administrative function as important and financially significant as medical care. As a result, Narkomzdrav managed to retain control over medical services for the insured throughout the 1920s. But eventually Vigdorchik's prediction that some form of insurance medicine would overtake and replace unified Soviet medicine was confirmed. By the late twenties insurance medicine would come back into favor as the organizational form that could address the pressing problems of accounting and control over specialized and privileged medical services for the working class.

The jurisdictional struggle that dominated the relations between Narkomtrud and Narkomzdrav throughout the twenties was thus much more than a simple question of who should oversee particular medical facilities. The profoundly political character of medical care that escapes our attention under normal conditions became explicit in the Soviet Union as the representatives of workers competed with health experts to define the class dimensions of Soviet medicine. Initially, there was an attempt to strike a compromise that would create special medical services for the insured while allowing Narkomzdrav to retain control over those services. The structure for such a compromise was worked out at the Fifth All-Russian Congress of Trade Unions, where an alternative proposal that would have empowered the newly established insurance kassy to organize their own medical aid was rejected, not only because it violated the principle of unified Soviet medicine, but also because the kassy had insufficient funds.[47] The compromise, while leaving insurance medicine under the jurisdiction of Narkomzdrav, required that commissariat to create rabmedy, that is, special organs for administering medical aid to the insured. Ironically, the rabmedy were structurally similar to the subdepartments Narkomzdrav had grudgingly created for the same purpose in July 1918 and then hastily liquidated in February 1919. Acknowledging the special links between social insurance and the working class, the compromise stipulated that the insurance kassy of Narkomtrud, along with union representatives, would have an active role in managing the *rabmedy*.

According to this compromise, Narkomzdrav retained control over the *rabmedy*, but Narkomtrud carried much of the financial burden for insured medical care. The insurance kassy struggled to collect the insurance taxes from extremely reluctant and hard-pressed local factories and then contributed a significant part of their budget, in what was called the ''g'' fund, to the local health departments. From 1924 to 1930, the insurance system contributed between 21 to 29 percent of its total budget to the health departments, making this one of its largest single expenditures,[48] while the importance of that contribution to the budget of the local health departments increased year by year. From 1924 to 1928, fund ''g'' was the single largest source of financing for local health departments, accounting for 47 percent of their total expenditures by 1926–27.[49]

Considering the weight of this financial responsibility, Narkomtrud wanted to see, first of all, that the insured workers under its jurisdiction actually received the full benefit of this insurance money. Second, it wanted to be in a position to control and monitor expenditures. It was not long before Narkomtrud representatives concluded that the special *rabmedy* under Narkomzdrav were not meeting these minimum requirements and initiated a campaign to transfer medical services from the *rabmedy* directly to the insurance kassy. This unofficial campaign gained momentum throughout the twenties, especially as workers themselves became increasingly vocal about the poor quality of their medical care.

When we examine this dispute between the two commissariats with the benefit of hindsight, it seems obvious that the early attempt to reach a compromise between Narkomtrud and Narkomzdrav was bound to fail. For as a heated debate in 1926 between the respective commissars, Shmidt and Semashko, revealed, there were two ways of interpreting precisely the same information about how the insured were faring in the hands of the health departments. Shmidt charged that the ''g'' fund contributed by Narkomtrud to the health departments was being used for the general population and not exclusively for the insured, while Semashko, angered by Shmidt's charge, was quick to assert that workers invariably received far better care than peasants. Citing figures from the region hosting the conference at which they spoke, Semashko pointed out that the yearly medical expenditure for each (uninsured) peasant was 45 kopecks, and for an insured family, 12 rubles and 78 kopecks. He also emphasized that the quality of medical care for the insured was significantly better than that available to peasants, who were forced to rely on feldshers for much of their care.[50]

Although L. P. Nemchenko, the head of the Narkomtrud insurance system, expressed skepticism about Semashko's figures,[51] one could hardly dismiss the latter's claims as a simple statistical distortion. In fact, there was no doubt that the insured benefited far more than any other group under the public health system. Christopher Davis has compared the per capita expenditures on the insured and the uninsured, and the former come out well ahead. Excluding from consideration the rural areas, where health care was poor and where relatively few insured workers lived, a comparison of urban groups shows that an insured person received 17.99

rubles worth of medical care as against 5.26 rubles for the uninsured in 1925–26.[52] Narkomzdrav built hospitals in areas with high concentrations of the insured, that is, in important industrial areas, which gave the insured better access to medical facilities. And where those facilities existed, the insured were required by the structure of the benefit system to visit them with some regularity in order to obtain a sickness certificate from a physician. Moreover, the insured as a group were more aggressive in demanding medical treatment of various sorts. Thus, relatively speaking, this group was certainly receiving what Davis calls "a disproportionate amount" of the available services.

Following this line of reasoning, Davis and others have suggested that the inegalitarian character of the Soviet health system in the twenties was one of its principal shortcomings.[53] But, as Shmidt's comments made in the course of his 1926 debate with Semashko reveal, a major complaint from unions and Narkomtrud at that juncture was that the health system was not sufficiently unequal. The workers may have been receiving better care than peasants, but that meant little when they compared their care to the services some kassy had managed to provide before the Civil War and to the care that "Nepmen and capitalists" could purchase at private clinics under Narkomzdrav jurisdiction. After describing the private clinics as cleaner and better equipped than state hospitals, Shmidt posed the question on the mind of many workers: "Why can't the workers have their own hospitals as well equipped? If we can agree with Narkomzdrav, we can fully satisfy the insured with medical aid."[54]

Thus, the principal objection raised by Shmidt in this debate, and the one that workers' organs were to repeat throughout the twenties, concerned the indiscriminate use of funds specifically earmarked for the insured. And this was the objection that Semashko was unable to refute effectively. According to a decree signed by Narkomzdrav and Narkomtrud in March 1924, all funds contributed by the insurance organs were supposed go into a special account, fund "g," that would be used strictly to satisfy the needs of the insured. Medical care would be offered either in treatment centers open only to the insured, or in general medical facilities. In the latter case, the insured were to be given priority over the general population. This was the law. In practice, the insurance organs and the unions in some areas, such the Ukraine and the Caucasus, were able to exert enough control over the *rabmedy* to approximate the guidelines set forth in the decree. But in other areas, especially in Russia, the influence of insurance organs was sporadic and medical care for the insured suffered accordingly.[55]

What frequently happened, much to the frustration of the insurance organs, was that money given to the *rabmedy* would disappear into the general budget of the health department. A 1924 study by the Russian Social Insurance Administration showed that 33.3 percent of the *rabmedy* did not control fund "g," and 16.6 per cent did not even keep a record of how fund "g" was spent. Furthermore, in 36.1 percent of the provinces the *rabmedy* had not furnished a single treatment facility for special service to the insured, and in 41 percent of the provinces where such services existed they were under the jurisdiction of the health departments instead of the *rabmedy*.[56] In other words, the *rabmedy*, organs designed specifically to give unions and insurance organs some control over medical services, were frequently powerless and sometimes even nonexistent. To make matters worse, the health departments themselves were virtually at the bottom of the local government hierarchy, so that fund "g" would often disappear into the impoverished general budget of the *ispolkom*.[57]

Despite Semashko's claims about the actual pattern of distributing insurance allocations, the fact remained that workers were increasingly dissatisfied with the quality of their medical care, and Narkomtrud was unable to exert sufficient pressure on the *rabmedy* to improve that care. From 1925 onward one finds frequent reference to the fact that medical care was the most backward sector of the Soviet insurance system. As workers became increasingly vocal about their discontent with the status quo during this period, Narkomtrud realized that its own reputation among the workers was suffering as the result of widespread dissatisfaction over medical care, even though that care was technically the responsibility of Narkomzdrav.[58] In 1926 a lead editorial in the national insurance journal carried the following pronouncement: "We must abandon the view that the insurance organs are not 'responsible' for medical aid. Workers consider, and will continue to consider, poor medicine not from the point of view of blaming one office or another, but as an essential inadequacy of Soviet social insurance."[59]

The growing impatience of workers with the quality of insurance medicine is borne out by the stenographic reports of several regional insurance conferences in 1925 and 1926, where workers were particularly eager to relate their medical horror stories about how long one had to wait for treatment, about unqualified physicians or the absence of physicians altogether.[60] At one such meeting a factory representative complained that many workers went blind because they could not get glasses, others needed teeth and the insurance kassa took several months to supply them. The health department representative explained that his department had prepared 21,000 teeth and was making the remaining 17,000 as quickly as it could. The kassa representative sought to distance his institution from specific problems by claiming that the whole structure was wrong, and he reiterated the demand that social insurance organs be entrusted with all medical care for the insured.[61] In the end, no one was satisfied with the state of medical care for the insured and most of the blame fell on the insurance organs.

Workers began to campaign for the privileged treatment they had historically expected, and a frequent refrain of these conferences was that "not one kopeck of 'g' should go to nonworkers."[62] In 1925 the All-Russian Congress of Metal Workers decreed that fund "g" should be utilized exclusively by the *rabmedy* with the strictest possible accounting. The decree also praised the example set by a recent Sovnarkom decision that authorized the Central Insurance Administration to build its own hospital in the Northern Caucasus.[63] In February 1926, the Third Plenum of VTsSPS issued a resolution to transfer fund "g" to Narkomtrud.[64] There were similar resolutions from other leading union organs.[65]

This campaign to strengthen insurance medicine at the expense of unified Soviet medicine was determined but cautious. The prerevolutionary workers' insurance movement, repressed but not forgotten, still formed the inescapable historical context for this campaign and, try as they might, its proponents could not ignore the political dimensions of that history. The unions and insurance organs were frequently accused of trying to revive the Menshevik campaign for a self-administered workers' insurance medicine.[66] It was an ever-present danger that Faingold had recognized when he first called for the revival of insurance medicine in 1923, and he was careful to insist from the outset that the link between insurance medicine and working-class control had been irrevocably broken:

> Two sides appear even today—insurance medicine and "unified" medicine. . . . For Mensheviks, insurance medicine meant removing it from the Soviet apparatus. But for a Marxist to defend this is different. We can't oppose this to unified medicine, but must turn unified medicine into workers' preventative, i.e. insurance medicine. With the help of the insurance organs, and especially with insurance physicians.[67]

Such was Faingold's rather convoluted attempt to sever the links between a concept and its history. Similarly, those who campaigned for insurance medicine in the late twenties were astute in their rhetoric when they chose as their political slogan "unified workers' medicine" rather than the traditional and more accurate slogan "workers' insurance medicine." They hoped this new slogan would draw on the revolutionary insurance tradition without either reviving politically undesirable associations or contesting too vigorously officially sanctioned slogans such as unified Soviet medicine. In this way, they tried to dissociate their campaign from long-standing demands for autonomous, self-administered medical services while emphasizing the class character of their own demand for privileged medical care for the insured.[68] But during the twenties it was still almost impossible to speak of working-class privileges without reviving revolutionary visions of working-class control. It is evident from the evolving politics of Soviet insurance medicine that the political ambitions of the proletariat simmered just below the surface calm of NEP, a fact which would figure dramatically in the coming cultural revolution.

The dangerous tendency of many workers to confuse the revolutionary enthusiasms of a bygone era with the adumbrations of Stalin's coming revolution may help explain why a March 1927 decree, which seems to have surprised and certainly dismayed the insurance organs and the unions, completely eliminated the *rabmedy* at the very time when Narkomtrud and the unions called for the strengthening of these working-class organs.[69] In response to concerned inquiries from the insurance organs, Health Commissar Semashko assured insurance representatives that the elimination of these "special fists" for medical aid to the insured would not weaken this aspect of insurance medicine, but no one could have taken much comfort from these assurances.[70] One possible explanation for the decree, of course, is that the campaign had gone too far in reviving the revolutionary tradition of "workers' insurance medicine," a legacy that lingered in the imaginations of its participants.

If the elimination of the *rabmedy* seemed like a victory for Narkomzdrav, in the end neither Narkomzdrav nor Narkomtrud emerged victorious from the lengthy jurisdictional struggle outlined here. It took a revolutionary transformation of dramatic proportions to break the hold of Narkomzdrav over medical care for the insured, and when this finally occurred many of the objectives and principles that had originated in the workers' insurance movement and had been promoted by Narkomtrud during the 1920s were indeed embraced. The government set out to reform radically the social insurance system in order to reestablish links between medical care and other insurance benefits, and, within that context, the elimination of the *rabmedy* may have been, paradoxically, a harbinger of the demise of Se-mashko's unified Soviet medicine. By 1930 an extensive system of factory-based ambulatoria and polyclinics began to replace regional hospitals, and the task of administering those services was entrusted to factory-based insurance organs.[71] In one of many articles on the importance of this shift, one finds the following en-thusiastic projection:

> Why is medical aid torn from production? Because of the system of the "*edino*" [unified] dispensary; [but] medicine ought to have a class-industrial character, serving the in-dustrial workers first. In Moscow dispensaries are torn from production. They serve the place of residence, not the workplace. . . . If now 75 percent don't receive medical aid at work, soon 80 percent will.[72]

Narkomtrud had been vindicated, but by this time it had come under attack for bureaucratism. The social insurance kassy, which had preserved a tenuous but unmistakable link to the insurance movement, also came under increasing attack after 1928 and were eliminated by 1933 when the administration of social insurance was transferred to the unions.[73] The rationale for that decision is yet another story. But in the present context one could argue plausibly that at least one goal of the workers' insurance movement had finally reached fruition, even if in a political and institutional setting far different from the one its leaders had envisioned. Although the kassa tradition was rejected, many workers would nevertheless receive privileged and specialized medical care at their factories. Yet, the all-encompassing category of "the insured" increasingly included the newly arriving peasants of a rapidly expanding work force and no longer served as a meaningful category for bestowing privileges on the hereditary working class. As a result, the entitlement criteria for receiving sickness benefits were changed in order to discriminate against these peasant workers, and new entitlement categories were created, this time embracing workers in the leading branches of Soviet industry so that relatively generous medical resources could be channeled to closed facilities serving the factories of these leading workers.[74] If the social insurance system as conceived by Narkomtrud during NEP no longer existed, that commissariat's conception of working-class medicine as a separate and superior branch of Soviet medicine had come of age during the second revolution. The revolution from above confirmed that the politics of entitlement would remain intact when other revolutionary aspirations had long since faded.

ACCOUNTING AND CONTROL: THE PHYSICIANS

From the account so far it would seem that, while Narkomtrud championed the cause of the working class by fighting to reserve insurance monies for the insured alone and by demanding special medical facilities, Narkomzdrav preferred to sacrifice the immediate interests of workers as a class to the long-term goal of creating a unified and relatively egalitarian health system. But such were the complexities of class medicine that the question as to which commissariat represented the best interests of the workers remained in dispute throughout the twenties. For in another context Narkomzdrav could legitimately claim to be defending workers against the excessively cost-conscious insurance organs of Narkomtrud. Precisely because Narkomtrud set aside so much of its budget for medical care, it was also concerned that those allocations be spent efficiently, which meant policing the doctors, who issued sickness certificates, and the workers, who received insurance benefits. In the aftermath of the Civil War, problems of accounting and control had become central in this, as in virtually every other branch, of Soviet administration.[75] Once again Narkomzdrav and Narkomtrud were divided over this issue, but this time it seemed that Narkomzdrav was more concerned to protect the health of insured workers whereas Narkomtrud was willing to sacrifice the individual worker's well-being in its efforts to control medical expenditures. This apparent discrepancy between the interests of the workers as a class, which seemed well served by Narkomtrud, and the interests of the worker as an individual patient, who seemed to prefer the physicians working in Narkomzdrav, was one of the unanticipated contradictions of this newly evolving social medicine.

The problem of control over working-class medicine was addressed, if not satisfactorily resolved, within the context of yet another jurisdictional struggle. Two institutions were in charge of medical expertise and control in insurance medicine, the Medical Control Commission (VKK) and the Medical Expert Commission (VEK). An insured patient passed through the various medical organs in the following sequence. To receive both sickness benefits for temporary incapacity and the appropriate medical care, the worker applied directly to a physician for a medical certificate confirming incapacity. If the condition lasted more than five days each time or two weeks altogether, the worker then applied to VKK, a commission which included one insurance physician, that is, a physician under the jurisdiction of the insurance system, and two Narkomzdrav physicians.[76] VKK determined both the nature and the seriousness of the incapacity and the most effective treatment. Finally, if the temporary incapacity seemed likely to become permanent, or if it were a case of permanent incapacity from the outset, VKK sent the patient to VEK, a commission made up of medical experts who would determine the type and degree of incapacity, which would lead to a particular health regime and an invalid pension.[77]

At the beginning of NEP this entire network of medical professionals was placed under the jurisdiction of Narkomzdrav, to the continuing frustration of the insurance administration. Narkomtrud strongly objected to the arrangement because the social insurance system paid for benefits and pensions that individual physicians, VKK, and VEK authorized, as well as for medical care, but it exercised no control over the physicians who determined these expenditures. Narkomzdrav countered that if the insurance organs gained control over VKK and VEK they would violate the rights of insured workers, illegally depriving them of benefits in the name of economic efficiency.[78]

According to Narkomtrud, the problem began with the physicians who examined patients and issued certificates for short-term illness. The social insurance system distributed generous sickness benefits, amounting to an average of almost ten sick days a year for each insured worker, with the benefits approaching full wage.[79] This meant that Narkomzdrav physicians spent much of their time certifying that the insured were entitled to sickness benefits, and Narkomtrud claimed that these physicians were indifferent to the expense that such certification implied. In the face of such indifference, it was left to insurance physicians to control expenditures by detecting malingering and thereby restricting certificates. As spokesmen for Narkomtrud complained repeatedly, the insured predictably viewed the insurance physician from the kassa as a "commissar who stands between the patient and the physician,"[80] whereas the physician from Narkomzdrav was *dobry* ("the good guy"), the defender of the individual worker.[81] Semashko contributed to this picture, portraying Narkomzdrav physicians as disinterested professionals who defended the interests of ailing workers against the purely economic concerns of insurance physicians, a picture largely confirmed by the experiences of the insured.[82]

At this time, not only the insurance physicians, but VKK as a whole had a poor reputation that could only get worse if that agency were transferred to Narkomtrud. One insurance activist, comparing the physicians in VEK to those in VKK, wrote that "[VEK] is staffed with highly qualified specialists while VKK is a fairly motley assortment of physicians, where along with experienced physicians there are those completely lacking in experience."[83] The nature of the work in VKK explains why competent physicians were unlikely to enlist. As one VKK physician complained, he and his colleagues were overworked and underpaid. "The physicians sit in VKK like machines. They swallow and then spew out decisions, in the majority of cases confirmations."[84] Another VKK physician from Leningrad complained of similar conditions, where a commission that should have seen twenty to twenty-five patients daily saw sixty-five, working six to seven hours without a break.[85] However poor the credibility of VKK as a whole, throughout the 1920s insurance physicians associated with VKK had a particularly unflattering reputation among the workers as they tried to reduce the number of certificates that Narkomzdrav physicians (who outnumbered them on the commission) dispensed with great liberality.[86]

It would seem, then, that in the case of individual physicians and VKK, the much heralded social aspect of Soviet medicine was reduced largely to addressing the pressing problem of controlling medical expenditures by controlling the physicians who provided medical services. This translated into a struggle between traditional conceptions of medical practice defended by Narkomzdrav and the restrictions on that practice that insurance medicine had inevitably to impose. For even as Commissar Semashko complained that medical schools were still training physicians in the old ways, producing physician-artisans rather than social physicians,[87] neither he nor the physicians themselves were prepared to abide by the constraints imposed on medical practice in an extensive social insurance system.[88] Once again it was Vigdorchik who tried to articulate and thus pave the way for the radically new role which insurance physicians would have to fill. Traditionally, the physician was obliged to take all the patient's complaints into account, distributing medicine on request and assuming that a person claiming to be ill was in fact ill, but with free medical care and generous sickness benefits physicians were expected to adopt a different stand toward their insured patients. As Vigdorchik wrote in 1921: "[T]he physician should be experienced, but also impartial. The expert to a significant extent serves as a judge between two sides—the applicant and the insurance organs."[89] These experts would assign patients to preestablished categories of illness and disability, determining entitlement and thus becoming important agents in an unmistakably political process.

If this was the perspective embraced by those who spoke for the insurance system, physicians themselves sought to preserve purely medical considerations as separate from and prior to such a politics of entitlement. As one insurance worker complained: "Sometimes a physician simply gives medicine at the request of the patient—this happens because he doesn't think about the interests of social insurance. He only heals, and for the rest, that is someone else's problem."[90] In the domain of insurance medicine, healing was not enough. Control of expenditures was equally important, and it was that fiscal responsibility that many physicians seemed determined to ignore during this transitional period. The result, at least as interpreted by insurance representatives, was excessively generous sickness benefits compounded with a rate of malingering allegedly on the rise and at times reaching epidemic proportions.[91]

If the problem had simply been that physicians were overly cautious in treating sick workers, this might not in itself have led to unmanageable sickness expenditures. For, as the physicians argued in their own defense, the aim of Soviet medicine was to prevent serious illness, and a cautious attitude toward workers' ailments would serve that end.[92] The insurance administration's more serious criticism, however, was that physicians were more concerned to maintain good relations with their patients by agreeing to all their requests than to ascertain the state of their health. "Physicians, not involved in the internal life of the kassa and not knowing its means . . . are generous. To preserve good relations with patients they give out certifications left and right."[93] One explanation for this was that physicians had not broken away from the habits of traditional medical practice, but beyond this was the fact that physicians were often intimidated by workers who used their privileged position to browbeat the less favored medical professionals.[94] In 1926, VTsSPS was forced to appeal to local union organs to put a stop to the "rude bearing of union members to medical personnel."[95]

By 1927 the weight of opinion about how to provide medical care for workers was shifting away from the perspective of Narkomzdrav. In this context the Central Insurance Administration of Narkomtrud finally achieved what it had demanded since 1921—VKK was transferred from Narkomzdrav to Narkomtrud.[96] But this did not necessarily resolve the problem of training a cadre of insurance physicians with the appropriate attitude toward medical care for the insured. In 1927 a new cadre of more than one thousand insurance physicians graduated,[97] but in 1928 the functions of VKK were reduced so that this organ was no longer a viable base from which to transform medical relationships with the insured.[98] A more dramatic restructuring of medical care for the insured was not far off, a transformation that would presumably help close the gap between the medical profession and the insurance system. But in the meantime Semashko did all he could to resist and reverse the decision to transfer VKK to the insurance organs. He claimed that the decision placed a purely medical matter into the hands of incompetent and bureaucratic insurance physicians, removing that responsibility from Narkomzdrav physicians who, as he put it, "entered the path of qualified medical care full of love, in order to serve the workers."[99] But this traditional image of the physician committed to "purely medical matters" and to the best interests of the patient was being undermined by the financial constraints of a system that provided free medical care and extensive sickness benefits for the insured.

The case of VEK introduced yet another set of factors into the dispute over insurance medicine, and here, as in the jurisdictional struggle over VKK, Narkomzdrav seemed to occupy the high ground, defending the integrity of medical science, whereas Narkomtrud focused on the more practical problems of expenditure, control, and labor productivity. Once again the scientific emphasis of Narkomzdrav prevailed during NEP, but by the late twenties a general impatience with theory for its own sake translated, in this context, into an endorsement of the insurance system's emphasis on categorizing invalids efficiently and exploiting their remaining labor capacity.

Unlike VKK, which was an organ of control with low prestige whose physicians were often poorly trained, VEK was a prestigious body and was considered the leading institution in the science of insurance medicine. Generally staffed by highly trained medical specialists, it was part of a network of institutions involved in studying labor incapacity, professional illness, and industrial accidents. There were numerous clinics devoted to the study and treatment of professional illness, one attached to Moscow State University, another in Leningrad, and the relevant periodicals of the time carried reports of detailed statistical studies attempting to establish links between illnesses and professions.[100] These studies, combined with the equally widespread investigations of industrial accidents, were part of a more general enthusiasm during these years for scientific investigations into all aspects of labor and life. The newly developing science of insurance medicine was to provide objective criteria for controlling various pathologies and for assigning benefits and services in cases of accident or illness.

Narkomzdrav retained jurisdiction over VEK during the twenties by emphasizing the scientific grounding of its medical expertise, while Narkomtrud objected that the commission specialists concentrated on purely biological measures of labor incapacity whereas the social causes of incapacity and the use of remaining labor capacity should have been their principal focus.[101] There was some substance to the claim that much of the sophisticated scientific research on labor incapacity, trauma, and professional illness had little practical relevance to the insurance function of VEK. For example, the commission was supposed to assign invalids to one of six categories, depending on the degree of incapacity. But until 1925 only invalids in the first three categories, ranging from complete incapacity to incapacity requiring transfer to another job, received pensions, so that an assignment to categories four through six had no practical significance at all.[102] In 1924 and 1925 legislation was finally introduced for invalidity resulting from industrial accidents or professional illness, and in this case invalids in categories four through six also received pensions. Only about 4 percent of VEK patients, however, were classified as professional illness or accident victims,[103] but VEK continued to classify all invalids according to the six categories, an exercise in futility which the more practically minded insurance system eliminated when it took control of VEK.[104]

Even when professional illness became a special criterion for invalidity in 1925, the specialized scientific investigations into the links between professions and illness were only indirectly relevant to the insurance functions of VEK. VEK operated with a predetermined list of illnesses which would qualify as professional illness, a list drawn up by the Professional Hygiene Department of Narkomtrud. In constructing that list, the department had begun with all the illnesses included in West European legislation but had then excluded many illnesses because of the limited material resources of the insurance kassy. Other illnesses had, in turn, been added under pressure from the relevant unions.[105] This suggests that economic and political concerns were at least as important in defining the scope of VEK expertise as were the isolated scientific investigations into professional illness carried on at specialized clinics.

Throughout the 1920s, the scientific investigations conducted at individual factories and laboratories were preliminary at best and could not provide a reliable scientific basis for labor policies, at least in the short term. In the end, VEK's attempt to establish "objective" scientific criteria for determining labor incapacity and entitlement did not pass the exacting test of political expediency. Under the difficult economic conditions of NEP, VEK was caught between the scientific ambitions of its medical experts, who aspired to contribute to a new and important branch of medical science, and the political and economic demands of the insurance system.

With the pressures of industrialization mounting in the late twenties, the officially mandated balance shifted unequivocally in favor of insurance constraints, and the scientific aspirations of VEK increasingly came under attack. The commission's experts were criticized for assigning invalids to groups according to lost labor capacity instead of concentrating on remaining labor capacity and retraining. This new orientation was obviously a direct result of the changing labor market. Under the conditions of high unemployment during NEP, invalid pensions were used to encourage the aged and the infirm to leave the factories, but, with the industrialization drive, labor shortages began to replace unemployment as the principal labor problem, and invalids became a valuable, and often skilled, labor pool that VEK, with its focus on incapacity, failed to exploit. According to figures of the Central Insurance Administration, in 1931, out of 767,000 invalids 40 percent were in the third group and could therefore work, while among all labor invalids 56 percent were workers, and often highly qualified. There were, for example, 57,000 metal workers, 15,000 miners, 72,000 textile workers, and 32,000 railroad workers, whose skills were extremely valuable during those years.[106]

As early as 1927, there were indications that changing economic conditions would strengthen the hand of Narkomtrud in its attempt to wrest VEK from Narkomzdrav jurisdiction. A 1927 decree announced that the head of VEK should be an insurance kassa representative, and it advised the commission to abandon the narrow biological methods of the past years and turn to the study of labor conditions.[107] By 1928, VEK in Leningrad and other localities had been transferred to the jurisdiction of the insurance system, but in Moscow, where Narkomzdrav had the most influence and where even the transfer of VKK was illegally resisted, the fight between Moscow insurance and health organs over VEK was prolonged and bitter. Health department representatives accused insurance workers of scientific illiteracy or worse. As one health department official admonished his insurance counterpart, "You understand nothing. The question [of insurance statistics] is very complex. Insurance workers are illiterate."[108] Insurance officials, in their turn, attacked VEK experts for assigning pensions casually and for operating from a "completely medical point of view." They also objected that VEK physicians worked as experts only incidentally, and not exclusively, as they would under Narkomtrud jurisdiction.[109]

The medical experts themselves joined the fray, circulating documents that accused the insurance organs of incompetence and even deliberate falsification in the use of statistical data. These experts did not want VEK to fall under the jurisdiction of the insurance system, but at the same time in the wake of the Shakhty affair they had to defend themselves against accusations of counterrevolutionary activity and failure to follow a class line in assigning patients to invalid categories.[110] It is interesting to note that during this dispute over VEK jurisdiction the insurance representatives themselves made a point of defending the medical experts against charges of counterrevolutionary activity, stressing that their own criticisms of VEK were directed at the Health Department rather than at the individual experts. An insurance representative expressed the hope that the experts, freed from the tutelage of the health department, would overcome their negative attitude toward the insurance organs.[111] The social insurance administration apparently hoped to win over a cadre of committed and respected experts to the cause of insurance medicine.

A 1929 Central Committee decree on social insurance, which began the process of restructuring the whole insurance system, set the stage for a new emphasis in this area of medical expertise. It called for the establishment of special institutes in Moscow and Leningrad to prepare new cadres of medical experts. These institutes, which remain active to this day, were to train experts to focus on labor capacity rather than incapacity.[112] This change in terminology indicated not just a shift in emphasis, but a basic reorientation in medical expertise, a reorientation that was in part the outcome of a maturing system of insurance medicine. In 1932 a SNK decree formally transferred VEK to the insurance organs, a move that the Ukrainian and Russian Commissariats of Public Health apparently resisted vigorously but unsuccessfully.[113] A contemporary account explained the transfer as follows:

On May 8, 1932, [VEK] was moved from the organs of health to insurance. Why? Because the work of [VEK] didn't change at all during the reconstruction period, on the basis of the Decree of [VEK] of August 25, 1931. They continued to establish invalidity only by anatomical signs, without considering functional ability and remaining

labor capacity of the patients or their social-production conditions. [VEK] worked as
of old, in quiet offices, without links to the workers, without studying production.[114]

At this juncture the physicians involved in insurance medicine were caught up
in the general wave of antiprofessionalism unleashed by the Shakhty affair, but this
brief history of VKK and VEK suggests that the insurance system was engaged in
a prolonged struggle against the medical practices of Narkomzdrav physicians
throughout the 1920s. It would take time to wear down the resistance of these
physicians, and, more important, to train new ones, but the special, so-called social,
demands of insurance medicine seemed to be the wave of the future.

CONCLUSION

The rivalry between Narkomtrud and Narkomzdrav was more than simply the embodiment of the bureaucratic tendency to increase the power of one's institution by
expanding its resources and responsibilities. Each commissariat was convinced that
medical services for the working class should be delivered in a specific institutional
and ideological context. Narkomtrud, operating within the framework of insurance
medicine, was concerned primarily with entitlement, control, and funding; Narkomzdrav was committed to unified Soviet medicine, including a certain standard
of professional autonomy for its physicians. If, in the early days of the Revolution,
no one was sure how the general commitment to working-class medicine would
translate into specific medical practices, it turned out that the concept of insurance
medicine promoted by Narkomtrud was a more realistic model for class medicine
than the medical order envisioned by Narkomzdrav. It was also some time before
the revolutionary expectations evoked by the notion of working-class medicine were
tempered by the harsh realities of administrative expediency that accompanied the
attempt to provide extensive medical care for the insured. As we have seen, working-
class self-administration of medical services was a slogan of the prerevolutionary
workers' insurance movement, but it never figured in Bolshevik plans for Soviet
medicine. Working-class privileges were another matter, however, and in this respect Narkomtrud clearly spoke for the workers it represented when it insisted that
the funds collected by the insurance organs for medical services should be spent
exclusively on the insured. Narkomzdrav chose instead to organize medical care
according to universal and egalitarian principles, and at first its policy prevailed,
but Narkomzdrav faltered when the working class began to demand the fruits of its
revolutionary sacrifices. If egalitarianism was a favorite theme throughout these
years, Narkomtrud for one never confused this with the pressing political task of
the day, which was to make reliable medical care available to the working class.

Perhaps the most important lesson of the dispute between Narkomtrud and
Narkomzdrav was that there were inevitable costs as well as benefits to the insurance
medicine promoted by Narkomtrud. Class medicine involved accounting and control
as well as privilege, and this meant that the individual worker was caught up in a
vast bureaucratic organization which determined entitlement according to its own,
allegedly objective but often painfully arbitrary, criteria and which was constantly

on guard against malingering and overly generous medical practitioners. From this standpoint, the worker might well have chosen to renounce his or her membership in the working class to become an individual patient served by the physicians of Narkomzdrav. But privilege and administrative control were inseparable, and however much Narkomzdrav and its physicians resisted the encroachment of insurance medicine, the class orientation was bound to prevail in one form or another. Eventually the Soviet medical system incorporated many of the features promoted by Narkomtrud under the rubric of what had now become ideologically defunct: "workers' insurance medicine."

Having explored this tension between working-class privilege and administrative control in early Soviet medical practice, one can easily see how writers like Titmuss and Foucault might differ in their assessments of the "social dimension" of medicine. The case of Soviet insurance medicine illustrates the redistributive dimension of social medicine that Titmuss advocates, while reinforcing Foucault's claim that medical knowledge serves as an important instrument for exercising power in modern society. The impulse to resolve this tension, that is, to redistribute social benefits without simultaneously extending the arm of the state into all areas of labor and life, has informed political debate throughout this century, and no obvious resolution is in sight.

NOTES

1. For example, see Richard Titmuss, *The Gift Relationship* (New York, 1971), p. 13; and *Social Policy* (New York, 1974), pp. 26–27.

2. Michel Foucault, "Two Lectures," in Colin Gordon, ed., *Power/Knowledge* (New York, 1980), pp. 107–8.

3. In *The Birth of the Clinic* (New York, 1975), Foucault has written an intriguing account of how, by the end of the eighteenth century, the modern clinic provided a context within which the individual became the object of what he calls the "medical gaze," or scientifically structured discourse. He defines clinical experience as "that opening up of the concrete individual, for the first time in Western history, to the language of rationality" (p. xiv). He argues that for two hundred years this discourse has "constituted the dark but firm web of our experience" (p. 199). One could argue that the Bolsheviks set out to unravel this web when they made class the object of their medical gaze.

4. E. Iakovenko, "O predmete i zadachakh sotsial'noi meditsiny," *Sotsial'naia gigiena,* 2 (1923), 9.

5. Christopher Davis refers extensively to the social insuarance system in "Economic Problems of the Soviet Health Service: 1917–1930," *Soviet Studies,* 35 (1983), 353.

6. See Alvin Gouldner, *The Dialectic of Ideology and Technology* (New York, 1976), for an interesting account of why social science is more political than we like to admit, and Marxism is more scientific than we are willing to acknowledge.

7. There were frequent references to the inadequacies of the existing arrangement, as in a 1907 report from a factory inspector showing that, out of 601 mills and factories in Petersburg, with 95,000 workers, 58% offered no medical aid and only one site had its own hospital. Nineteen factories had agreements with private and city hospitals and the others provided ambulatory aid: Viv', "Kak fabrikanty lechat rabochikh," *Voprosy strakhovaniia,*

no. 6 (1913), p. 5. In all of Russia, 61% of the factories offered no medical aid and only 7.8% had hospitals while 23% provided ambulatories: "Kak budet' postavleno lechenie rabochikh po zakonu 23 Iulia 1912g," *Strakhovanie rabochikh*, no. 1 (1912), p. 4. According to some 1911 data, in the Petersburg province 74% of the factories provided no medical aid. Moscow province, however, fared better. Out of 411 factories with 206,000 workers, 19% had hospitals (with 157,000 workers), 64% had agreements with other hospitals, and only 16% had no medical aid: Viv', "Kak fabrikanty," p. 5.

8. I. M. Rubinow, *Studies in Workmen's Insurance: Italy, Russia, Spain* (New York, 1911), 3:2228.

9. A. I. Vishnevetskii, *Razvitie zakonodatel'stva o sotsial'nom strakhovanii v Rossii*, 2d ed. (Moscow, 1926), pp. 27–28.

10. See Ruth Amende Roosa, "Workers' Insurance Legislation and the Role of the Industrialists in the Period of the Third State Duma," *Russian Review* 34 (October 1975), for a detailed discussion of the Duma debate. She emphasizes that industrialists themselves were divided over who should pay for medical care, especially in earlier discussions.

11. See M. K. Korbut, "Strakhovye zakonoproekty v tretei gosudarstvennoi dume," in B. G. Danskii and B. T. Miliutin, *Materialy po istorii sotsial'nogo strakhovaniia* (Moscow, 1928); and "Strakhovye zakony 1912 goda i ikh provedenie v Peterburge," *Krasnaia letopis*, no. 1 (1928).

12. B. G. Danskii, "Pered strakhovaniem," *Pravda*, 166 (1912). In *Bol'shevistskaia pechat'* (Sbornik materialov): *Vypusk* III (1907 g.-fevral' 1917g.) (Moscow, 1961), p. 261.

13. Korbut, "Strakhovye zakonoproekty," p. 36.

14. Ibid., p. 21.

15. I. Chistiakov, *Strakhovanie rabochikh v Rossii* (Moscow, 1912), pp. 291–93.

16. See B. G. Danskii, *Rabochii ustav bol'nichnoi kassy* (St. Petersburg, 1913).

17. The first such facility, created for the families of kassa members but technically off-limits to the members themselves, opened in April 1914 in the province of Tul'skii and was apparently popular. In 1915 five sickness kassy in St. Petersburg united to open a hospital, and from 1914 to 1917 four such *raion* hospitals opened in St. Petersburg and one opened in Nikolaev, Saratov, Kiev, and Rostov on the Don. See N. A. Vigdorchik, "Kassovaia meditsina," *Teoriia i praktika sotsial'nogo strakhovaniia*, 4 (1923), pp. 119–22.

18. See I. Stetsovskii, "Rabochee strakhovoe dvizhenie v period Fevral'skoi revoliutsii," in Danskii and Miliutin, *Materialy*, p. 193; and Solomon Schwarz, *Sotsial'noe strakhovanie v Rossii v 1917–1919 godakh* (New York, 1968), p. 51.

19. Vigdorchik, *Teoriia i praktika*, p. 132.

20. Schwarz, *Sotsial'noe strakhovanie*, p. 67.

21. Ibid., pp. 86–87.

22. Ibid., p. 31; G. I. Osipov, "Strakhovaia kampaniia v Peterburge: rabota v pravlen-iiakh bol'nichnykh kass," in Danskii and Miliutin, *Materialy*, p. 31.

23. Vishnevetskii, *Razvitie*, p. 49.

24. V. Shmidt, "O vzaimootnosheniiakh NKT s VTsSPS," *Vestnik Narkomtruda*, nos. 2–3 (1918), p. 25.

25. This set of decisions clearly corresponded to the prevailing Bolshevik policy in regard to other working-class organizations. By January 1918 the factory committees, which had played an important role as factory-based organs for working-class self-administration, came under attack as Lenin distinguished between workers' control in the popular sense of workers directly running factories and a form of working-class participation in administration where workers would "kontrol" by monitoring the actions of administrators to see that they fulfilled their responsibilities. At the First All-Union Trade Union Congress in January 1918 the factory committees were subordinated to the unions and those who advocated complete autonomy for local workers' organs were condemned as syndicalists. See Margaret Dewar, *Labor Policy in the USSR* (New York, 1956), p. 33.

26. Vigdorchik, *Teoriia i praktika*, p. 132; Vishnevetskii, *Razvitie*, p. 49.

27. Vigdorchik, *Teoriia i praktika*, p. 138.

28. Ibid.

29. Schwarz, *Sotsial'noe strakhovanie*, p. 155.

30. *Izvestiia*, June 29, 1918. Cited in Schwarz, *Sotsial'noe strakhovanie*, p. 158.

31. S. Kolokol'tsev, "K voprosu o vzaimootnosheniiakh komissariatov truda i sotsi-al'nogo obespecheniia," *Vestnik Narkomtruda*, nos. 4–7 (1918), p. 20.

32. A. Vinokurov, "Novyi zakon o polnom sotsial'nom obespechenii trudiashchikhsia," *Zhurnal NKSO*, no. 2 (1918), p. 5.

33. The jurisdictional battle between Narkomtrud and Narkomsobes continued throughout the Civil War, with various categories of pensioners shifting back and forth between them. In March 1919, Narkomtrud dealt with incapacity through work or daily life, and Narkomsobes dealt with poverty. But these distinctions were increasingly vague since need rather than employment status became the determining factor for the receipt of benefits. A November 1919 decree, which remained unpublished, merged Narkomsobes and Narkomtrud into one commissariat, Narkomtrud and Sotsial'noe Obespechenie (SO) (Vishnevetskii, *Razvitie*, p. 92). By then, however, Narkomtrud itself was becoming largely superfluous, a process that was hastened in 1920 with the creation of the Glavkomtrud to direct labor matters (see Dewar, *Labor Policy*, p. 48). After this reform, Narkomtrud and Narkomsobes were separated again in April 1920 and Narkomsobes had jurisdiction for all social welfare functions except unemployment. In December even that function went to Narkomsobes and the final link between insurance and the working class organs was broken (Vishnevetskii, *Razvitie*, p. 93).

34. Vishnevetskii, *Razvitie*, p. 82.

35. B. I. Faingol'd, "Blizhaishie zadachi v rabote otdela s.o. i o.t. NKT," *Vestnik Narkomtruda*, nos. 1–2 (1919), p. 60.

36. Vishnevetskii, *Razvitie*, p. 86.

37. Z. Tettenborn, "Sotsial'noe obespechenie v periode voennogo kommunizma," in Danskii and Miliutin, *Materialy*,p. 264.

38. Z. Tettenborn, "Sotsial'noe obespechenie i sotsial'noe strakhovanie," *Voprosy sot-sial'nogo obespecheniia*, nos. 5–6 (1921), p. 13.

39. The trade-union debate centered on whether or not there was a place for autonomous workers' organizations, namely, the unions, in a proletarian state like the Soviet Union. Trotsky and Bukharin argued that there was no need for organs separate from the state, whereas the Workers' Opposition wanted to transfer the administration of economic organs to union control. Lenin settled the debate with the compromise position that unions were necessary to defend workers against arbitrary bureaucratic rule, but they should not interfere in the administration of the economy. In spite of Lenin's declaration, the role of unions in the Soviet system remained ambiguous and controversial, and the same can be said of the territorial kassy. They were administrative organs under the jurisdiction of Narkomtrud and thus technically state organs, but they were also workers' organs with considerable autonomy. Their exact status remained controversial throughout NEP.

40. N. A. Miliutin, *Proekty, postanovki sotsial'nogo obespecheniia trudiashchikhsia*, 4 (St. Petersburg, 1920), p. 28. Miliutin became the head of the NKF RSFSR in 1922. See N. A. Miliutin, "Vospominaniia," *Voprosy strakhovaniia*, no. 26 (1927), p. 4.

41. I. Segalovich, "Ne predreshaia," *Voprosy strakhovaniia*, no. 45 (1926), p. 7.

42. Ibid.

43. There were even rumors in 1922 that the Larinskaia Commission for simplifying the Soviet apparatus had recommended liquidating Narkomsobes and transferring its functions to Narkomtrud and Narkomzdrav. G. Levin, "Ob odnom 'proekte'," *Vestnik sotsial'nogo obespecheniia. Kharkov*, no. 4 (1922), p. 14.

44. Vigdorchik, *Teoriia i praktika*, pp. 43, 139.

45. Ibid., p. 42.

46. Vishnevetskii, *Razvitie*, p. 207.

47. Ibid.

48. Jack Minkoff, "The Soviet Social Insurance System since 1921" (Ph.D. diss., Columbia University, 1960), p. 326.

49. Davis, "Economic Problems," p. 353.

50. *Voprosy strakhovaniia*, no. 7 (1926), p. 3.

51. He especially objected to Semashko's attempt to compare the individual peasant to an insured family with an unspecified number of members. Ibid., p. 5.

52. Davis, "Economic Problems," p. 351.

53. Ibid.

54. "Rech' Shmidta na Brianskom gubs''ezde profsoiuza," *Voprosy strakhovaniia*, no. 7 (1926), p. 1.

55. *Sotsial'noe strakhovanie v 1924–1925* (Moscow, 1925), pp. 24–25; Vishnevetskii, *Razvitie*, p. 190.

56. *Sotsial'noe strakhovanie v 1924–1925*, p. 87.

57. Ibid., p. 86.

58. Sheila Fitzpatrick has explored the far-reaching ramifications that this working-class restlessness and discontent had for Stalin's revolution from above. In the realm of social insurance, as in areas she has explored, the workers themselves were instrumental in hastening radical reforms that Stalin and others were preparing to initiate. See "The Cultural Revolution as Class War," in S. Fitzpatrick, ed., *Cultural Revolution in Russia, 1928–1931* (Bloomington, Ind., 1978).

59. "Nashi blizhaishie zadachi v 1926g.," *Voprosy strakhovaniia*, no. 1 (1926), p. 3.

60. *Mezhsoiuznaia strakhovaia konferentsiia Rogozhsko-Simonovskogo raiona* (Moscow, 1925), p. 16; *Mezhsoiuznaia konferentsiaa po sotsial'nomy strakhovaniiu Vasileostrovskogo raiona, noiabr' 1925* (Leningrad, 1926), pp. 32, 43–44; *Mezhsoiuznaia konferentsiia po sotsial'nomy strakhovaniiu Vyborskogo raiona, dekabr' 1925* (Leningrad, 1926), pp. 5, 43; *Mezhsoiuznaia konferetsiia po sotsial'nomy strakhovaniiu Tsentral'nogo gorodskogo raiona, dekabr' 1925* (Leningrad, 1926), p. 23.

61. *Mezhsoiuznaia konferentsiia Vasileostrovskogo raiona*, pp. 43–44.

62. *Otchet pervoi Luganskoi okruzhnoi mezhsoiuznoi strakhovoi konferentsii* (Lugansk, 1926), p. 16.

63. Vishnevetskii, *Razvitie*, p. 208.

64. "VTsSPS: III Plenum, VI Sozyv," *Voprosy strakhovaniia*, no. 7 (1926), p. 7.

65. Vishnevetskii, *Razvitie*, p. 208.

66. "K VII Mosk. Gubs''ezdy Profsoiuza," *Voprosy strakhovaniia*, no. 8 (1926), p. 1.

67. B. I. Faingol'd, "Rol' organov sotsial'nogo strakhovaniia v dalneishem razvitii sovetskoi meditsiny," *Voprosy strakhovaniia*, nos. 29–30 (1923), p. 3.

68. *Otchet Luganskoi konferentsii*, p. 20.

69. "VSNK RSFSR," *Voprosy strakhovaniia*, no. 30 (1927), p. 25.

70. "Novoe polozhenie o medpomoshchi zastrakhovannym," *Voprosy strakhovaniia*, no. 15 (1927), p. 2.

71. Henry Sigerist, *Medicine and Health in the Soviet Union* (New York, 1947), p. 107.

72. *Voprosy strakhovaniia*, no. 10 (1931).

73. "III Plenum VTsSPS," *Voprosy strakhovaniia*, nos. 7–8 (1933), pp. 10, 13.

74. "Na novom etape," *Voprosy strakhovaniia*, no. 5 (1931), p. 3; *Voprosy strakhovaniia*, no. 6 (1931), p. 9.

75. Much as Lenin had foreseen in 1918: "widespread, general, universal accounting and control, the accounting and control of the amount of labor performed and of the distribution of products—is the *essence* of the socialist transformation, once the political rule of the proletariat has been established and secured." Lenin, *The Lenin Anthology*, ed. by R. Tucker (New York, 1975), p. 428.

76. Insurance doctors were also called *doverennyi* doctors. See Vigdorchik for history of the two types of doctors, referred to as *lechashchii* and *kontrol'nyi*, in Europe. *Teoriia i Praktika*, p. 35.

77. Vishnevetskii, *Razvitie*, p. 156. In fact, during the early period VKK ended up deciding cases of permanent incapacity in those areas where no VEK had been established.

See M. V. Verzhblovskii, *Ocherki istorii vrachebno-trudovoi ekspertizy v RSFSR,* 30 (Leningrad, 1971), p. 29.

78. An insurance worker outlined the dilemma: "The argument for keeping VKK and VEK (for invalidity) under Narkomzdrav is that the insurance organs, as economic organs, wouldn't be objective. And the argument that insurance organs are also elected organs, standing on the side of the legal interests of the workers, is not convincing (according to Narkomzdrav) because economic interests, as more powerful, prevail over ideological interests. But NKZ is not only neutral, it is indifferent to the material reserves of the insurance organs, and given the soft-hearted doctors, there is the danger of the tendency of VKK and VEK to satisfy the interests of the workers without sufficient foundation." Dondarov, "VKK i BVE," *Vestnik sotsial'nogo strakhovaniia: Zakavkazia,* no. 11 (1924).

79. L. V. Zabelin, *Sotsial'noe strakhovanie v zhizni rabochego SSSR* (Moscow, 1930), p. 25; "2-e Vsesoiuznoe strakhovoe soveshchanie," *Voprosy strakhovaniia,* no. 16 (1926), p. 4.

80. Ia. Ia. Katsman, "O doverennykh vrachakh s kass," *Voprosy strakhovaniia,* no. 32 (1923), p. 4.

81. L. Litvinov, "VKK i lechaschie vrachi," *Voprosy strakhovaniia,* no. 37 (1925), p. 12.

82. "Obzor pechati," *Voprosy strakhovaniia,* no. 15 (1928), p. 15. Even Vigdorchik, a strong supporter of kassa medicine, admitted that European experience with the two types of doctors had shown that the *lechashchii* doctor was "far superior" to the *kontrol* doctor. "The *kontrol* doctor becomes a dry bureaucrat. The sick look on him as an investigator, searching for deception." *Teoriia i praktika,* p. 35. See ibid., chap. 6, for a detailed discussion of the difficult relations between doctors and the sickness kassa in Europe.

83. V. N. Katin-Iartsev, "O vzaimootnoshenii mezhdu BVE i VKK," *Voprosy strakhovaniia,* no. 29 (1924), pp. 11–12.

84. *Soveshchanie Prezidiumov Moskovskikh strakhovikh kass,* Stenograficheskii otchet (Moscow, 1924), p. 97.

85. Katin-Iartsev, "O vzaimootnoshenii," p. 14.

86. L. Bronshtein, "Nuzhen reshitel'nyi perelom," *Voprosy strakhovaniia,* no. 28 (1929), p. 13.

87. N. A. Semashko, "Meditsina na sluzhbe trudiashchikhsia," *Sotsial'naia gigiena,* 3–4 (1924), p. 5.

88. This controversy surrounding medical practitioners was not unique to Soviet medicine. It figured just as prominently in Europe where a system of kassa medicine was an integral part of an expanding network of social insurance systems. As insured workers began to receive medical care directly from their kassy, doctors were pressured to leave their private practices and join the kassy, where they sacrificed their financial and vocational autonomy to the kassa administration. Kassy insisted on having their own doctors in order to avoid bankruptcy, and doctors in various countries went on strike in response to pressures to join the kassy (Vigdorchik, *Teoriia i praktika,* pp. 35–36). Vigdorchik describes an interesting incident in Leningrad itself in mid-1918 when a special union of doctors was formed with the intention of voluntarily joining the all-city kassa. But no agreement was reached with the kassa and the union quickly dissolved (ibid., p. 134). Soon after that the whole concept of kassa medicine was supplanted by unified Soviet medicine.

89. N. A. Vigdorchik, *Vrachebnaia ekspertiza pri nerabotosposobnosti, Rukovodstvo dlia ekspertov* (Moscow, 1921), pp. 27, 36.

90. Zharkovskii, "Eshche o simuliatsii i kontrol'," *Vestnik sotsial'nogo strakhovaniia: Zakavkazia,* nos. 6–7 (1924).

91. "VII S"ezd Profsoiuza," *Voprosy strakhovaniia,* no. 51 (1926), p. 4. Zabelin reported that for 1924–25 the number of sickness days was 986.49 for every 100 insured, and 1,069.70 days for 1925–26. The year 1926–27 was one of financial crisis for social insurance, and there was an intense struggle against truancy, which was reflected in the drop in sick

days to 967.6. The figure rose again by 1927–28 to 994.6 (preliminary data) and he gave the projected 1928–29 figure as 980 (Zabelin, *Sotsial'noe strakhovanie v zhizni*, p. 25). In fact figures from that year were 1,020 per 100 workers (Kotov, "Ocherednye zadachi sots-strakha," *Voprosy strakhovaniia*, no. 28 [1929], p. 4).

92. *Soveshchanie Prezidiumov Moskovskikh kass*, p. 89.

93. Ibid., p. 84.

94. Zharkovskii, "Eshche o simuliatsii."

95. "Na zashchity medrabotnikov," *Voprosy strakhovaniia*, no. 36 (1926), p. 1.

96. "Bor'ba s progulami," *Voprosy strakhovaniia*, no. 5 (1927), p. 1.

97. G. Iniutin, "Novye kadry doverennykh vrachov," *Voprosy strakhovaniia*, no. 25 (1927), p. 2.

98. "Postanovlenie NKRKI po obsledovaniiu organov sotsstrakha," *Voprosy strakhovaniia*, no. 21 (1928), p. 4.

99. "Obzor pechati," *Voprosy strakhovaniia*, no. 15 (1928), p. 15.

100. See *Sotsial'naia gigiena*, 8 (1926), for a review of the work of these clinics from 1923 through 1925; also M. Ia. Lukomskii, "Klinika i poliklinika professional'noi boleznei," *Gigiena truda*, nos. 1–2 (1923), p. 47; B. B. Koiranskii, "K metodologii izucheniia pro-fessional'noi vrednostei," *Gigiena truda*, no. 7 (1923), p. 3; M. Ia. Lukomskii, "Pervye shagi tsentral'noi laboratorii po izucheniiu profboleznei na transporte," *Gigiena truda*, nos. 7–8 (1926), p. 108.

101. Vainshtein, "Vrachebnaia ekspertiza invalidov," *Voprosy strakhovaniia*, no. 34 (1923), p. 11.

102. Verzhblovskii, *Ocherki*, p. 34.

103. Zabelin, *Sotsial'noe strakhovanie v zhizni*, p. 46.

104. Verzhblovskii, *Ocherki*, p. 35.

105. "Sotsial'noe obespechenie invalidnosti ot professional'noi boleznei," *Gigiena truda*, no. 9 (1924), p. 136.

106. K. Vasil'evich, "V poriadke diskussi," *Voprosy strakhovaniia*, no. 13 (1931), p. 21.

107. Verzhblovskii, *Ocherki*, p. 32.

108. *Vrachebnaia ekspertiza invalidnosti*, prilozhenie k biulleteny Mosgubkomsots-strakha, nos. 17–18 (Moscow, 1929), p. 16. See also ibid., p. 5.

109. Ibid., p. 14.

110. In March 1928 a group of engineers from the Shakhty region was tried for sabotage, the first in a series of trials which called a dramatic halt to Lenin's policy of tolerating, and fully exploiting the valuable skills of, bourgeois experts.

111. Ibid., pp. 6–8.

112. The Moscow institute, the Central Institute for Expertise in Labor Capacity (TsIET), merged in 1937 with the Central Institute for Invalid Labor (TsITIN) to become the Central Institute for Invalid Expertise and Labor (TsIETIN), which is its name today. A similar merging in Leningrad created the Leningrad Scientific Institute of Expertise on Labor Capacity and the Organization of Labor of Invalids (LIETIN). Verzhblovskii, *Ocherki*, p. 50.

113. "O peredache VTEKa," *Voprosy strakhovaniia*, nos. 16–17 (1932), p. 1; "Bol'she vnimaniia vrachebno-trudovoi ekspertize," *Voprosy strakhovaniia*, nos. 23–24 (1932), p. 1.

114. *K voprosam vrachebno-trudovoi ekspertizy* (Voronezh, 1933–34), p. 3.

N E I L   B.   W E I S S M A N

Origins of
Soviet Health Administration

Narkomzdrav, 1918–1928

> Every social system has its own medicine.
> The organization of health care for the
> population is among those ideological
> "superstructures" which rest on a definite
> socioeconomic foundation and are defined
> by it.
>
> N. A. Semashko, 1928

On June 16, 1918, some sixty delegates from local soviets in nineteen provinces gathered in Moscow for the First All-Russian Congress of Medical-Sanitary Sections. The moment was hardly opportune for such a gathering. General political uncertainty, unfolding civil war, and spreading epidemics all threatened the new Soviet regime. Moreover, most physicians continued to denounce cooperation with the young Bolshevik government. Yet the majority of delegates, inspired by utopian visions of a new "revolutionary" medicine, threw themselves enthusiastically into the work of the congress. Indeed, the assembled representatives of central and local health institutions defined what were to become the chief characteristics of the medical "superstructure" of the emerging socialist system.[1]

N. A. Semashko gave the most succinct statement of the new principles in a report to the congress entitled "Fundamental Tasks of Soviet Medicine on the Local Level." First, the future commissar of health argued, there was the "urgent organizational task" of unifying Soviet medicine by overcoming bureaucratic divisions in the administration of health care. Second, treatment was to be provided to all by qualified professionals free of charge. Finally, a heavier emphasis was to be placed on sanitation and other social measures aimed at alleviating disease and improving the living conditions of the poor.[2] These three concepts—unity, universally available professional care, and preventive medicine through sanitation— were to remain the cornerstones of Soviet health care. Indeed, Semashko's report, devoted as it was to provincial medicine, omitted only one major point which emerged at this meeting as a founding principle of Soviet health policy. It was left to Bolshevik physicians Z. P. Solov'ev and E. P. Pervukhin to present to the congress plans for a commissariat of public health (*Narodnyi komissariat zdravookhraneniia*, or Narkomzdrav). This new institution, the first in Russia's history to unify control over health care administration, would be the chief vehicle for the realization of the high hopes of the congress majority for the creation of the socialist system's "own medicine."

This essay investigates the development of the Commissariat of Public Health in the first decade of its existence. The central concern is an evaluation of Narkomzdrav's efforts to implement the principles outlined by Semashko and other leaders of Soviet medicine in the summer of 1918. This approach reveals the fundamental institutional dynamic of Soviet health care in the 1920s—the effort to combine centralized direction with heightened professionalism in an attempt to overcome the formidable obstacles to the establishment of a modern medical system in Russia.

THE BIRTH OF NARKOMZDRAV, 1917–1918

The traditional political and administrative order of tsarist Russia would appear to offer fertile ground for a highly centralized, unified health care system. Over the centuries tsarist rulers and civil servants had demonstrated a distinct preference for organizational forms based on state direction from the center and an equally strong hostility toward those based on the concept of local autonomy. Consequently, the authorities in St. Petersburg had often initiated in Russia social developments that elsewhere were dominated by private groups or local self-government.

This was certainly true of medicine. The tsarist government played the leading role in introducing professional health care in the empire and guided medical developments thereafter. Physicians in Russia typically received their training in government institutions, practiced medicine within the context of an extensive system of bureaucratic regulation, and carried on their careers as members of an official estate. Moreover, a substantial majority were employed in various government-related medical institutions rather than in private practice. In an 1889 article on rural practice, Professor of Medicine M. Kapustin aptly drew the following contrast which highlighted Russian physicians' self-conception:

> Medical care has been dealt with as a *personal* transaction between the patient and the doctor, established on the same basis as commerce or a trade. Zemstvo medicine is essentially a public institution. Here the ministration which the physician gives the patient is not a personal service, nor is it an act of charity, it is a public function which he fulfills. . . . The doctor is a public servant.[3]

Despite extensive state intervention and the public nature of medicine, the tsarist authorities failed to develop a unified health care system. The government's difficulties were of an internal and external nature. Within the state apparatus, tsarist bureaucrats had not matched their proclivity for centralization with a knack for coordination. Administration in many vital areas, such as factory inspection or agrarian reform, suffered from the division of jurisdiction among competing ministries and departments, with conflict often intensified by personal rivalries and animosities. In the field of health, the list of agencies participating in administration included the Imperial Court, the ministries of internal affairs, education, finance, agriculture, and trade and industry, and even the Holy Synod. Within the leading institution alone—the Ministry of Internal Affairs (MVD)—activity and authority was further divided among the Medical Council, chief medical inspector, and Main Administration for Local Affairs.

The external obstacles to a well-integrated centralized medical system were, if anything, more formidable. The last decades of the tsarist era saw the emergence of a broad movement among the educated public in favor of popular self-government, a development which could hardly fail to touch medical institutions. During the 1890s, for example, liberals were active in defeating a proposed hospital statute which would have extended state bureaucratic control over zemstvo medicine and its physician employees. Physicians themselves participated in the growing movement for autonomy, their demands for independence from state regulation fueled by a heightened sense of medical professionalism. The chief vehicle for their self-assertion was the Pirogov Society of Russian Physicians, a professional organization which drew on the traditions of zemstvo health care to develop an ethos of public service free of centralized control.

The depth of opposition to medical centralization in tsarist government and society was demonstrated clearly by the fate of the single most determined effort to overcome it. In the wake of a severe cholera epidemic in southern Russia in 1910, G. E. Rein, head of the MVD's Medical Council, set out to establish a new ministry of health. Although the would-be reformer had the sympathy of the tsar, he was unable to overcome resistance from within the state bureaucracy and a drumbeat of criticism from the Pirogov Society before the outbreak of war in 1914. Two years later Rein finally secured approval for the idea, but only on the basis of the government's special emergency powers. When it was presented to the health commission of the Fourth Duma for confirmation, Rein's plan was rejected, forcing withdrawal of the legislation in early 1917.[4]

What was the Bolshevik attitude toward the administration of health care? In the years before 1917 those in the party who were responsible for health administration had said little about the details of the future organization of medicine beyond calling for comprehensive social insurance in the hands of the working class. Instead, the Bolsheviks preferred to link specific change to the broader issue of fundamental social revolution. As Bolshevik editorialists wrote in the party periodical *Zvezda* in an article on the particular question of health conditions in St. Petersburg published in 1910, "true sanitation (and with it also the realization of the idea of self-government) will come only when transferred into the hands of those for whom it is literally a matter of life and death."[5]

Almost immediately after the October Revolution, Bolshevik physicians took steps to give more precise organizational form to the demand for a radical transformation of health care. Initially, the new authorities placed medicine in the hands of the Military Revolutionary Committee (MRC). Within the MRC, party leaders created a medical-sanitary section headed by Bolshevik physician M. I. Barsukov to mobilize medical resources to aid Red Guard units and handle other emergency tasks. As early as mid-November, however, Barsukov joined with party physicians A. N. Vinokurov and I. S. Veger to propose the creation of a new organ, the Committee for the Protection of the People's Health (*Komitet po okhrane narodnogo zdraviia*).[6] This body, working through other commissariats and the medical-sanitary sections of local soviets, would serve as a more permanent vehicle for centralized direction of health care.

According to the memoirs of Barsukov and Vinokurov, Lenin responded positively to the principle of unifying medical administration under a single agency.[7] But the leader also insisted that the proposal was premature. He argued that practical considerations demanded that nothing be done before a proper network of local medical-sanitary sections was established and the masses were educated on the need for a central body. In a more political vein, Lenin voiced fear that the proposal would spark charges of reviving Rein's plans for an oppressive bureaucratic apparatus and pointed to the need to undermine the staunch opposition of the Pirogov Society to the new regime.

That Lenin's reservations were perceived as provisional is clear from the determination with which Barsukov and his colleagues continued to work toward the centralization of medical administration. The government established "collegia" of Bolshevik medical personnel to direct health activities within separate commissariats and in January 1918 created the Council of Medical Collegia (*Sovet vrachebnikh kollegii*) as the "highest medical organ of the Worker and Peasant Government."[8] Throughout the new regime's chaotic first spring, council members extended coordination of medical administration and campaigned for the organization of a commissariat of health. One crucial component of the effort in this direction was the planning for a national congress of Soviet medical personnel. The inability of Barsukov and his coworkers to convene such a gathering in politically stormy November 1917 had been a significant factor in persuading Lenin and the Council of People's Commissars to postpone centralization of health administration.[9] Success in this venture now would provide a powerful impetus for carrying the unification process to its conclusion.

The composition of the First All-Russian Congress of Medical-Sanitary Sections told much about the future leaders of Soviet medicine. Of the seventy-five delegates who ultimately attended congress sessions, a clear majority of forty-five were physicians. The others included fourteen feldshers, seven pharmacists, four medical students, and a nurse. Although only twenty-eight participants were Bolsheviks, they dominated the gathering. In the meeting's heated debates, for example, the Bolsheviks were able to have a representative of the feldshers' union expelled from the congress for what were described as anti-Soviet views. Moreover, Bolsheviks controlled the congress presidium, far outnumbering the adherents of other parties. Bolshevik physicians Solov'ev, Pervukhin, and Semashko served as the reporters on the most vital policy issues.[10]

Chief among these issues was the organization of medical administration in the new, postrevolutionary era. On this question the congress fully realized the expectations of its conveners, recommending "the creation of a single central organ—

the Commissariat of Public Health —to direct all medical-sanitary affairs.'' With this resolution in hand, the proponents of the new agency returned to the Council of People's Commissars to press their case. On July 11 the government decreed the establishment of a commissariat of public health, responsible for ''leadership of all medical-sanitary institutions of the country.''[11]

Viewed retrospectively, the process by which the commissariat was created appears to be a unilinear march toward centralization. Although correct in its broadest terms, this interpretation risks minimizing the considerable opposition to the establishment of the commissariat. There had always been a great deal of hostility to the centralization of medical affairs, usually voiced in terms of a defense of independent zemstvo medicine. The dual revolutions of 1917 had done much to intensify the sentiment. Although no stenographic records of the June congress are extant, we do know that the Solov'ev and Pervukhin reports aroused bitter debate. Even after the congress, the membership of the Council of Medical Collegia remained divided on the establishment of the commissariat, voting only four to two in favor of the measure. During deliberations in the Council of People's Commissars, physicians I. S. Veger and M. G. Vecheslov argued heatedly against the new institution, denouncing Semashko for ''Rein-like belching.'' Their view reflected the firm sentiment of the Pirogovtsy, whose official journal—*Obshchestvennyi vrach*—had carried a denunciation of the June congress resolutions as the ''funeral of zemstvo medicine.'' Semashko's own recollections make it clear that only Lenin's firm support carried the day for the proponents of the commissariat.[12]

Given the substantial resistance—especially among the medical community—to the creation of a unifying central agency, why did Semashko, Barsukov, and their colleagues persist in their efforts and ultimately succeed? One obvious answer is the general commitment of the Bolsheviks to centralized administration. As one leading Western specialist on Soviet medicine has argued:

It is a characteristic trait of the Bolshevik mentality . . . not to leave anything to chance, even in areas as distant from the political scene as medicine and public health. Almost from the day they seized power, the Bolsheviks proceeded to reshape medical services along lines calculated to bring maximum benefits to the regime and its supporters, and to be used as an instrument against their opponents and detractors.[13]

Evidence in support of this view abounds. From the first the Bolsheviks demonstrated active hostility toward autonomous organizations of the medical professions (a sentiment fueled by a corresponding animosity of groups including the Pirogov Society toward the new regime). Lenin's thinking on the timing of the unification of health administration in the months after the October Revolution was clearly influenced by concern over the political strength of the Pirogovtsy. When the Bolsheviks did create the commissariat in the summer of 1918, they certainly intended the agency to serve as a primary vehicle for the extension of party control over a recalcitrant medical profession. Solov'ev admitted as much in his report to the June medical congress. The establishment of a commissariat, he insisted, ''is demanded by our entire administrative experience and by our struggle with the counterrevolutionary bourgeois rot penetrating so many institutions."[14]

Yet as Solov'ev's words also indicate, beyond the political task of combatting "bourgeois rot" there was a positive administrative rationale for the agency. The Bolsheviks had always argued that revolution would fundamentally transform the conditions of health care. In the view of Semashko, Barsukov, and their colleagues, nothing epitomized this transformation more than the creation of the commissariat. Such an institution was not to be feared—as it had been under tsarism—as a vehicle for oppressive bureaucratic regulation. Rather, it would be a tool, forged in the fires of revolution, for placing state power at the disposal of the Bolshevik physicians. The commissariat would make it possible to remold the framework of health care in Russia. As Semashko argued in his summary of sentiment at the June congress, a centralized approach was "extremely desirable and rational."[15] The ends to which state power would be applied—or, put differently, the definition of "rationality" offered by Semashko and his colleagues—emerged clearly during the Civil War era.

THE CIVIL WAR ERA, 1918–1921

The period immediately following Narkomzdrav's creation was hardly propitious for the establishment of a new order in medicine. Even before 1914, health care in tsarist Russia lagged sadly behind that available in almost all other European nations. The First World War only made matters worse. Extensive combat created an enormous demand at the front for medical care for soldiers and the many civilian evacuees. Moreover, the war effort drained supplies of food and fuel, contributing to a deterioration in living conditions in the rear. The violent Civil War which commenced in earnest in the summer of 1918 further disrupted the economy and brought the tribulations of combat from the periphery into the heart of Russia. Streams of soldiers, deserters, refugees, and bagmen flooded the nation's railroads and waterways, carrying with them chaos and infectious disease. Between the start of 1918 and mid-1920, for example, Soviet authorities registered almost five million cases of typhus alone.

Under these conditions Narkomzdrav's operations became a seemingly endless series of emergency measures, shock campaigns mounted to meet crisis after crisis. The exigencies of the Civil War did not, however, force the abandonment of the basic principles of the new health system. The three goals elaborated in June 1918— unity, universally available qualified care, and social measures aimed at preventing disease—continued to drive official policy. Indeed, in certain respects, the demands of war reinforced rather than weakened the commitment of Narkomzdrav's leadership to these ends.

The first task—and central principle of all Narkomzdrav activity through the 1920s—was the concentration of health care in the hands of the commissariat and its local agents, the soviets' medical-sanitary sections (soon renamed health sections, or *zdravotdely*). Although the Council of People's Commissars had explicitly charged Narkomzdrav with "unification of all medical and sanitary affairs of the

RSFSR," it was apparent from the outset that there would be resistance from other agencies. Representatives of both the Commissariat of Transportation and Main Military Sanitary Administration, for example, refused outright to attend the initial meetings on unification.[16]

In the face of determined opposition, Narkomzdrav had to make some concessions. The extraordinary crisis on the epidemic-ridden railroads coupled with the political power of railway authorities (who included, for a time, Cheka chief Felix Dzerzhinskii), for instance, forced the creation of semiindependent transportation health sections. In most spheres, however, Narkomzdrav prevailed. Take the case of health care for students, a matter originally assigned to the Commissariat of Enlightenment. Most delegates at the First All-Russian Congress of School Sanitation Physicians in March 1919 reported that their activity had already been transferred to *zdravotdel* control, an organizational state of affairs confirmed in principle by a formal congress vote.[17]

Even more striking was the organizational outcome of a controversy over the provision of health care to insured workers. In the wake of the October Revolution, the government had placed control over factory medical facilities in the hands of hospital funds (*bol'nichnye kassy*). This approach had strong ideological justification, for the funds could be viewed as a vehicle of proletarian democracy. Institutionally, the idea of a separate "insurance medicine" had the support of the funds' supervising agency, the Commissariat of Labor. Narkomzdrav, for its part, was determined not to allow this fundamental violation of the principle of unified health care. As Semashko argued in 1919 in an article published in *Izvestiia*, "To counterpose or even separate insurance medicine . . . from Soviet medicine is purely absurd, an anachronism devoid of any real basis. To whom are workers counterposed in a workers' republic? Parasites and exploiters? But the Soviet republic knows none. . . . " Practically, he continued, an independent insurance medicine would lead only to parallelism, the dissipation of resources, and conflict.[18] The government's decision largely reflected Semashko's view. A decree of February 21, 1919, transferred medical care for the insured to Narkomzdrav and its agencies, though sanitary supervision over factories remained outside their control.[19]

A variety of factors contributed to the "gathering of medicine," as Semashko characterized it. The close ties among the small group of Bolshevik physicians involved in directing health care in the government, for example, was undoubtedly a factor. Yet the decisive force behind the process was clearly support by the party leadership, and particularly Lenin, for Narkomzdrav. "Only thanks to the assistance of V. I. Lenin," Semashko later recalled, "was the arduously initiated unification carried through successfully."[20]

Why would Lenin and other party leaders consistently side with Narkomzdrav in this matter? The reasons emerge clearly in the rebuff of the single greatest challenge to the commissariat's authority in the health field—the claims to prominence of the new All-Russian Medical-Sanitary Workers Union. Vsemedikosantrud, as the union was called, was organized in March 1919 to represent some 134,000 feldshers, nurses, and other medical workers.[21] Its goal, the democratization of medical affairs, was to be achieved through both equal status for all health workers and extensive union participation in the management of health institutions. Neither principle was acceptable to Narkomzdrav. As early as May 1918 the Council of Medical Collegia had ruled that feldshers could only be seen as assistants to physicians and called for steps to curtail further training of feldshers.[22] Semashko again in 1919 presented the Narkomzdrav view in a fierce attack on Vsemedikosantrud. To act on the union's principle of "bakeries by bakers, hospitals by orderlies, Narkomzdrav by feldshers," he argued, "means falling into petty bourgeois (*meshchanskii*) syndicalism." Control over health care could be placed only in "the hands of the 'specialists', i.e., physicians, absolutely forbidding anyone from interfering in any way."[23] Once more Semashko had his way. At the second Vsemedikosantrud congress in February–March 1920—a gathering addressed personally by Lenin— union leaders were forced to accept "energetic work to increase discipline and productivity among medical-sanitary workers" rather than meaningful participation in the direction of health care as their chief function.[24]

It would be easy to ascribe the support of the party leadership for Narkomzdrav in this and the related struggles for unity in health affairs to the general determination of the Bolsheviks to monopolize political power. Certainly the decision against Vsemedikosantrud was consistent with the party's fear of syndicalism and overall policy of curbing union autonomy. Indeed, the decisive congress of medical workers only preceded by a matter of days the Ninth Party Congress in which all unions were forced to accept one-man management. Similarly, independent "insurance medicine" was partially discredited by its Menshevik roots.

Yet there was another, more positive factor at work in Narkomzdrav's favor— the attraction of Lenin and other Bolshevik leaders to specialized scientific knowledge. Early on, in contradistinction to the feelings of many of his supporters, Lenin recognized the importance of tapping the expertise of Russia's professionals. As he put it at the Eighth Party Congress in March 1919, the new government would require the cooperation of the large stratum of "bourgeois physicians, engineers, agronomists and cooperative specialists." Bolsheviks, he insisted, must "learn humility and respect for the work of specialists in science and technology."[25] In the field of medicine, it should be noted, this emphasis on a scientific approach paralleled thinking in other countries such as Germany, France, England, and the United States.

Of course, it could be argued that this willingness to rely on bourgeois specialists was, in E. H. Carr's phrase, a "temporary evil" forced by the exigencies of the Civil War.[26] In the case of physicians, however, the commitment was longterm. As Lenin proclaimed in his address to the second Vsemedikosantrud congress, "The collaboration of the representatives of science and of the proletariat—only this collaboration will be able to eradicate all the weight of poverty, illness, filth. . . . No dark force can stand before the united representatives of science, the proletariat and technology."[27] The organizational embodiment of specialized scientific knowledge in the field of medicine—and, therefore, the beneficiary of party support—was, of course, physician-dominated Narkomzdrav.

The combination of the two strands—the demand for political control and the respect for technical knowledge—was evident in the Bolshevik approach to the medical profession at large. A substantial majority of Russia's physicians rejected the October Revolution, and some (if not the majority, as the Bolsheviks alleged) actively engaged in sabotage against the new regime. The government was unwilling to tolerate such opposition. The authorities quickly took steps to liquidate the institutional bases of physicians' autonomy, such as the medical bodies of the zemstvos and town dumas or the health agencies of the Provisional Government, and launched a bitter rhetorical assault on professional organizations like the Pirogov Society as hotbeds of counterrevolution and sabotage. With the outbreak of the Civil War, party leaders had no compunction about drafting physicians; in fact, mobilization of medical professionals outlasted that of any other occupational category. Narkomzdrav orders were backed by the guns of the Cheka and Revolutionary Military Council.

Simultaneously, however, the new government took steps to win over physicians. Working through Narkomzdrav, the authorities resisted efforts to equalize wages among medical workers.[28] Special decrees guaranteed material privileges not only to physicians cooperating with the regime's military and anti-epidemic efforts but also to their families. Bolshevik physician I. V. Rusakov articulated the reigning sentiment in March 1918 when he insisted that the regime's medical opponents could be converted for "if they find themselves on the opposite side of the barricades from us, it is only through misunderstanding."[29]

The lengths to which the regime would go to clear up this misunderstanding— and the way in which unification of Soviet medicine was informed and even driven by a concern for specialized knowledge—was evident in the organizational structure of Vsemedikosantrud. The authorities pressed physicians to join the union, a goal largely achieved in 1920 when the All-Russian Union of Professional Associations of Physicians (*Vserossiiskii soiuz professional'nykh ob'edinenii vrachei*) agreed to amalgamate. Yet the government rejected the full equalization of physicians with other union members by allowing the creation of a semi-independent physicians' section within the organization. When delegates at Vsemedikosantrud's Third Congress in October 1921 voted to abolish the section, the All-Russian Trade Union Council overruled them.[30] Even more striking, a 1922 resolution of the physicians' section calling for the independence of medical institutions from the soviets prompted the Politburo to direct Semashko and Dzerzhinskii to take measures to eliminate "unhealthy" tendencies within the organization. But the section itself was not liquidated.[31]

The insistence on specialized knowledge as a key to first-rate medical care also informed the regime's effort to achieve its second fundamental goal of health care for all classes, especially the proletariat. Indeed, in the eyes of both Narkomzdrav's physician-administrators and the party leadership universal accessibility (*obshche-dostupnost'*) and professionalized knowledge were integrally connected. N. Krupskaia stated the relationship explicitly in an *Izvestiia* article which appeared, significantly, one day after the formal establishment of Narkomzdrav.[32] Describing the health care system of tsarist Russia, she argued

Zemstvo and municipal medicine . . . proclaimed as its basis free and universally accessible [care]. . . . But it was unable to realize its aspirations. For the wealthy medicine remained paid, with its quality corresponding to its price. Only unqualified medicine, the medicine of independent feldshers, was universally accessible. And no matter how much the leaders of zemstvo and municipal medicine repeated the harm of feldsherism and the need for broad availability of qualified care, the latter seemed unnecessary to the ruling classes and was not extended to wide circles of the toiling masses.

Conversely, the defining characteristic of Soviet medicine would be the availability for all of first-rate care by well-trained physicians.

In the best circumstances, the achievement of such a goal in doctor-poor Russia would have been difficult. At a time of civil war and epidemic, it was simply impossible. By 1920 approximately 40 percent of the nation's physicians had been mobilized for Red Army service; both military and civilian medical personnel found their attention focused primarily on combatting disease.[33] Although relatively few physicians emigrated in this era, their ranks were painfully thinned by exposure to typhus, cholera, and the like. Indeed, casualty rates for physicians often far exceeded those of Red Army soldiers. For its part, Narkomzdrav struggled bravely to fill the inevitable gaps in the provision of qualified health care. Training facilities for nurses, orderlies, and even feldshers were established in nearly all provincial centers, but primary emphasis was on the education of physicians. By 1920, the number of medical faculties had expanded from seventeen to twenty-five. Virtually all physicians were pressed into state service, either in the military or in nationalized civilian health care institutions.[34]

Despite these efforts, Narkomzdrav was clearly running a losing race against war and disease. On the eve of the First World War tsarist Russia possessed some 24,000 civilian physicians (or, more accurately for purposes of comparison, at the end of 1914 approximately 18,300 in the area outside Poland and the western provinces). By 1921, Narkomzdrav's estimate was just over 11,000, though admittedly the Ukraine and White Russia were excluded from the calculation. Statistics on health care in these years are unreliable, marred by haphazard bookkeeping and inflated by emergency treatment of epidemic victims. Nevertheless, the available data suggest a general decline in visits to clinics for treatment. Worse yet, in the official reports, the proportion of care provided by feldshers increased.[35]

What of the third basic principle of Soviet medicine, the improvement of health conditions through a systematic program of prophylaxis and sanitation? The new regime was explicit about its goals in this area. The program adopted at the Eighth Party Congress in March 1919 indicated, ''As a basis for its activity in the area of public health, the RCP above all proposes the implementation of broad sanitary measures aimed at preventing the spread of disease. The dictatorship of the proletariat has already made possible an entire range of hygienic and curative measures unachievable within the context of bourgeois society.''[36] Making good on this promise, the government introduced sweeping legislation in sanitation (Narkomzdrav officials boasted, for example, that Soviet Russia was the first country in the world to establish hygienic inspection of housing across all its territory). The authorities also mandated systematic preventive measures, such as obligatory vaccination against smallpox. As a final component of the prophylactic dimension of Soviet medicine, the government declared an all-out assault on "social diseases," among them tuberculosis, venereal disease, and alcoholism. In this context especially, health officials elaborated a program of "dispensarization" in which clinics and other medical facilities would not only provide care but also serve as vehicles for sanitary education and preventive measures against disease.

Here, too, war and epidemic disrupted the regime's effort. The authorities had hoped to undertake a major campaign against tuberculosis based on the dispensary concept, for example, but by 1921 only fifteen dispensaries had been established.[37] Similarly, at a time of pressing demand for scant supplies little could be done to implement meaningful inspection of foodstuffs. Yet while the emergencies of the Civil War era inhibited the elaboration of a full system of social prophylaxis, they also reinforced the regime's determination to move in this direction. In the case of the Red Army, health officials launched an active campaign of hygienic propaganda to keep the fighting forces free of disease. In the first ten months of 1920 alone, attendance at sanitation lectures reached nearly four million.[38] In a like fashion, military authorities established an extensive network of disinfection detachments and attempted to vaccinate all soldiers against cholera and typhus. On the home front, the government initiated a series of shock campaigns against unsanitary conditions which encouraged epidemics. As Lenin dramatically proclaimed at the Seventh Congress of Soviets in December 1919, "Either lice will defeat socialism, or socialism will defeat lice!"[39] In order to guarantee implementation of necessary measures to control such threats, the Council of Worker-Peasant Defense established special supervisory commissions including both health officials and Chekists within Narkomzdrav and the *zdravotdely*.

In a 1920 report to the Eighth Congress of Soviets, the commissariat characterized medical work in the Civil War era as the product of "two contradictory forces: favorable social conditions, unlimited scope for curative-sanitary work, energetic leadership of this work by the laboring masses themselves; on the other side—difficult economic conditions, blockade, civil war."[40] The statement aptly characterizes Narkomzdrav's early experience. Through the nationalization of the health care system and the relative concentration of control in the hands of the commissariat, the regime had established the institutional framework for a new, socialist medicine. The commissariat could serve as the instrument for the creation of a health care system that was "rational" in the sense of being both comprehensive and informed by technical expertise. All that was required, in the eyes of Narkomzdrav officials, was a period of peace and economic recovery.

THE NEP ERA, 1922–29

Although the close of the Civil War and the inauguration of the New Economic Policy brought relief to the populace of the USSR, these events did not immediately reduce the challenges confronting the officials of Narkomzdrav. Epidemics proved more difficult to halt than military conflict, particularly in the face of postwar famine.

Equally important, the introduction of NEP brought new threats to the institutional framework of the nationalized health system. As part of a general effort to balance the extraordinarily strained national budget, the central authorities in May 1922 abruptly transferred financing of most medical facilities to local government.[41] The immediate result was a frantic rush by resource-poor Soviet executive committees to curtail the network of hospitals and clinics and, in some cases, to abolish *zdravotdely* by merging them into administrative sections. Outside the Narkomzdrav apparatus, proponents of "insurance medicine" again called for the creation of separate health institutions for the working class. In an even more radical departure, delegates at the May 1922 congress of Vsemedikosantrud's physicians' section passed a resolution in favor of autonomous "public" *(obshchestvennyi)* medical institutions, free of Soviet control.[42] Although the authorities dealt quickly with dissent within the physicians' section, the legalization of private health facilities under NEP made the emergence of a sizeable independent health sector a distinct possibility. The private practices and clinics which began to appear in the nation's major cities signaled that an era of peace and ideological relaxation could be as much a challenge to Narkomzdrav's policies as civil war.

Narkomzdrav's leaders responded by reaffirming the basic principles of Soviet medicine elaborated in 1918 and defended throughout the Civil War era. Despite the depth of the changes brought about by the adoption of NEP, the commissariat was successful in maintaining, and even extending, the new health care system after the crisis of 1922. Organizationally, this meant a continuing emphasis on unified control over medical institutions. In the case of care for the insured, for example, Narkomzdrav officials firmly rejected both the reestablishment of hospital funds and the creation of a semiautonomous division of workers' health within the commissariat, going so far as to suggest that such ideas were Menshevik-inspired. The initial outcome was a March 1924 compromise, which favored Narkomzdrav by placing insurance care under special divisions within the *zdravotdely*.[43] At the beginning of 1927 the government gave the commissariat a "good present" for the new year, as Semashko put it, by liquidating the divisions.[44] Narkomzdrav was also able to blunt the threat of private practice, at least in regard to institutional development. Official surveys reported relatively few private clinics and hospitals, with almost all of them located in Moscow and Leningrad.[45]

Narkomzdrav's success in warding off outside challenges was paralleled by progress in the enhancement of the commissariat's own capabilities. The budget crisis of 1922 prompted deep cuts in the staff and an administrative shake-up aimed at simplification of the apparatus.[46] Although efforts at structural "rationalization" continued throughout the decade, personnel reduction did not. Despite the steady emphasis of government leaders on bringing the size of the state apparatus under control, the commissariat's staff grew significantly. By one official calculation, Narkomzdrav's contingent of employees expanded by 65 percent (from 230,911 to 381,836) between 1924 and 1928, outpacing the growth of every other major branch of Soviet government.[47]

Equally significant, the quality of leading administrative cadres also improved markedly. From the first, Semashko and his colleagues emphasized the importance of a contingent of highly professional, experienced administrators. In keeping with this view, the commissariat directed local soviets not to shuffle *zdravotdel* executives and extracted a promise from the party not to reassign Communist physicians without informing Narkomzdrav.[48] The insistence on continuity and training produced results, as evidenced by a 1927 survey of 464 leading medical administrators.[49] These senior and middle officials—both in the center and the provinces—were most often physicians with more than five years' experience in the health field. Indeed, 202 of them had been employed in health before the Revolution. Even more impressive in a state apparatus notorious for high turnover, more than half (262, or 56 percent) had occupied their positions for more than three years. The party was well represented among all senior officials (59 percent) and local middle-level officials (31 percent), strong testimony to Narkomzdrav's ability to convert non-Communist physicians and to lay claim to the services of Old Bolshevik professionals.

These findings were confirmed in a broader survey of the entire state apparatus conducted at the end of the decade.[50] At the central level, Narkomzdrav's personnel were characterized by their relatively advanced age, high level of education, and middle- and upper-class social backgrounds. More than three-quarters fell into the most senior age group (thirty-five and older); similar proportions reported higher education degrees and "white collar" (*sluzhashchie*) social status. In the provinces, too, health administrators remained older, better educated, and less proletarian than employees of any other branch of government. Although senior Narkomzdrav officials were largely Communists (more than three-quarters, for example, at the *okrug* level), the large number of nonparty scientific specialists employed by the commissariat reduced it to a low standing overall in this category.

The development of an effective, unified apparatus dominated by physicians helped Narkomzdrav advance toward its second goal of universally accessible, qualified care. A variety of statistical indices can be employed to chart the commissariat's progress. At the Sixth All-Russian Congress of Zdravotdely, for example, Narkomzdrav official Miskinov reported the following data on hospital care in the territory of the RSFSR.[51]

	1913	1926
Population per bed	756	615
Population per maternity bed	21,889	8,783
Rural hospital stations	—	2,656

Available figures on care outside hospitals in clinics and the like are no less impressive.[52]

	1913	1926	1928
Urban medical facilities	1,230	—	5,673
Rural medical facilities	4,367	—	7,531
Factory aid points	*	1,064	

*isolated cases

According to the views expressed by Narkomzdrav spokesmen, qualitative improvement in treatment kept pace with the quantitative expansion of medical facilities. Health officials took particular pride in outlining the development of various forms of specialized care, such as dentistry or physiotherapy. Moreover, in the post-Civil War era the commissariat was finally able to make headway in its determination to replace feldshers with physicians.[53]

Finally, although approximately three-quarters of the health budget was devoted to the expansion of treatment facilities, the commissariat did not forget its fundamental commitment to preventive medicine. Indeed, as A. N. Sysin—Narkomzdrav's recognized leader in sanitation policy—argued in 1928, "In no area of health protection did the historic date of 11 July 1918 . . . have as much significance as in the nation's sanitary affairs."[54]

The commissariat's determination to make prevention the distinguishing characteristic of Soviet medicine was made evident in 1922. While almost the entire network of medical facilities was transferred to local financing (even in Moscow, Semashko argued, "you can count our institutions on one hand!"), the basic agencies of sanitation and of the campaign against social disease remained on the state budget. Consequently, both areas experienced significant development. A government decree of September 15, 1922, set obligatory norms for sanitation agencies throughout the RSFSR. The legislation mandated a minimum of 1 sanitary physician for every 50,000 urban residents and 1 physician and 1 assistant for 200,000 rural citizens (or a total staff of more than 900 physicians). Dissatisfied with the impact of this measure, the authorities on February 19, 1927, stiffened the norms and made them dependent on the degree of economic development in a given locality, overall nearly doubling the required contingent of physicians.[55] State intervention was also central in the effort to defeat social disease. By 1927, for example, Narkomzdrav had supervised the extension of a network of 262 tuberculosis dispensaries, serving all cities with a population in excess of 50,000 and most from 20,000 to 50,000.[56] Admittedly, there was much less dramatic progress in the fight against venereal disease and alcoholism.

Statistics such as these—particularly when measured against the indicators for tsarist health care—are impressive. Yet it would be incorrect to interpret them as evidence of unqualified success in Narkomzdrav's policies in the 1920s. Certainly many health officials of that era were quick to criticize the results. Some argued that the proper standard of comparison was not prewar Russia but the medical accomplishments of Western Europe. Here, the USSR lagged sadly behind. Others made a more pointed critique, contending that aggregate figures often disguised serious shortcomings in the quality of care. In his report to the Sixth Congress of Zdravotdely, for example, Miskinov admitted that facilities in district cities and factory settlements were "especially old, shabby, and in need of repair" and rural conditions were worse still.[57] Even in the sphere of sanitation, the decade ended with an angry debate over a "crisis" in preventive medicine. In sum, Soviet medical administrators were discovering that the elaboration of new, "rational" principles of health care was one thing but effective implementation was something else altogether.

The gap between theory and practice was clear in regard to the central Narkomzdrav principle of organizational unity. On paper, the concentration of most health matters in the hands of the commissariat's local agencies—the *zdravotdely*—ought to have made it easy to reach out from Moscow into the provinces. In reality, medical affairs at the grass roots proved difficult to control.

One barometer of the commissariat's troubles—a "clear and impartial reflection of the correct state of health organization in this or that province," as Narkomzdrav specialists V. Goriushin and S. Cherniak put it—was the budget.[58] Although health funding increased throughout the decade, Narkomzdrav officials argued that resources remained insufficient to meet the crying demands of the populace for proper care. The decentralization of finance in 1922 meant that the commissariat was heavily dependent on the generosity of local soviets. This was particularly so at the end of the decade as a result of a decline in the other major source of income—namely, contributions from the social insurance fund.

Health Expenditures RSFSR (millions of rubles)[59]

	1924/25	1925/26	1926/27	1927/28
State budget	22.0 (10.0%)	32.3 (10.6)	40.2 (10.3)	46.4 (11.4)
Local budget	83.3 (39.9)	113.0 (37.0)	146.2 (38.3)	170.0 (42.0)
Insurance fund	90.8 (43.5)	143.1 (46.9)	180.6 (47.3)	174.1 (42.9)
Other	12.7 (6.1)	16.9 (5.5)	15.0 (3.9)	15.2 (3.7)
Total	208.8	305.3	382.0	405.7

The response of local authorities to pleas for aid from the center was sluggish at best. The relative weight of funds assigned to health in local budgets declined steadily across the decade. When there was a revenue shortage, health allocations often went unfulfilled. Between 1924/25 and 1925/26, for example, the health share of local budgets in the RSFSR fell from 13.2 to 12.8 percent, and actual outlays were 11.3 percent and 10.8 percent respectively.[60] By some calculations local funding for health in mid-decade lagged behind that of the prewar zemstvos and town dumas.[61] The difference in the perspectives of Narkomzdrav and local soviets on the issue of spending for medical care was evident in the variance of norms established. The commissariat's guideline for proper annual outlay for a hospital bed in 1925/26, for example, was 700 rubles. Average local expenditure was 440 rubles.[62]

In the budgetary battle with local authorities, Narkomzdrav possessed few effective weapons. Plans for an all-citizen tax for medical care were scuttled by the Commissariat of Finance. The concept of a state-mandated percentage of local budgets for health needs ran aground on the principle of Soviet self-government. Proposals of minimum norms for individual types of treatment had to be abandoned for fear that those local soviets exceeding the standards would cut back their budgets. Even direct intervention with state funds proved to have its limits. Initially, the commissariat sought to help meet emergency needs by offering subsidies *(dotatsii)* to cover local deficits. The practice in the provinces of intentional deficit spending to acquire extra state monies forced Narkomzdrav in 1924 to shift to a system of matched grants *(subventsii)*, but even this failed to end the cat and mouse game. When grants were made available for wage hikes, local authorities ignored hospital construction in order to amass the required matching funds. The commissariat's response of directing grants to construction did increase building, but it also led to local cutbacks in expenditures for medication.[63]

Narkomzdrav's difficulty in bringing its authority to bear in the provinces extended beyond budgetary matters. When the central authorities moved to implement greater planning in health protection at the end of the decade, for instance, they discovered a sorry state of affairs. As Gosplan spokesman M. Donskoi complained in 1928, a significant number of *zdravotdely* had yet to submit their reports for 1926 to the commissariat. Referring to the statistical work planned by Narkomzdrav's State Institute of Social Hygiene, he insisted that only through a more coherent approach would the activity of local health officials "lose its at times primitive *(kustarnyi)* character, its lack of system, its palliative nature, and acquire a scientific-planned base."[64]

In the commissariat's eyes the chief problem was simply a lack of responsiveness by local officials to central direction. Actually, the matter was more complex. In 1926, for example, health authorities were scandalized by a series of highly publicized fatal accidents in state hospitals, particularly birthing facilities in Moscow. Investigators uncovered a series of shortcomings in hospital operations ranging from overburdening of staff to a failure of the medical union to maintain discipline. Yet debate also centered on the excessively "bureaucratic" control system in which centralized supervision by Narkomzdrav and the *zdravotdely* sapped the authority of hospital administrators. The commissariat admitted the problem. In December 1926, after hearing a report from Semashko, the medical union central committee passed a series of resolutions including a call for "the granting of greater independence to curative-hygienic facilities in their work, liberating them from the daily petty tutelage of the health organs."[65] As the issue suggests, overcentralization could be as much a threat to a properly "unified" Soviet medicine as local autonomy.

Narkomzdrav's difficulty in translating principle into practice was also painfully apparent in regard to the establishment of universally accessible qualified treatment. The most vocal criticism of Narkomzdrav policy in this sphere came from labor officials, who accused the commissariat of a peasant deviation in excessively diverting insurance funds from the proletariat to care of the general populace. The accusations certainly had little substance. One official calculation placed per capita spending on insured and uninsured in 1924/25 at 24 rubles 35 kopecks and 2 rubles 40 kopecks respectively; the following table gives data on treatment from Miskinov's report to the Sixth Congress of Zdravotdely.[66] These statistics, if anything, minimize the advantage of the insured, who had access to the best facilities and nearly monopolized specialized treatment. The persistence of these criticisms in the face of evidence from Narkomzdrav and the Worker-Peasant Inspectorate to the contrary can only be explained by lingering bitterness over subordination of medical insurance to the health organs.

Labor officials' characterization of Narkomzdrav policy was accurate in only one sense. As an agency of the Communist government, the commissariat did give

	Clinic Visits		Bed-Days	
	1924	1925	1924	1925
RSFSR:				
Per capita	1.2	1.4	0.3	0.4
Insured	6.3	6.8	1.7	1.8
Uninsured	0.7	0.9	0.2	0.2
District, *okrug* cities:				
Per capita	0.9	1.2	0.2	0.3
Insured	4.7	5.4	1.1	1.2
Uninsured	0.6	0.8	0.2	0.2

priority to the proletariat. In announcing Narkomzdrav's 1927 victory on the insurance issue, for example, Semashko denounced the idea of equal care for town and country as "politically dangerous, practically senseless."[67] Yet the Narkomzdrav staff was aware of the interconnection between urban and rural health conditions and of necessity devoted much effort to achieving precisely the kind of "leveling" that the commissar rhetorically renounced.

Concern over well-being in the countryside was certainly justified. The drastic contraction of medical facilities caused by the transfer of finance to local budgets in 1922 hit the rural network hardest, exacerbating an already difficult situation. Although the authorities eventually were able to halt the contraction of rural facilities and even begin a gradual process of expansion, the provision of care to the peasantry lagged far behind that available to other citizens. Narkomzdrav studies in mid-decade indicated that 42 percent of all *volosts* lacked hospital beds and 21 percent were without physician's points *(punkty)*; per capita expenditures on urban and rural areas could diverge by a factor of ten or more.[68] At the Sixth Congress of Zdravotdely, Semashko admitted "shame over what is still occurring in our rural network." Miskinov made the same point more dispassionately in reporting, "The rural network of physicians' points has one-third of the normal bed capacity [and] forty percent of the normal clinical capability, and specialized care is in a completely rudimentary condition."[69]

As a part of the government's "Face to the Countryside" policy, the central authorities did order local soviets to allocate greater resources to rural medicine. But compliance remained elusive. Semashko sarcastically opened his address to the Sixth Congress of Zdravotdely with the "modest request" that local officials carry out government decrees, rectifying a situation in which improvements in rural funding "often remain on paper."[70]

In its effort to strengthen health care in the villages, the commissariat experienced difficulties that extended beyond the recalcitrance of provincial soviet executives to the medical profession at large. During the 1920s the number of physicians in the RSFSR expanded rapidly, but with strikingly modest impact on rural areas. Whereas the overall ratio of citizens to doctors fell from 6,900:1 in 1913 to 2,590:1 in 1926, the corresponding rural figures were 20,300:1 and 18,900:1.[71] The chief cause for the discrepancy was a simple refusal of physicians to practice in the countryside. In 1924, eighty percent of all physicians resided in large cities (more than one-third in Moscow and Leningrad alone), despite high levels of urban unemployment. Three years later Semashko denounced a situation in which 1,500 unemployed physicians lived in Moscow while one-fifth of the posts in rural physicians points went vacant.[72]

Low pay and poor working conditions had much to do with physicians' "mass psychosis of urbanism," as one health official rather cynically put it.[73] So, too, did a system of medical education that emphasized professionalism and specialization. "Excellent as this system may be for the complicated medical service of a city," reported the sympathetic American observer Anna Haines, "one is somewhat appalled at the dilemma of a rural community unable to afford more than one doctor, and forced to choose among pediatricians, surgeons, psychiatrists and dentists"[74]—if, one might add, such physicians could be recruited at all. Even family ties gravitated against rural practice. A significant number of unemployed physicians were married women, unwilling to separate from spouses or children.

Many argued, however, that urbanism also reflected a serious loss of idealism in the profession. An article by A. Lepukaln published in 1927 in Narkomzdrav's official bulletin attacking the "unhealthy, craven, decadent" spirit undermining the Russian medical tradition of service to the people brought forth a chorus of criticism of young physicians as crass cowards devoid of revolutionary commitment.[75] One commentator, for example, contrasted the materialism of recent medical students who traveled from village to village in search of higher pay with the self-sacrifice of the "old populists" of the zemstvo era.[76] Of course, such nostalgic references to the virtues of bygone days must be taken with a grain of salt, especially in an era of postrevolutionary stabilization. Yet there is similar evidence of an unwillingness of physicians to respond to the high principles of the new Soviet medicine in another vital area of health care, public sanitation.

Narkomzdrav officials repeatedly proclaimed the prophylactic emphasis to be the key distinguishing characteristic of socialist health care. And they explicitly associated the preventive approach with central control through the commissariat, in contrast to the local emphasis of prerevolutionary zemstvo medicine. The establishment of state norms for sanitation and the retention of the core cadre of sanitary physicians on the central budget, in the Narkomzdrav view, made possible for the first time in Russian history a systematic approach to the prevention of disease. Yet here, too, reality failed to conform to expectations in familiar ways. A lack of funding, and consequent staff shortages, undermined the willingness of health officials to concentrate on public hygiene. In the countryside especially, the enormous demand for immediate treatment robbed overburdened physicians of time or energy for preventive activities.

Directives from Moscow urging more attention to sanitation produced but modest results. By one official calculation, local soviets in 1926 devoted a mere 1.9 percent of health budgets to combatting social disease. Between early 1925 and the start of 1927 the number of sanitary physicians in the RSFSR increased only modestly, from 1,102 to 1,246 (or, to count posts actually filled, from 958 to 1,116), and the rural contingent actually declined from 644 to 607. Many of the urban physicians were seriously underpaid and were forced to occupy other positions simultaneously or engage in private practice. Some cities lacked sanitary physicians altogether.[77] Ironically, when local authorities like the provincial agencies of the Worker-Peasant Inspectorate or Commissariat of Finance responded to central directives at all, it was to use calls for a "regime of economy" to cut back facilities for prophylactic medicine. The Council of People's Commissars attempted to address the issue through the upward revision of sanitation norms in 1927. Yet as the Narkomzdrav authority on sanitation Sysin reported bitterly, many local authorities continued to reduce staffing, even to the point of replacing *zdravotdel* sanitary-hygienic subsections with a "completely unsanctioned" skeletal system of sanitation inspectors.[78]

Narkomzdrav's difficulties in inculcating a preventive orientation to health care extended beyond local officialdom to the medical profession at large. Semashko and his colleagues in Moscow repeatedly bemoaned the low esteem in which personnel working in public hygiene were held. Sanitary physicians writing to the journal *Gigiena i epidemiologiia,* for example, complained of being dismissed as "specialists in bazaars, backyards and toilets," rather than the bearers of a new form of socialist medicine. In the area of budgetary allocation, they alluded to the existence of a form of "class conflict," in which regular physicians took the role of the "propertied" and sanitation personnel the dispossessed.[79]

In the struggle for status, the close relationship of the workers in preventive medicine to the authorities in Moscow could be a distinct liability. As one Saratov health official argued, many provincial physicians regarded prophylactic measures as "an unavoidable tribute" that had to be paid the center.[80] The potential for resentment on these grounds was demonstrated in 1927 in a conflict over responsibility for the "commanding heights" of preventive medicine—the fight against social disease. Reacting to Narkomzdrav's insistence that this task be assigned to the state-supported sanitation apparatus, leading health authorities of the Ukraine and White Russia campaigned for transfer of the responsibility to the regular staff of local *zdravotdely*. Significantly, Narkomzdrav's critics associated the regular physicians with the high ideals of zemstvo medicine. Conversely, they denounced the sanitation personnel as "bureaucrats" and the aspirations of the commissariat to concentrate prophylaxis in the sanitation apparatus as "chauvinism."[81] Narkomzdrav leaders vigorously defended the sanitary physicians and the commissariat's own leading role. Yet they also admitted in terms similar to those of Sysin that much needed to be done to change the sanitary physicians from the unwanted "stepchildren" of local *zdravotdely* to "favorite sons."[82]

The inability of the central authorities to transform attitudes on sanitation when coupled with the failure to popularize medical practice in the countryside suggests a concluding evaluation of Narkomzdrav's experience in the 1920s. The commissariat was established to "unify" health care in the new socialist system. In part, this meant the pursuit of a political end, the imposition of government control in the field of medicine. Yet centralization was also seen as a necessary prerequisite for a fully rational approach to health care that could transform Russian conditions in utopian ways. As in the economic sphere, Bolshevik leaders defined rationality in terms of nationwide planning, universally obligatory norms, and technical specialization. The commissariat was to be the vehicle for consistent application of this definition.

During the 1920s, the leaders of Soviet medicine discovered that Russian reality would not easily yield to such redefinition. Much of the problem flowed from the enormous gap between the health needs of the impoverished, war-torn nation and the resources available to meet them. Despite significant achievements, Russia continued simultaneously to run far ahead of its European neighbors in mortality and disease and to lag far behind in numbers of physicians and hospitals. Under these conditions, new approaches to health care were extremely difficult to initiate. How, for example, could preventive medicine be emphasized in the face of the pressing human need for immediate care? Soviet health authorities repeatedly complained of the vicious cycle in which prophylaxis seemed the only way to make a dent in disease rates, but the very extent of illness made it nearly unconscionable for *zdravotdely* and individual physicians to divert time and energy from treatment.

Some of the shortcomings in the Soviet system of health care, though, did not result from a bitterly recalcitrant reality. Rather, they were the consequences of the approach to medicine adopted by the regime and defended by the commissariat. The heavy emphasis on technical expertise undoubtedly foreclosed policy options. In regard to rural medicine, for example, Narkomzdrav vetoed the extension of independent feldsher stations as a transition step toward more professionalized facilities, thus defending the primacy of physicians but leaving many peasants without care. Even the resort to trained midwives in rural areas as a means of reducing high mortality rates during birth had to be implemented over the strenuous insistence of many within the Narkomzdrav apparatus that hospitals were the only proper place for deliveries.[83]

The commissariat's insistence on unity, defined ultimately as central control over health care, was equally problematic. The policy not only proved hard to implement, but also, it can be argued, sapped the enthusiasm of the medical profession. In explaining the reluctance of *zdravotdely* and regular physicians to respond more positively to the call for preventive medicine, for example, Narkomzdrav's critics pointed to the close association of sanitation with central intrusion in local affairs. They explicitly identified the recalcitrant provincial medical personnel with the earlier zemstvo physicians, implying a shared resistance to state supervision.

Narkomzdrav's leaders replied to such criticisms by doggedly reaffirming centralized state direction of health care and rejecting appeals to the zemstvo tradition. Semashko made the point in prophetic terms in 1928 in an article on the shortage of rural physicians.[84] Although he defended the younger generation, the commissar went on to make a stark observation about solving the problem. "Socialist organization of the economy," he argued in searching for principles for Soviet medicine, "differs from capitalist above all by being planned while the latter is anarchistic." And planning, he continued, is based on service as an obligation or "duty" (*po-vinnost'*)—"not philanthropy and not fulfillment of a populist debt but a duty to the state." This call to duty, for physicians and indeed all Soviet citizens, was soon to be issued in terms far harsher than Semashko could have imagined.

NOTES

1. For details on the congress see M. I. Barsukov, et al., *Ocherki istorii zdravookhraneniia SSSR (1917–1956 gg.)* (Moscow, 1957), pp. 86–92; and A. I. Nesterenko, *Kak byl obrazovan Narodnyi komissariat zdravookhraneniia RSFSR: Iz istorii sovetskogo zdravookhraneniia (oktiabr' 1917 g.-iiul' 1918 g.)* (Moscow, 1965), pp. 68–75.

2. B. D. Petrov and B. M. Potulov, *N. A. Semashko* (Moscow, 1974), pp. 62–63.

3. Mark G. Field, "Medical Organization and the Medical Profession," in Cyril E. Black, ed., *The Transformation of Russian Society* (Cambridge, Mass., 1967), p. 544. For employment patterns see Nancy M. Frieden, *Russian Physicians in an Era of Reform and Revolution, 1856–1905* (Princeton, N. J., 1981), pp. 211–12, 323.

4. On Rein, see J. F. Hutchinson, *The Cleansing Hurricane: Politics and Public Health in Revolutionary Russia, 1900–1918* (Baltimore: Johns Hopkins University Press, forthcoming); Nesterenko, *Kak byl obrazovan*, pp. 3–7; and Peter F. Krug, "Russian Public Physicians and Revolution: The Pirogov Society, 1917–1920" (Ph.D. diss., University of Wisconsin, 1979), p. 55.

5. Nesterenko, *Kak byl obrazovan*, pp. 5–6.

6. Ibid., p. 17; and M. Barsukov, "Neskol'ko slov o sovete vrachebnikh kollegii," *Voprosy zdravookhraneniia* [hereafter, *VZ*], no. 19 (1928), p. 7.

7. Barsukov, "Neskol'ko slov," pp. 7–8.

8. *Postanovleniia KPSS i sovetskogo pravitel'stva ob okhrane zdorov'ia naroda* (Moscow, 1958), p. 2.

9. Nesterenko, *Kak byl obrazovan*, pp. 17–18.

10. Ibid., pp. 68–76. Congress resolutions are reproduced in M. I. Barsukov, *Velikaia oktiabr'skaia sotsialisticheskaia revoliutsiia i organizatsiia sovetskogo zdravookhraneniia (oktiabr' 1917 g.-iiul' 1918 g.)* (Moscow, 1951), pp. 300–5.

11. *Postanovleniia*, pp. 27–28.

12. Nesterenko, *Kak byl obrazovan*, pp. 82–83.

13. Field, "Medical Organization," p. 541.

14. Nesterenko, *Kak byl obrazovan*, p. 71.

15. Petrov and Potulov, *Semashko*, p. 66.

16. Ibid., p. 69.

17. Barsukov, *Ocherki*, p. 144.

18. *Izvestiia*, 46 (February 28, 1919), p. 4.

19. Ibid., 40 (February 21, 1919), p. 4.

20. Petrov and Potulov, *Semashko*, pp. 69–70.

21. On the organization of the union, see E. I. Rodionova, *Ocherki istorii professional'nogo dvizheniia meditsinskikh rabotnikov* (Moscow, 1962), pp. 89–94. On feldshers, the chief rivals to physicians, see Samuel Ramer, "Who Was the Russian Feldsher?" *Bulletin of the History of Medicine*, no. 50 (1976), pp. 213–25.

22. The text of the resolution is given in Barsukov, *Velikaia oktiabr'skaia sotsialisticheskaia revoliutsiia*, pp. 297–98. The view was confirmed at the June medical congress. See ibid., p. 301.

23. *Izvestiia*, 69 (March 30, 1919), p. 1.

24. Rodionova, *Ocherki*, p. 100; and Krug, "Russian Public Physicians," pp. 253–56.

25. Quoted in Kendall E. Bailes, *Technology and Society under Lenin and Stalin* (Princeton, N. J., 1978), p. 51. On the Bolshevik attitude toward science and specialization, see also Thomas F. Remington, *Building Socialism in Bolshevik Russia* (Pittsburgh, 1984), chap. 5.

26. E. H. Carr, *The Bolshevik Revolution* (London, 1966), 2:189–90.

27. B. M. Potulov, *V. I. Lenin i okhrana zdorov'ia sovetskogo naroda* (Leningrad, 1969), p. 86.

28. Krug, "Russian Public Physicians," pp. 240–51.

29. Barsukov, *Ocherki*, pp. 71–72.

30. Rodionova, *Ocherki*, pp. 94–95, 101–2; and Krug, "Russian Public Physicians," chap. 8.

31. Rodionova, *Ocherki*, pp. 109–112; and S. A. Fediukin, *Bor'ba s burzhuaznoi ideologiei v usloviiakh perekhoda k nepu* (Moscow, 1977), pp. 81–82.

32. *Izvestiia*, 149 (July 17, 1918), p. 2. It is possible to overemphasize the regime's positive attitude toward the physicians. See the critique of Barsukov in Krug, "Russian Public Physicians," pp. 297–311.

33. Narodnyi komissariat zdravookhraneniia, *Otchet narodnogo komissariata zdravookhraneniia k 8-mu s'ezdu sovetov* (Moscow, 1920), p. 20.

34. Narkomzdrav, *Otchet*, p. 20; and *Statisticheskie materialy po sostoianiiu narodnogo zdraviia i organizatsii meditsinskoi pomoshschi v SSSR za 1913–1923 gg.* (Moscow, 1926), p. xxi.

35. Narkomzdrav, *Statisticheskie materialy*, pp. xi-xiii and xix-xxii.

36. *Postanovleniia*, p. 39.

37. Narkomzdrav, *Otchet*, p. 15; and *Statisticheskie materialy*, p. xvii.

38. Narkomzdrav, *Otchet*, p. 26. Barsukov goes so far as to claim that the Soviet effort in sanitation education actually began on the eastern front. Barsukov, *Ocherki*, p. 131.

39. Quoted in Barsukov, *Ocherki*, p. 127.

40. Narkomzdrav, *Otchet*, pp. 6–7.

41. On the panicked reaction of local officials to this "bombshell," see N. Semashko, "O perekhode na mestnye sredstva," *Biulleten' narodnogo komissariata zdravookhraneniia* [hereafter, *BNKZ*], no. 9 (1922), p. 1.

42. On the revival of the Pirogov Society see Krug, "Russian Public Physicians," epilogue. For the commissariat's response to the resolutions, see *Izvestiia narodnogo komissariata zdravookhraneniia*, nos. 3–4 (1922), pp. 1–2.

43. *BNKZ*, no. 6 (1924), p. 2.

44. *BNKZ*, no. 1 (1927), p. 5.

45. See, for example, Narkomzdrav, *Statisticheskii obzor sostoianiia zdravookhraneniia i zabolevaemost' zaraznymi bolezniami v RSFSR v 1927 g.* (Moscow, 1931), pp. 572–77.

46. N. Freiberg, "Narodnyi komissariat zdravookhraneniia za 10 let," *BNKZ*, no. 20 (1927), pp. 10–15, and G. Karanovich, "Etapy razvitiia mestnykh organov zdravookhraneniia," *BNKZ*, no. 20 (1927), pp. 15–20.

47. Cited in Stephen Sternheimer, "Administration for Development," in W. M. Pintner and D. K. Rowney, *Russian Officialdom* (Chapel Hill, N. C., 1980), pp. 324–25. Only the tiny theater, film, and publishing bureaucracies grew more rapidly.

48. *Tsentral'nyi ispolnitel'nyi komitet SSSR, Stenograficheskii otchet, tretiia sessiia, deviatyi sozyv* (1922), p. 125; and *BNKZ*, no. 23 (1922), pp. 6–7.

49. *VZ*, no. 19 (1928), pp. 29–30.

50. Ia. Bineman and S. Kheinman, *Kadry gosudarstvennogo i kooperativnogo apparata SSSR* (Moscow, 1930), pp. 48–49.

51. Narkomzdrav, *Trudy shestogo vserossiiskogo s''ezda zdravotdelov* (Moscow, 1927), p. 87.

52. Data cited in H. E. Sigerist, *Medicine and Health in the Soviet Union* (New York,

1947), pp. 34–35, and D. Gorfin, "Lechebnoe delo na poroge 2-go desiatiletiia sovetskoi meditsiny i blizhaishie perspektivy," *VZ*, no. 19 (1928), pp. 62–67.

53. Gorfin, "Lechebnoe delo," p. 63, and Narkomzdrav, *Statisticheskie materialy*, p. xiii.

54. A. Sysin, "Na poroge novogo desiatiletiia," *VZ*, no. 19 (1928), p. 34.

55. The legislation is reviewed by I. A. Dobreitser in *Vestnik sovremennoi meditsiny*, no. 8 (1927), pp. 509–513; and by Sysin in *BNKZ*, no. 8 (1927), pp. 15–19; and *Gigiena i epidemiologiia*, no. 10 (1927), pp. 22–26.

56. *Gigiena i epidemiologiia*, no. 10 (1927), pp. 61–62.

57. Narkomzdrav, *Trudy*, p. 92.

58. V. Goriushin and S. Cherniak, "Zdravookhranenie v mestnom biudzhete," *BNKZ*, nos. 13–14 (1926), p. 19. On the issue of finance see Christopher Davis's fine essay "Economic Problems of the Soviet Health Service: 1917–1930," *Soviet Studies*, 35, no. 3 (1983), pp. 343–61.

59. A. Rozova, "Finansirovanie dela zdravookhraneniia v RSFSR," *VZ*, no. 8 (1928), p. 13. A similar calculation is made in Davis, "Economic Problems," p. 348.

60. Narkomzdrav, *Trudy*, pp. 57–59.

61. Goriushin and Cherniak, "Zdravookhranenie," p. 20; and G. Dreisin, "Narodnoe zdravookhranenie v mestnom biudzhete SSSR na 1925–26 g.," *BNKZ*, no. 17 (1926), p. 14.

62. *BNKZ*, nos. 13–14 (1926), p. 24.

63. V. Goriushin and N. Poliakov, "Subventsiia na 1926–27 biudzhetnyi god," *BNKZ*, no. 2 (1926), pp. 4–9. The matching grant principle had the further drawback of rewarding the richest, rather than the neediest, provinces.

64. M. Donskoi, "Ocherednye zadachi planirovaniia zdravookhraneniia," *VZ*, no. 1 (1928), p. 14.

65. *Vestnik sovremennoi meditsiny*, no. 1 (1927), pp. 64–65. On the issue generally, see M. Gliuzman, "O bol'nichnykh neuriaditsakh," *BNKZ*, no. 22 (1926), pp. 3–4; N. Bakhmutskii, "Neobkhodimo uporiadochit' rabotu v lechebnykh uchrezhdeniiakh," no. 4 (1927), pp. 5–7; and Narkomzdrav, *Trudy*, p. 30.

66. M. Donskoi, "Kontrol'nye tsifry po zdravookhraneniia na 1926–27 g.," *BNKZ*, no. 19 (1926), p. 6; Narkomzdrav, *Trudy*, p. 89, and Davis, "Economic Problems," pp. 350–52.

67. *BNKZ*, no. 1 (1927), p. 5.

68. M. Ginsburg, "Finansovye perspektivy sel'skoi meditsiny," *BNKZ*, no. 21 (1925), pp. 12–13; and Davis, "Economic Problems," p. 350.

69. Narkomzdrav, *Trudy*, pp. 22, 92.

70. Ibid., p. 22.

71. *Vestnik sovremennoi meditsiny*, no. 18 (1927), pp. 1158–60.

72. B. Ivanovskii, "Skol'ko u nas vrachei i kak oni raspredeleny," *BNKZ*, nos. 2–3 (1924), pp. 3–4.

73. K. Volkov, "Otchego pustuiut uchastki," *BNKZ*, no. 21 (1927), p. 25.

74. Anna J. Haines, *Health Work in Soviet Russia* (New York, 1928), p. 20.

75. See *BNKZ*, no. 11 (1927), pp. 3–5; no. 21 (1927), pp. 23–32; *VZ*, no. 2 (1928), pp. 29–31; and no. 3 (1928), pp. 14–18.

76. Sanvrach, "K voprosu o prichinakh pustovaniia sel'skikh uchastkov," *VZ*, no. 2 (1928), pp. 24–25.

77. *BNKZ*, nos. 13–14 (1926), pp. 21–22; and *Gigiena i epidemiologiia*, no. 10 (1928), pp. 8–10.

78. *Gigiena i epidemiologiia*, no. 1 (1928), pp. 5–6.

79. Ibid., no. 4 (1927), pp. 59–60.

80. L. Mukoseev, "K voprosu o sostoianii meditsinskoi pomoshchi v derevne," *BNKZ*, no. 20 (1926), p. 48.

81. See Sysin's review of the issue in *Gigiena i epidemiologiia,* no. 3 (1927), pp. 21–31.

82. Ibid., no. 1 (1928), p. 7.

83. Narkomzdrav, *Trudy,* pp. 93, 117, 120–27.

84. N. Semashko, "Obsluzhivanie derevni i zadachi vrachei," *VZ,* no. 3 (1928), pp. 14–15.

SAMUEL C. RAMER

Feldshers and Rural Health Care in the Early Soviet Period

The city was the Soviet regime's original political base. During the 1920s Bolshevik administrative activity was most effective in urban areas. The countryside, by contrast, was governed for the most part by the resurgent peasant commune, the leaders of which tenaciously defended their parochial interests with little regard for Bolshevik goals or ideology.[1] In public health, as in other fields, the peasantry in the countryside posed a tremendous challenge, not only to the limited human and material resources of the new regime but also to its declared mission of building socialism in Russia.

For the young Soviet regime, as for its tsarist predecessor, extending modern medicine into rural areas was a formidable task. This essay examines the difficulties associated with improving rural medicine by focusing on the role that feldshers, or paramedics, played in rural health care systems. The efforts made by early Soviet health planners to replace feldshers with physicians illuminate not only the kind of medical system they sought to create in the countryside, but also the obstacles they faced in doing so. To place their plans in perspective, it is helpful to review the role that feldshers played in rural health care during the fifty years prior to the revolution.

"FELDSHERISM" IN PRE-REVOLUTIONARY RUSSIA

One of the most intractable problems that local public health authorities faced prior to 1917 was that of providing the countryside with enough physicians to serve the needs of the peasantry. Physicians could only survive in rural areas as salaried employees, and the number of salaried positions which local governments could afford was comparatively small. Statistics fluctuated over time, but at best only 30 percent of Russia's civilian physicians practiced in rural areas during the pre-1914 period, while almost 80 percent of the country's total population lived in the countryside.[2] The shortage of physicians was thus an almost exclusively rural problem, a fact that absolute figures illustrate better than percentages. In 1913, for example, there were only about 7,000 civilian physicians employed in rural practice throughout the empire.[3] Here they were expected to serve a rural population in excess of one hundred million people. In cities, the ratio of physicians to population in 1913 was 1:1,400, which was roughly equivalent to that in other European cities. In rural areas, however, the average ratio was 1:20,300. In many outlying provinces, of course, this ratio was much larger.[4]

This unsatisfactory ratio does not even fully reflect problems of the availabilty of health care in the countryside. In the Russian empire peasants were scattered over such enormous expanses of territory that travel between villages even a few miles apart was arduous, especially in the spring and fall seasons of muddy roads. Peasants who lived more than fifteen miles from a physician were unlikely to call on him except in the most dire circumstances, and usually too late for him to provide effective help.

Most observers believed that the day when all peasants would have ready access to a physician's care was decades away. Local governments charged with providing medical care in rural areas therefore hired various auxiliary medical personnel to assist physicians and, in many cases, to act in their place. The most common and numerous of these auxiliary practitioners in the prerevolutionary era was the feldsher, or physician's assistant.[5]

Russian law licensed feldshers to treat patients only under a physician's direct supervision. In practice, however, many feldshers were stationed at remote rural outposts where they were essentially on their own. The nearest physician might be several hours or more away, and visit only infrequently. Even feldshers who worked in the same rural clinic with a physician treated many emergency patients independently, since the physician was often absent on other business. As late as the beginning of the twentieth century, almost one-third of the patients in rural areas were treated by feldshers rather than physicians; in poorer and more remote provinces this percentage commonly exceeded one-half.[6] Reality thus made nonsense of the law.

As early as the 1860s, zemstvo physicians active in developing rural medical programs vigorously opposed any legitimization of this independent feldsher practice, which they called "feldsherism." As they correctly pointed out, even the best-trained feldshers had not been adequately prepared to practice on their own. Moreover, they feared that any explicit legitimization of "feldsherism," even as a temporary necessity, might encourage local authorities to content themselves with hiring feldshers as cheaper—and implicitly satisfactory—substitutes for physicians. Were this to happen, they argued, peasants would be condemned to second-class medical care which differed little from that provided by the traditional healers or znakhari whose influence physicians sought to displace.[7] Finally, physicians contended that feldshers practicing alone gave the peasantry a distorted vision of modern medicine, thereby complicating the already difficult task of making its principles part of the peasantry's way of life.[8]

There was, of course, no practical way to end feldsherism quickly, and local health administrators tacitly recognized this when they assigned feldshers to independent posts. In 1890, for example, there were 2,800 independent feldsher stations in the zemstvo provinces alone, as opposed to only 1,440 physicians' bailiwicks (uchastki). During the quarter century prior to World War I significant progress was made in providing more physicians for the countryside and in reducing, if only slightly, the number of independent feldsher stations. Thus by 1910 the number of independent feldsher stations in the zemstvo provinces had declined to 2,620, whereas the number of physicians' bailiwicks had grown to 2,686.[9] Although these figures attest to a significant expansion in the number of rural physicians, they also illustrate the continued importance of independent feldsher practice in rural areas.

If there was any consolation to be derived from the feldsher's prominent role during the prerevolutionary period, it was that the quality of feldsher school graduates had increased dramatically. The primary cause of this improvement was a radical transformation in the social origins and overall educational qualifications of feldsher students. Whereas semiliterate peasant boys had been virtually the only feldsher students in the 1860s, by the 1890s feldsher schools had begun to enroll increasing numbers of urban youth, predominantly women, many of whom had completed a substantial part of a classical gymnasium education. In 1910, for example, almost 15 percent of all feldsher students were women who had graduated from gymnasia. An additional 43 percent, almost all women, had completed four to seven years of gymnasium education. (More than 70 percent of all feldsher students in 1910 were women.) The higher quality of matriculating students enabled the burgeoning number of feldsher schools created before 1914 to offer more sophisticated medical courses.[10]

Trained midwives were another important group of auxiliary medical personnel who worked in rural areas. Peasant women, however, rarely called on them for assistance in childbirth. Such midwives were generally outsiders, often young, and did not fare well in the competition with traditional village midwives for the confidence of peasant women. Physicians concerned with reducing the high level of infant mortality in the countryside urged that the positions of midwife and feldsher be combined. By working as a feldsher, they argued, the midwife would have a better chance to win the peasants' trust, since women who had been treated successfully by a feldsher-midwife for minor injuries or diseases would be far more likely to call on this same feldsher-midwife during childbirth. By the early twentieth century, the majority of feldsher students, most of them young women of urban origin, were training to become precisely such feldsher-midwives.[11]

The argument that female feldsher-midwives would be better rural practitioners than either midwives or feldshers proved difficult to test, since the best-educated feldsher-midwives did not go to the countryside in large numbers. As the most cultured and best qualified graduates of feldsher schools, they had their pick of the best urban jobs. Thus rural obstetric care did not improve much, and most independent feldsher posts continued to be held by male feldshers, whose medical skills and overall cultural attainments were generally inferior to those of their female counterparts.

So feldsherism was all the more repugnant to physicians because they knew that, on the whole, the feldshers who engaged in independent practice were those least qualified to do so. Many were *rotnye* feldshers whose training as corpsmen in the army did not prepare them for civilian practice, much less for the role of independent practitioners. Physicians considered these *rotnye* feldshers to be the equivalent of *znakhari*, a characterization given substance by the extent to which *rotnye* feldshers and *znakhari* borrowed from one another's techniques and medicinal armories in order to maintain or augment their peasant clientele.[12]

FELDSHERS AND PROFESSIONALIZATION PRIOR TO 1917

Prior to 1890, feldshers and midwives in Russia were a scattered group of medical workers with many common grievances but few vehicles for communicating with one another and no forum in which to share their views. In 1891, Dr. Boris Oks created such a forum by founding the journal *Fel'dsher,* which he edited and published for the next twenty-five years. Dr. Oks was more active as an entrepreneurial publisher than as a physician. He identified himself totally with the cause of improving feldshers' professional status. Until 1905 he was the acknowledged leader of the feldsher movement, and his passionate articles on various aspects of feldshers' professional existence left a clear stamp on the journal.

Unlike its editor, most contributors to the journal were themselves practicing feldshers. The journal's wide circulation enabled feldshers from across the empire to compare their problems and consider their professional goals. These goals were set forth in the articles and letters that they wrote for *Fel'dsher* and the numerous other feldsher journals that appeared after 1905.[13] Almost all contributors sought to improve their working conditions, repeatedly pointing to their low pay, inadequate housing, and lack of holidays. Their most heated criticism, however, was directed at the way physicians and hiring authorities treated them on the job. Many of the better educated civilian feldshers had absorbed quasi-populist attitudes in feldsher schools and looked forward to working with physicians as partners in healing the Russian people. Once in practice, however, they found that even sensitive physicians regarded them as useful subordinates at best. To most physicians, feldshers were social as well as professional inferiors, and it was not unusual for a physician to treat a feldsher almost as a personal servant. Such treatment, especially when coupled with predictable workaday conflicts, understandably bred resentment among the more proud or idealistic of these young feldshers.

Written in the language of "the insulted and the injured," articles and letters by feldshers were an ongoing plea for physicians—and society in general—to accord them the respect to which they believed their education and the value of their work entitled them. They urged that the law define clearly the feldsher's rights vis-à-vis the physician and sanction explicitly the independent role that they were forced to play in the countryside because of the shortage of rural physicians.

Feldshers understood that the only sure way to improve their professional status was to enhance their medical skills. They therefore urged that feldsher education be reformed, that refresher courses be established for those already in practice, and finally that the university medical faculties be opened to feldshers who had proved themselves capable medical practitioners. Tsarist health officials consistently refused to make this latter concession, insisting that only those who had completed a classical gymnasium were prepared to become physicians. In their view, the breadth of a gymnasium education was an indispensable part of a physician's training. Lacking such an education, most feldshers were effectively barred from becoming physicians. In the democratic ethos of an increasingly revolutionary age, many feldshers came to regard this insistence on a gymnasium diploma as social discrimination.

In the wake of the 1905 revolution, two rival national organizations competed for the loyalty of feldshers, feldsher-midwives, and midwives. The most influential of these was the Union of Societies of Physicians' Assistants, whose journal *Fel'dsherskii vestnik* was the single most important feldsher publication between 1906 and 1918. Its explicit concern with broader social and political questions and their impact on public health mirrored that of the Pirogov Society of Russian Physicians. Its rival was the Organization of Russian Feldshers, whose journal *Fel'dsher,* still edited by Dr. Oks, insisted that professional organizations and their journals should confine themselves strictly to the discussion of professional problems.[14] The feldsher congresses held during these years at the district, provincial, and even national level testify to a growing professional consciousness among feldshers as well as to the continuing frustration of their professional aspirations. The records of these conferences were published and circulated to an audience much larger than those actually in attendance and helped set off further discussions in feldsher journals.[15]

In order to improve their professional standing, feldshers made every effort to gain a voice in the medical councils and societies that physicians dominated. They sought membership in the provincial and district sanitary bureaus which sprang up at the turn of the century. They urged that delegates from their societies be admitted as voting members to Pirogov congresses. In short, they wanted physicians to recognize them as junior partners—not simply subordinates—in the improvement of public health.[16] Not many did so. In the immediate aftermath of 1905 there was a tendency to accommodate some feldsher demands, but most physicians rejected the idea of giving feldshers any voice in medical decisionmaking. For most physicians, feldsher practice was a necessary evil to be endured, but not endorsed.[17]

THE FELDSHER PROFESSIONAL MOVEMENT AND THE REVOLUTIONS OF 1917

The revolutionary events of 1917 triggered an explosion of professional activity among feldshers. Whereas only 54 societies for feldshers trained in civilian schools (*shkol'nye* feldshers) existed prior to 1917,[18] more than 300 new local and provincial societies of *shkol'nye* feldshers were created during 1917 alone. Almost all of these new societies became affiliates of the All-Russian Union of Unions of Physicians' Assistants, the renamed successor to the Union of Societies of Physicians' Assistants and publisher of *Fel'dsherskii vestnik.* By mid-1918 the Union of Unions embraced over 350 local and provincial *shkol'nye* feldsher societies.[19] Its leaders were primarily concerned with improving the social status and professional position of *shkol'nye* feldshers. Although they claimed in mid-1917 that their organization stood "outside parties," they went on to recognize "the socialist parties" as their "ideological representatives."[20] Their political stance was that of moderate socialists, less wedded to any party than to a general enthusiasm for the Revolution, democracy, and socialism. Thus they supported the Provisional Government and urged all socialist parties to unify their tactics.[21]

Rotnye feldshers organized themselves for the first time in the wake of the February Revolution. Almost 75,000 of these combat medics, most of them peasants, had been trained during the war. Their very numbers and the political climate within the army, where they remained throughout 1917, invited action. The first organizational meeting of *rotnye* feldshers was held in Petrograd on March 5, 1917, and the formation of a national union was immediately proposed. The first national congress of *rotnye* feldshers was held in June 1917, with 700 in attendance. This congress created the All-Russian Union of Physicians' Assistants (*lekarskikh pomoshchnikov*), which by 1918 boasted a membership of 80,000.[22] In early 1918, a second union of *rotnye* feldshers who worked for the railroad was established.[23]

Both these *rotnye* feldsher unions published journals in which they sought to improve their professional position.[24] Embittered by the long-standing refusal of *shkol'nye* feldshers to admit *rotnye* feldshers into their organizations, neither of these new unions established ties with the older *shkol'nye* feldsher union. The generally egalitarian atmosphere of 1917–18 fanned *rotnye* feldshers' resentment of the professional exclusivity of their *shkol'nye* rivals, and tense relations between the two feldsher groups persisted even after they merged with others into a single health workers' union in 1919.[25]

Although the Union of Unions of Physicians' Assistants accepted "socialism" as the revolution's ultimate goal, its leaders—particularly the editors of *Fel'dsherskii vestnik*—immediately opposed the Bolshevik seizure of power. The Bolshevik program of building socialism in Russia overnight, they argued, would lead inevitably to dictatorship, violence, and a reaffirmation of the old regime's worst qualities.[26] The editors of *Fel'dsherskii vestnik* were arguably even more militant in their opposition to Bolshevik power than the Pirogov physicians.[27] Initially, at least, a large number of *shkol'nye* feldshers shared their hostility to the Bolshevik regime.[28]

But the leaders of the Union of Unions of Physicians' Assistants were in fact more divided in their attitude toward the Bolshevik regime than *Fel'dsherskii vestnik's* inflammatory editorials indicated. More important, many rank-and-file *shkol'nye* feldshers welcomed the October Revolution, as did the mass of *rotnye* feldshers who were demobilized in 1918. They hoped that its initial social egalitarianism would spill over into the professional arena, bringing them both wages equivalent to those of physicians and full participation in public health bodies. These goals were a clear challenge to physicians' claims to exclusive competence in medical questions.

The organizational center of this "feldsher challenge," to use Peter Krug's phrase, was Vsemediksantrud, the trade union which the Bolsheviks organized in late 1918 to represent all "medical workers," from physicians, feldshers, and midwives to nurses, sanitary personnel, carpenters, and cooks.[29] *Shkol'nye* feldshers took the lead in organizing Vsemediksantrud. In October 1918, after a year of vacillation, the leadership of the Union of Unions of Physicians' Assistants voted to disband their independent union and enter the newly formed Vsemediksantrud.[30]

The role of the Union of Unions of Physicians' Assistants in the formation of Vsemediksantrud was crucial, since *shkol'nye* feldshers were the only medical practitioners with extensive organizational experience who favored a mass health workers' union. *Rotnye* feldshers and sanitary personnel followed the *shkol'nye* feldshers' lead in joining Vsemediksantrud.[31] Neither group had a long tradition of separate organization, and both saw affiliation with Vsemediksantrud as the most promising way to improve both their material position and their professional status.[32]

Physicians—who had recently formed their own separate union—would have been outnumbered in this large production union had they entered it without special provisions to guarantee their autonomy in matters of medical expertise. The leaders of Vsemediksantrud espoused a syndicalist vision repugnant to physicians and, as Peter Krug has shown, ultimately unacceptable to the Soviet regime. Both Lenin and physicians such as N. A. Semashko, who headed the Commissariat of Public Health (Narkomzdrav), insisted that criteria of social class should be subordinate to expertise in the administration of health care, a vision that coincided with Lenin's more general belief that the young Soviet republic needed to make use of existing technical specialists. The physicians' union eventually entered Vsemediksantrud as an autonomous section, thus maintaining the dominance of physicians in the administration of public health. As Krug makes clear, Narkomzdrav's rejection of the "feldsher challenge" of 1919 facilitated its cultivation of a working relationship with the Pirogov physicians.[33]

THE SOVIET REGIME AND THE FUTURE OF FELDSHER PRACTICE

The First World War brought a halt to the gradual improvement that local institutions had made in rural health care. Large numbers of physicians and feldshers were drafted into the army, depleting an already inadequate supply of modern medical practitioners. As the war dragged on, followed by the turmoil and dislocations of the Revolution and the collapse of local authority, the state of medical care in the countryside became ever more desperate. It was in this situation of crisis that the Soviet regime came to power.

The institution which ultimately took the lead in framing Soviet public health policies was Narkomzdrav, created in mid-1918. Both its early leaders and the rank-and-file physicians who cooperated in building Soviet medicine, were committed to creating a revolutionary new system of public health which would embody the most advanced principles of preventive medicine while providing the best possible therapeutic care to all members of the population. The sheer ambitiousness as well as the egalitarian nature of these goals evoked admiration.[34] Given the chaos of the Civil War and the general deterioration of life under War Communism, however, Narkomzdrav officials made major policy decisions long before they had either the manpower or the finances to implement them.

One of the most crucial of these decisions concerned the kinds of medical practitioners needed by the young republic and the way in which they should be educated. To train enough physicians it was essential not only to increase the number of medical faculties, but also to expand the pool of potential physicians. Here the demands of public health coincided with the Bolsheviks' goal of democratizing higher education. On August 2, 1918, the Council of People's Commissars ruled that institutions of higher education were open to all over the age of sixteen, regardless of whether they had completed secondary school. Entrance exams and tuition were also abolished.[35] In the wake of this ruling, *shkol'nye* feldshers and persons who would earlier have gone to feldsher schools now became eligible for the medical faculties.

Narkomzdrav, which had inherited the Pirogov Society's legacy of opposition to feldsherism, was committed from the outset to eliminating feldshers altogether and to replacing them with various other auxiliary personnel. In May 1918, even before the creation of Narkomzdrav, the First All-Russian Congress of Health Boards (*zdravotdely*) voted to end admission to all feldsher schools in the fall of 1918.[36] Although this resolution reflected the preferences of leading Bolshevik physicians, it was not acted on. A more comprehensive discussion took place in late 1919 at the All-Russian Congress on Medical Education in Moscow.

The main report on feldsher education at this congress was presented by Dr. L. F. Raukhvarger, head of the Department of Medical Schools of Narkomzdrav. In his report, which the congress adopted verbatim in its resolutions, Raukhvarger recommended the gradual elimination of the position of feldsher. Modern medicine, he argued, required that medical practitioners be classified strictly by their level of competence. This being the case, the confusion between the feldsher's training as a physician's assistant and his frequent role as a de facto physician was intolerable. Nevertheless, Raukhvarger recognized that "the extreme shortage of physicians and nurses precludes any haste in liquidating the feldsher's position. Similar caution is essential in the matter of eliminating feldsher schools."[37] In adopting this ambivalent stance, the congress remained true to the principles cherished by physicians without ignoring the realities of rural medicine in the early 1920s.

If the feldsher's position was to be gradually eliminated, what medical roles did health planners envision for those already trained and practicing as feldshers? In the first place, Narkomzdrav encouraged *shkol'nye* feldshers to enter medical faculties and become physicians.[38] Initial hopes that *shkol'nye* feldshers who had been admitted directly into the third year of medical school would be able to complete their studies proved too optimistic. Overwhelmed with clinical work in their medical school courses, most of them never succeeded in making up the biology and chemistry they lacked when they were admitted. Taking another approach, several universities decided to admit *shkol'nye* feldshers to medical school programs that required them to finish two years of study in one calendar year. These efforts were also for the most part unsuccessful.[39]

A number of special, accelerated medical faculties were established specifically for *shkol'nye* feldshers, and some feldshers did manage to earn their physicians' diplomas through them. The most successful of these courses was established at the Moscow Medical Institute in 1921. Of the 350 feldshers who entered in 1921, 228, or about 65 percent, graduated as physicians in 1924. Most of the dropouts occurred amid the hunger and cold of the first trimester in 1921.[40] Such accelerated courses for feldshers were, however, abolished in 1925. Subsequently 400 places were set aside annually in ordinary medical faculties for feldshers who could pass the entrance exams, which by then had been reinstated. (There was opposition to this on the grounds that reserving any places for feldshers would lower the overall quality of the entering medical school class.)[41]

The Moscow Medical Institute's example is impressive precisely because it was exceptional. Most feldshers in practice at the time of the Revolution never became physicians. Because of family obligations and financial need, few could afford the luxury of returning to medical school, even under advantageous conditions.[42] During the 1920s, the regime also encouraged practicing feldshers to acquire a physician's degree by going to school part-time at night. The number who did so was small: many feldshers worked in remote areas where there were no night courses, and urban feldshers were usually too exhausted by their regular work to take advantage of this opportunity.

In its earliest discussions of the feldsher's role, therefore, Narkomzdrav and its officials accepted the fact that feldsherism would exist in rural areas for some time to come. Despite their commitment to abolish the feldsher's position altogether at some time in the future, those concerned with rural health care thought it imperative to continue training feldshers. As late as October 1921, the Third All-Russian Congress of Health Boards (*zdravotdely*) reaffirmed the need to train more feldshers in schools adapted to produce feldsher-midwives.[43]

THE FIRST ALL-UNION CONFERENCE ON AUXILIARY MEDICAL EDUCATION: OCTOBER 1922

The reluctant recognition of the short-term need to continue training feldshers was dramatically reversed in October 1922, at the First All-Union Conference on Auxiliary Medical Education. Dr. A. S. Sholomovich, a psychiatrist who was head of the Department of Auxiliary Medical Education of Glavprofobr, delivered the major conference report.[44] He began with an overview of rural medicine in the wake of the Civil War, in which he emphasized the radical decline in the number of rural physicians. In 1922, for example, 78 percent of Russia's physicians lived in cities. One-third of the young Soviet republic's physicians lived in Moscow alone, more than in all of rural Russia.

These statistics represented a stunning retreat from prewar figures. More than 6,300 physicians had been working in the countryside in 1914; by 1921 there were only about 3,800. Despite an abundance of unemployed physicians in cities, more than 45 percent of rural physicians' posts stood vacant. In Sholomovich's view, the main reason for the scant number of physicians in rural practice was the destitute condition of the peasantry in the wake of the Civil War. "Physicians cannot go to work in the countryside even if they want to," he argued. "The village has become too impoverished to support them."[45]

With physicians thus concentrated in cities, independent feldsher practice flourished in the countryside to a degree unprecedented in recent Russian history. Whereas only 3,800 rural physicians' posts were occupied throughout the country, the number of independent feldsher posts had grown to 3,850. This widespread postrevolutionary feldsherism differed from that which had existed prior to 1914 because many of the feldshers practicing independently were recently demobilized *rotnye* feldshers who had received only the most superficial training before serving as corpsmen in the war. Such *rotnye* feldshers flooded the countryside when the Civil War ended, most returning to their home villages where they supplemented their income by practicing medicine. As of 1920, approximately one-third of the feldshers in the country were *rotnye* feldshers.[46]

In many provinces these *rotnye* feldshers constituted a majority of all feldshers in rural practice. Having surveyed five different provinces, Sholomovich found the following:[47]

Province	Shkol'nye	Rotnye	Total Feldshers
Gomel'	120	220	340
Viatka	108	142	250
Samara	140	320	460
Bashkir Republic	230	330	560
Perm'	61	360	421

Given such figures, he argued that over half of all the feldshers practicing in rural Russia as of 1922 "were *znakhars,* without the slightest medical education."[48] His conclusion was that "a new category of social medicine—subfeldsherism—has become widespread in the countryside."[49]

Sholomovich cited social and cultural as well as economic reasons for this "total degradation of rural medicine."[50] War, famine, and the shortage of physicians with established reputations in a given locality had created a situation in which the practitioners who could prosper best in the countryside were traditional healers, whose magico-religious belief system the peasantry tended to share, and demobilized *rotnye* feldshers, who were usually known in the village. As Sholomovich put it, "not only a physician, but even a trained civilian feldsher would be driven out of the countryside, since they don't have the roots there that the subfeldsher does."[51]

Despite this crisis in rural medicine, Sholomovich believed that improvement was imminent. He thought economic recovery would spur peasants to demand better medical personnel; this, in turn, would open up rural jobs for physicians who were unemployed or underemployed in cities. He was confident that "physicians will go to the countryside without compulsion. There are enough of them in Russia now, and their numbers will grow with every year. Feldshers will become superfluous, even as physicians' assistants, and will be replaced by nurses."[52] To guarantee an adequate corps of rural physicians, he suggested that one-third of each year's graduating physicians be sent to the countryside to serve an obligatory three or four years. Feldsher schools, no longer necessary, could be gradually revamped to train sanitary assistants and raise the qualifications of *rotnye* feldshers.[53]

The debate which followed Sholomovich's report captures the sharply divergent views that early Soviet physicians had of the feldsher's role. Most shared his conviction that feldsherism, and even the position of feldsher, should eventually be eliminated. But many also emphasized the need for feldshers, at least for the fore-seeable future. As L. M. Filippova, representing the Central Committee of Vse-mediksantrud, stated: "We've been talking about liquidating [the feldsher] for a long time, but in practice we haven't done it because life is more powerful than we are and demands for the countryside a medical worker with qualifications that are precisely those of the feldsher, whatever we choose to call him."[54]

A Voronezh physician argued that the feldsher's existence could not be elimi-nated

> because the conditions of life in Russia that brought feldsherism into existence are just as they were. It is impossible to imagine that even unemployed physicians will soon go into the impoverished countryside. We have a contentious and difficult battle ahead with *rotnyi* feldsherism. And feldshers, however undesirable as independent practi-tioners, are necessary as physicians' assistants. Therefore schools for feldsher-midwives should continue to exist and be closed only when all positions in the countryside are occupied by physicians. And that won't be soon.[55]

One's views on the need to train feldshers depended largely on one's assessment of how readily physicians would go into the countryside, even if it had been eco-nomically rejuvenated. By no means all conference delegates shared Sholomovich's optimism on this point. Dr. I. S. Ruzheinikov, director of Glavprofobr's Department of Medical Education, was particularly skeptical. However desirable in theory, he thought it impossible to compel one-third of all newly graduated physicians to serve in rural areas. "Last year," he recalled, "they wanted to send physicians [to rural areas] to fight the famine. Nothing seemed to work. Of four actually sent three didn't get there, while the fourth arrived and 'got sick'. It all boils down to the fact that physicians don't go to the countryside."[56]

Dr. V. A. Polubinskii, from Petrograd, agreed that physicians, who had never gone to the Russian countryside in massive numbers, were unlikely to do so in the foreseeable future. Closing feldsher schools thus struck him as the opposite of what was really needed, which was to upgrade them so that their graduates would be better qualified to replace the physician in remote areas. In essence, Polubinskii advocated the resurrection of the prerevolutionary feldsher school and thought that the crisis in rural health-care delivery could be substantially relieved if such schools—which would admit only those who had completed seven years of edu-cation—were established in every provincial capital.

Despite a forceful minority argument that feldsher training and practice were essential for the time being, the conference majority concluded that it was both necessary and possible to "liquidate feldsherism" in the coming years. It recom-mended that the short-term demand for feldshers and midwives in remote areas be met by adapting some existing feldsher-midwife schools for the supplementary training of *rotnye* feldshers. These upgraded *rotnye* feldshers, together with feldshers and feldsher-midwives already in practice, would ensure a plentiful supply of rural feldshers during the transition period in which enough physicians were being trained to make the feldsher entirely superfluous.[57] Although the conference stopped short of calling for an immediate end to all feldsher training, the sense of its recommendations was that feldsher schools should be gradually eliminated.[58] This decision to phase out feldsher schools was soon embodied in practice. By 1924 virtually all exclusively feldsher schools had ceased to exist, though a few schools for feldsher-midwives remained.[59]

THE TRANSFER OF PUBLIC HEALTH
TO LOCAL BUDGETS IN 1922

For the large number of feldshers who remained in rural practice throughout the 1920s, Narkomzdrav's public commitment to phase out feldsher practice was a serious blow. The two central goals of the feldsher movement had been to legitimize feldshers' professional activity and to enhance public appreciation of their work. By targeting the position of feldsher for extinction, Narkomzdrav transformed it into a professional dead end. Feldshers now had to endure the ordinary difficulties of everyday practice in the countryside without hope of recognition or advancement. Wherever cuts in medical personnel were necessary, they became prime targets.

The most immediate crisis for most feldshers, as indeed for the entire system of rural health care, was the decision of the Soviet government on May 1, 1922, to transfer the funding of public health to local budgets. Unable to sustain the existing commitment to public health and medical services, local governments resorted to a variety of measures. In many areas payment for medical treatment was introduced, undermining the zemstvo tradition of medical care without fees that had done much to build respect for it among the peasantry. Fees were generally followed by a decline in visits by peasants and a corresponding increase in the popularity of traditional healers.[60] In addition, the introduction of fees fueled a popular suspicion of medical personnel. As one feldsher reported, ''The population is beginning to regard us as robbers.''[61]

The typical response of most local governments, however, was to cut expenses. Medical personnel at all levels were laid off, and many hospitals and clinics were closed. Salaries were cut, often when several months in arrears.[62] Financing for physicians' visits to the various corners of rural bailiwicks was often eliminated, thus further isolating remote villages and feldsher posts.[63] The overall reduction in rural medical services in 1922 alone was on the order of 20 to 25 percent.[64] It is important to remember that this retreat occurred during one of the worst periods of famine and epidemic disease in modern European history.[65]

Feldshers were usually the first personnel to be cut, since local governments tried to retain what few physicians they had; 825 independent feldsher posts, or 18 percent of all such posts in the RSFSR, were abolished in the first six months of 1922. (Only 3 percent of rural physicians' posts were eliminated.[66]) The exact number of feldshers who were laid off is not known, but there were immediate complaints of ''wholesale dismissals.'' Another common tack was to reclassify feldshers as nurses without changing their duties, which amounted to a salary reduction.[67] Although the Conference on Auxiliary Medical Education had merely established guidelines, its commitment to ending feldsher practice tended to legitimize this kind of dismissal even after the budgetary crisis of 1922 abated, and reports of indiscriminate firings were widespread throughout the 1920s. In many cases feldshers were apparently dismissed without a physician to take their place.[68] This practice specifically violated Narkomzdrav's injunction that qualified feldshers in independent practice should not be removed until there was a physician to replace them.[69] Both Narkomzdrav and Medsantrud (Vsemediksantrud was shortened to Medsantrud in the mid-1920s) protested such indiscriminate dismissals and demotions,[70] but could do little to prevent them since local governments paid almost the entire salary of their medical workers.[71]

WHO SHOULD REPLACE THE FELDSHER?

If feldshers were to be eliminated, what kind of auxiliary medical practitioners were to take their place? In 1924 Narkomzdrav outlined four types of auxiliary personnel that it believed Narkompros should train in the coming years. The early Soviet medical system's emphasis on preventive medicine is evident in the descriptions of both the duties that these auxiliary personnel would perform and the qualifications they would need to do so.

Narkomzdrav first sought to develop a corps of "social assistance nurses" (*sestry sotsial'noi pomoshchi*). They were to work within the framework of the dispensary system, which lay at the heart of the system of preventive medicine envisaged by early Soviet health planners. The dispensary was an institution which ideally would have integrated the functions of therapeutic and prophylactic medicine in the most rational fashion possible. It was to be staffed by physicians who had special training in sanitation, sanitary education, and problems of early diagnosis. Most important, the dispensary and its staff were to be an integral part of community life.

As Narkomzdrav saw it, the role of the social assistance nurse in the dispensary system was "to connect what is done within the dispensary with what goes on in the family, the dormitory, the factory or the studio where the patient works, and to give the work of the dispensary a broad prophylactic character."[72] In brief, the social assistance nurse was to serve primarily as a source of sanitary and general preventive medical education. She (female identity was assumed) was to have mastered subjects such as hygiene (from home to workplace), childrearing, physical education, and sanitary legislation.[73] The very description of the social assistance nurse's sphere of activity outside the dispensary as "the family, the dormitory, the factory, or the studio" reveals Narkomzdrav's assumption that the dispensary system would initially be urban-based.

The second auxiliary position which Narkomzdrav defined in 1924 was the obstetric and pediatric nurse (*sestra po okhrane materinstva i mladenchestva*). This nurse, who was not a midwife, also had extensive duties concerned with preventive and sanitary medicine. Her work was to include everything from caring for infants in maternity wards to monitoring parental care of infant children at home. Narkomzdrav emphasized that such nurses should be gifted in struggling against the prejudices and superstitions that dominated popular attitudes toward maternal and infant care alike.[74] While trained pediatric nurses would have been invaluable in rural areas, the casual mention of maternity wards and the tacit assumption that their numbers would permit them ready access to the infant population indicates that Narkomzdrav planned to deploy them first in urban areas.

Hospital nurses (*sestry dlia lechebnykh uchrezhdenii*) were the third category of auxiliary personnel that Narkomzdrav sought to train. Their primary role was to care for the hospitalized patient, keeping track of his condition and summoning a physician when necessary. This job description closely corresponds to what the feldsher had done, except that the possibility of independent practice was not contemplated. Since most hospitals were either in provincial or district capitals, it was taken for granted that these nurses would be predominantly urban practitioners, although their role in rural medicine would clearly grow as the number of rural hospitals and clinics expanded.

The fourth type of auxiliary practitioner that Narkomzdrav sought to develop as of 1924 was the midwife. Echoing the sense of urgency that characterized pre-revolutionary obstetricians, Narkomzdrav's health planners emphasized that "providing the population with the most qualified possible obstetric care is an immediate, integral, and fundamental task of state power."[75] The chief reason for this urgency was the generally shared perception that, because of the distances involved, it would be decades before all parturient peasant women in Russia had reasonable access to an obstetric physician or maternity ward. Given this prognosis, Narkomzdrav sought to train a large corps of qualified and dedicated midwives who would "be able to work effectively not only in cities, in well-structured maternity wards, but on the periphery, in the conditions of rural life."[76] Narkomzdrav wanted midwives who, in addition to being able to manage normal deliveries on their own, could also diagnose abnormal circumstances quickly and either call for help or move the expectant mother to a hospital. In cases requiring immediate intervention, they were to deliver the child on their own (without, however, using any instruments). Like prerevolutionary health planners before them, Narkomzdrav officials looked to the midwife to reduce infant mortality in the countryside. She was also expected to know the principles of asepsis and antisepsis and to teach them to her peasant clientele. In the words of Narkomzdrav's planners, she "should be a sufficiently cultured worker, educated in the fields of biology and medicine, in order to serve as an authority amidst the surrounding ignorance, and be capable of struggling with the influence of *znakhari, znakharki, povitukhi* [traditional peasant midwives], and other exploiters of popular benightedness."[77]

Despite this emphasis on training qualified midwives for rural practice, so reminiscent of the zemstvo period, the condition of obstetric care in the countryside remained "catastrophic" throughout the 1920s.[78] In 1930, almost 90 percent of peasant women still gave birth either alone or with the help of a traditional midwife or *znakharka,* and prenatal consultations of any kind were rare.[79] This contrasted with considerable improvement in urban obstetric services. By 1927–28 there was prenatal care for almost 70 percent of urban Soviet women, a huge increase over the prewar figure. Almost 90 percent of urban births took place in a clinic or hospital.[80] Narkompros was unable to change overnight the kinds of schools and auxiliary medical personnel it was training, but it moved quickly to eliminate feldsher education. By 1928, exclusively feldsher schools no longer existed; of the 137 institutes preparing auxiliary personnel, only 5 were training feldsher-mid-wives.[81] There were also only five courses in the whole country in which *rotnye* feldshers could raise their qualifications to those of *shkol'nye*. The overwhelming majority of these auxiliary courses were training midwives, nurses, and pediatric nurses. Only two, however, were training "social assistance nurses," one in Mak-hach-Kala and the other in Simferopol'. The virtual absence of courses for such nurses suggests that local authorities, even in the capitals, did not consider them essential.[82]

During the early 1920s specialized medical *tekhnikumy* existed to train each category of auxiliary medical personnel. Gradually, however, the belief gained currency that, since such personnel all needed the same basic medical training, it would be more efficient to offer auxiliary medical education in large polytechnical medical institutes (*politekhnikumy*). In these institutes future midwives and nurses of all sorts would begin a common track of medical coursework; they would spec-ialize only later. Such an approach logically implied fewer but larger schools, each having sophisticated laboratories and equipment. This goal of establishing such auxiliary medical polytechnical institutes could not be implemented immediately, but, as of 1927, it became the official policy of Narkompros. By the early 1930s, such polytechnical institutes had become the main training ground for auxiliary medical personnel.[83]

PHYSICIANS AND FELDSHERS IN THE COUNTRYSIDE IN THE 1920s

In 1922, Sholomovich and other physicians had expressed confidence that physicians would willingly go to the countryside as soon as the rural economy improved, thereby rendering feldsher practice unnecessary. Several prominent physicians dis-puted this assumption, as we have seen, and time was to prove them correct.

Data collected in 1926 and 1929 illustrate the difficulty of attracting physicians to rural areas. On October 1, 1926, for example, out of 46,979 physicians in the country at large, only 6,471, or slightly under 14 percent, were practicing at rural posts. Almost 35 percent (16,298) were living in republic or provincial capitals, and 4,201, or almost 9 percent, were unemployed.[84] By April 1, 1929, the number of physicians in the country as a whole had grown impressively to 61,555. Of these, however, only 8,937, or slightly over 14 percent, were in exclusively rural practice. Just over 30 percent (18,650) of the country's total number of physicians worked in republic or provincial capitals, and 4,800, or about 8.5 percent, continued to be unemployed.[85]

These same statistical surveys illustrate the feldsher's ongoing importance in rural practice. In 1926, for example, with only 26,282 *shkol'nye* feldshers and feldsher-midwives employed in the country at large, 8,378 (almost one-third) were working at rural outposts. In addition, there were 4,972 *rotnye* feldshers in rural practice, out of a national total of 10,688. Thus in 1926 there were about 13,350 feldshers in exclusively rural practice.[86] These figures did not increase dramatically by 1929, but neither did they decline. On April 1, 1929, for example, there were 27,571 *shkol'nye* feldshers and feldsher-midwives employed in the whole country, of whom 8,589 (just over 31 percent) were assigned to rural posts. The number of *rotnye* feldshers in the country had also grown slightly, to 11,299, of whom 5,451, or almost half, were working in rural positions.[87] An even better indicator of the persistence of feldsherism was the fact that there were still 3,470 independent feldsher stations in rural areas in 1930.[88]

Why were physicians so reluctant to go to the countryside in the 1920s? Even more to the point, why was it so difficult to get physicians who were unemployed in cities to take up rural jobs? The difficulties that rural physicians faced were, after all, not new. In addition to the exhausting routine of treating patients, the psychological isolation, and the lack of cultural outlets that physicians had always endured in rural areas, a number of factors in the early Soviet period made rural service especially unattractive.

To begin with, the overall isolation which had always characterized the life of the rural intelligentsia had become much worse in the wake of the Civil War and remained so throughout the 1920s. On a more mundane level, throughout most of the 1920s physicians' salaries in rural areas were significantly lower than they were in cities.[89] Rural salaries were often not paid on time because of local budgetary difficulties, and physicians' financial problems were exacerbated by the difficulty of finding housing in many rural areas. Particularly in the early 1920s, the problem of salary had a direct impact on the physician's access to food. The rural physician endured the same shortages as the rest of the population, and in his weakened condition he was more vulnerable to the diseases he daily encountered.[90]

Commissar Semashko argued that the main reason physicians avoided the countryside was not low pay (although he conceded that pay was important) but, rather, the indifference and even outright hostility which many local authorities showed for the rural physician's professional as well as personal needs.[91] The physician arriving at a rural outpost was dependent on local authorities for housing and for the means of transportation which would allow him to visit patients living in outlying areas. When local authorities refused to provide an apartment, a horse, and other essential equipment, the physician was forced to acquire them using his own meager resources.[92] These working conditions contributed to the rapid turnover of medical personnel in the countryside, an endemic problem in the prerevolutionary period as well.

The dynamics of medical school recruitment also contributed to the shortage of physicians in the countryside. By the late 1920s, a large proportion of medical students were women, many of whom were bound to the city by family ties. This made it extremely difficult to dispatch them to the countryside for rural work. The feminization of the medical profession, a phenomenon which was well under way by the late 1920s, thus had a direct negative impact on rural medicine. Feminization, however, was only part of a more general underenrollment in medical schools in the late 1920s. The reason that young men in particular were not attracted to medical school was that they could attain a "more decent existence" by going to technical schools.[93] Becoming engineers and taking part in production was both more profitable and more in keeping with the Soviet regime's emphasis on industrial growth than was a career in medicine. Peasants were usually not sufficiently qualified for higher technical schools, but they could enter farming institutes. In any case they were not likely to become physicians.[94]

Physicians and feldshers also faced the threat of violence in the countryside. Peasant beatings or murders of medical personnel do not seem to have been related to the "specialist-baiting" so widespread in urban industrial settings during the late 1920s.[95] Instead, the peasantry's traditional suspicion of physicians had been exacerbated by the failures and shortcomings of the rural medical system in the 1920s. Here it is important to recall that peasants dealt with healers of all kinds in primarily personal terms. Thus physicians who had managed to win the confidence of the peasantry by virtue of long and successful practice were not likely to become targets of popular violence. But the general dearth of physicians in the countryside in the 1920s, coupled with the high turnover rate of those who were there, meant that peasant communities often did not know their local physician well. Where peasants lacked the trust that develops from such sustained ties, they tended to question the physician's performance whenever treatment failed or seemed to have resulted in death. Their periodic dissatisfaction was often well founded, and by no means "irrational." Many physicians in the countryside in the 1920s were recent graduates of medical school whose inexperience was compounded by a superficial training. They were overburdened, whatever their qualifications, and often lacked essential medications, bandages, and equipment. Their auxiliary and sanitary personnel were frequently involved in drunken and otherwise unprofessional behavior.[96]

The circumstances in which medical personnel were beaten or murdered varied from case to case, but on numerous occasions popular violence against medical personnel seems to have been provoked by newspaper articles or malpractice suits brought against a particular physician or feldsher. Medsantrud urged that frivolous malpractice suits and unfounded press attacks on medical personnel be stopped (without suggesting how one determined what was "frivolous" or "unfounded"), since they tended to undermine the authority that physicians needed in order to work effectively with a peasant population.[97]

Given the difficulty and disadvantages involved in rural practice, physicians who were employed in cities in the 1920s had no incentive at all to go to the countryside. Even many unemployed physicians refused to leave cities for rural jobs.[98] Some clearly dreaded the isolation of the provinces and the rigors of rural practice. Others preferred to remain close to large medical centers in the hope that a more appealing professional opportunity would turn up. Of those who chose to remain unemployed in cities rather than take a rural post, over 70 percent were women whose family ties and obligations bound them to the city.[99]

During the 1920s Narkomzdrav made a concerted effort to improve the living standards of physicians in the countryside and thereby to attract more physicians into rural practice. By a decree of 1925, for example, rural physicians were guaranteed free apartments, household services, and a 20 percent raise in salary every three years. Their children were to be given preferred status in admission to higher educational institutions. Most important, after three years of rural service they were to receive preferred treatment when applying for any vacant urban positions.[100]

In addition to these incentives, the Soviet regime tried a number of mechanisms to coerce physicians to go to the countryside. After 1925, it required all graduating medical students who had received a stipend to spend a year in rural service.[101] Unemployed physicians who refused rural employment were removed from the labor market, denied unemployment benefits, and dismissed from Medsantrud. In theory, they were ineligible for whatever urban jobs became available.[102] Yet, in order to be fully effective, these coercive measures required more coordination in enforcement than apparently existed, and a large number of unemployed urban physicians simply refused to go to the countryside no matter what the sanctions. Even among those who went, the turnover rate was extremely high, contributing to one physician's comment that physicians worked in the countryside "as if it were a military obligation, and flee their posts after a year at best."[103] In this regard, the early Soviet regime's tendency to glorify the urban proletariat while disparaging the peasantry as *petit bourgeois* doubtless curtailed what in earlier decades had been a populist instinct to go to the countryside to aid the peasantry.[104]

Both Narkomzdrav and Medsantrud recognized that, in the long run, the only way to attract qualified medical personnel to the countryside and keep them there was to create a more attractive life in rural areas. For the moment, it was essential to improve working conditions and protect medical personnel against the indifference and arbitrariness of local authorities.[105] Little was done in this regard during the 1920s, since local governments paid almost the entire salary of medical personnel and could treat them as they wished. In practice, neither Narkomzdrav nor Medsantrud possessed any effective means by which to protect medical personnel in the countryside.

THE RESURRECTION OF THE FELDSHER

During the 1920s it proved impossible to provide all rural residents with consistent access to a physician. The "face toward industrialization" that accompanied the First Five-Year Plan, together with the impoverishment of the village brought about by forced collectivization, made it even more difficult to supply the countryside with physicians. In particular, the famine in the Ukraine caused everyone who could to take refuge in the city.[106]

The feldsher's position in the countryside in the 1930s was also not an enviable or easy one. Rural feldshers not only witnessed the violence of collectivization, but also suffered from the same general deterioration in rural life that collectivization brought about. They were obliged in theory to take part in the assault on religion which was a major part of the "Great Break."[107] To the extent that they did, they drew on themselves the hostility of the majority of the community they served. Hungry, overburdened with work, and hopeful that the city might offer either a better job or an opportunity to requalify themselves as physicians, many feldshers simply left rural practice.[108]

Those who remained complained constantly that efforts to limit their authority in everyday practice seriously compromised their ability to serve the peasantry. In an effort to restrict the sphere of the feldsher's independent activity, for example, Narkomzdrav denied feldshers the right to write or renew prescriptions, to certify that peasants were unable to work because of illness or injuries sustained in fistfights, or even to possess common popular medicines. A feldsher's inability to testify to injuries or illness fundamentally undermined his authority in the village and could elicit popular hostility. As one feldsher complained: "No one can believe that a feldsher doesn't have the right to certify beatings, to dispense iodine salt, cod liver oil, turpentine, and so on, when private persons are selling these medicines right and left, when every citizen except the feldsher can buy and possess these items."[109]

Tacitly recognizing the impossibility of providing rural areas with adequate numbers of physicians within the immediate future, in the early 1930s the Soviet regime gradually resumed feldsher training within the framework of the *politekhnikum* system.[110] On September 8, 1936, it officially abolished these auxiliary medical polytechnical institutes, for whose advantages Narkomzdrav had argued with such force in the late 1920s, and resurrected feldsher schools.[111] The new law projected the recruitment of 44,770 students into feldsher schools in 1937 alone. While their training included emphasis on preventive medicine, many of those assigned to remote rural areas functioned—and continue to function today—as independent medical practitioners.[112]

Less than two decades after the Revolution, the regime that initially sought to eliminate feldshers and their practice now reversed itself. D. V. Gorfin, a participant in Soviet efforts to improve rural health as well as their chronicler, writes simply that "the task of liquidating feldsher stations, as the later development of rural medicine was to show, proved unrealizable."[113] This renewed commitment to training feldshers was a genuine defeat for those early Soviet physicians who had insisted that it was possible gradually to provide even remote peasants with access to a physician's care, and in the process to phase out feldsher practice altogether. From our own vantage point, the legislation of 1936 appears as a "reconciliation with reality" which would not have surprised those who had argued that the feldsher would be a necessary part of rural medicine in Russia for many years to come.

CONCLUSION

The fate of the feldsher mirrors the larger contours of early Soviet history. The idealistic and ambitious goal of providing a physician's care for every member of the Soviet population and eliminating the feldsher altogether conformed perfectly to the revolutionary enthusiasm of the early 1920s, as did the tendency to minimize the obvious practical difficulties involved. Those who insisted that the goals set forth were impossible to achieve in a short time—and there were many—were simply outvoted and ignored. During the New Economic Policy the status of health care in the countryside remained precarious, despite the emphasis that Narkomzdrav placed on it in theory. Finally, with the Great Break the countryside and the peasantry came to occupy a permanently second-rate position in Soviet society. The resurrection of the feldsher as a legitimate rural practitioner was but one recognition of this fact.

NOTES

I would like to thank the following organizations for their generous support in the writing of this article: the Tulane University Committee on Research, the National Endowment for the Humanities, the International Research and Exchanges Board, the Fulbright-Hays Fellowship Program, the Kennan Institute for Advanced Russian Studies of the Wilson Center, and the University of Illinois.

1. For a general discussion of the role of the commune in the 1920s see Moshe Lewin, *Russian Peasants and Soviet Power: A Study of Collectivization* (New York, 1975), pp. 81–106; Yuzuru Taniuchi, *The Village Gathering in Russia in the Mid-1920s* (Birmingham, 1968); D. J. Male, *Russian Peasant Organisation before Collectivisation: A Study of Commune and Gathering, 1925–1930* (Cambridge, 1971); E. H. Carr, *Foundations of a Planned Economy, 1926–1929*, 2 vols. (New York, 1969–71), 2: 236–49; Teodor Shanin, *The Awkward Class: Political Sociology of Peasantry in a Developing Society; Russia 1910–1925* (Oxford, 1972), pp. 162–99; and Dorothy Atkinson, *The End of the Russian Land Commune, 1905–1930* (Stanford, Calif., 1983), pp. 295–312.

2. Narkomzdrav RSFSR, *Statisticheskie materialy po sostoianiiu narodnogo zdraviia i organizatsii meditsinskoi pomoshchi v SSSR za 1913–1923 g. g.* (Moscow, 1926), p. xix.

3. Ibid.

4. Ibid.

5. The word *feldsher* was adapted from the German term for a military corpsman or paramedic. On the origins of feldsher practice in Russia, see Samuel C. Ramer, "Who Was the Russian Feldsher?" *Bulletin of the History of Medicine*, 50 (1976), pp. 213–25.

6. B. B. Veselovskii, *Istoriia zemstva za sorok let*, 4 vols. (St. Petersburg, 1909–11), I: 429. By 1921, in the wake of the Civil War, the portion of ambulatory patients treated by feldshers rather than physicians had risen to 38 percent, after which it began to fall. Narkomzdrav RSFSR, *Statisticheskie materialy*, p. xiii.

7. On the varieties of traditional peasant healers in Russia and the sources of their popular appeal see Samuel C. Ramer, "Traditional Healers and Peasant Culture in Russia, 1861–1917" in Esther Kingston-Mann and Timothy Mixter, eds., *Peasant Economy, Culture and Politics in European Russia, 1800–1917* (Princeton, N. J., 1990).

8. On "feldsherism" see Samuel C. Ramer, "The Zemstvo and Public Health," in Terence Emmons and Wayne S. Vucinich, eds., *The Zemstvo in Russia: An Experiment in Local Self-government* (Cambridge, 1982), pp. 292–98.

9. Z. G. Frenkel', *Ocherki zemskogo vrachebno-sanitarnogo dela* (St. Petersburg, 1913), pp. 121, 125.

10. *Spisok srednykh i nizshikh meditsinskikh shkol grazhdanskogo vedomstva v Rossii* (St. Petersburg, 1910), pp. xvi-xvii. For the reasons behind this transformation see Samuel C. Ramer, "The Transformation of the Russian Feldsher, 1864–1914," in Ezra Mendelsohn and Marshall S. Shatz, eds., *Imperial Russia, 1700–1917: State, Society, Opposition; Essays in Honor of Marc Raeff* (DeKalb, Ill., 1988), pp. 136–60.

11. Contrary to what health planners frequently asserted during the early Soviet period, the consolidation of these posts in the late tsarist period owed little to economic considerations. On efforts to improve rural obstetric care see Samuel C. Ramer, "Childbirth and Culture: Midwifery in the Nineteenth-Century Russian Countryside," in David L. Ransel, ed., *The Family in Imperial Russia: New Lines of Historical Research* (Urbana, Ill., 1978), pp. 218–35.

12. Nikolai Rudinskii, "Znakharstvo vo skopinskom i dankovskom uezdakh Riazanskoi gubernii," *Zhivaia starina*, 6, no. 2 (1896), pp. 174–77. Rudinskii's observations derive from his experience as a zemstvo physician during the 1880s.

13. The most important of these were *Fel'dsherskii vestnik* (1906–18), *Lekarskii pomoshchnik* (1906–7), and *Fel'dsherskaia mysl'* (1913–14).

14. *Fel'dsher* ceased publication in 1916 following Oks's retirement. At that point the Organization of Russian Feldshers merged with the larger Union of Societies of Physicians' Assistants.

15. Of these, the most influential were the three national congresses sponsored by the Union of Societies of Physicians' Assistants. For records of these congresses' deliberations see *Trudy pervogo Vserossiiskogo s"ezda fel'dsherov, fel'dsherits i akusherok s 20-go po 25-oe ianvaria 1907 goda v g. Moskve* (Moscow, 1907); *Trudy vtorogo Vserossiiskogo s"ezda fel'dsherov, fel'dsherits i akusherok s 10-go po 17-oe iiunia 1909 goda v g. Kieve* (Moscow, 1909); *Trudy tret'ego Vserossiiskogo s"ezda fel'dsherov, fel'dsherits i akusherok s 21-go po 27-oe iiunia 1912 goda v S-Peterburge* (Moscow, 1913).

16. P. A. Kalinin, "Doklad obshchemu sobraniiu Saratovskogo fel'dsherskogo obshchestva ob uchastii delegatov ot fel'dsherov v sanitarnykh sovetakh i v soveshchaniiakh vrachei," *Vrachebno-sanitarnaia khronika Saratovskoi gubernii*, 5–6 (May–June 1903): Prilozhenie k *Saratovskoi zemskoi nedeli*, 5 (May 1903), pp. 229–31.

17. For one physician's opposition to such feldsher participation see S. Igumnov, "Fel'dsherizm i sanitarnye sovety," *Vrachebnaia khronika Khar'kovskoi gubernii*, 10, no. 9 (September 1906), pp. 485–89. Igumnov was chairman of the Khar'kov provincial zemstvo's sanitary bureau.

18. For a list of these societies see P. Kalinin, *Profdvizhenie srednego meditsinskogo personala v Rossii. Istoricheskii ocherk* (Moscow, 1927), pp. 180–82.

19. *Dvenadsatyi delegatskii s"ezd Vserossiiskogo Soiuza soiuzov pomoshchnikov vrachei (8–14 maia n. st. 1918 g.)* (Moscow, 1918), pp. 5–6. Kalinin's figures are somewhat lower. He records that 279 new societies were established in 1917, bringing the total number of feldsher societies at the end of 1917 to 327. Kalinin, "Doklad," p. 49.

20. *Odinadtsatoe sobranie delegatov Vserossiiskogo Soiuza soiuzov pomoshchnikov vrachei (30 aprelia–4 maia 1917 g.). Rezoliutsii* (Moscow, 1917), p. 3.

21. Ibid.

22. A. Aluf, *Kratkaia istoriia professional'nogo dvizheniia medrabotnikov*, 3d ed. (Moscow, 1927), pp. 46–47.

23. *Vserossiiskii Soiuz zh.-d. rotnykh fel'dsherov.*

24. For the All-Russian Union of Physicians' Assistants this periodical was *Izvestiia Vserossiiskogo soiuza lekarskikh pomoshchnikov*, which ceased publication in late 1918. The All-Russian Union of Railroad *Rotnye* Feldshers published the *Vestnik zh.-d. fel'dsherov* briefly in 1918.

25. Kalinin, "Doklad," p. 50.

26. N. Popov, "1917-y god," *Fel'dsherskii vestnik*, 11, nos. 47–48 (December 15–23, 1917), pp. 586–87.

27. S. A. Fediukin, *Velikii Oktiabr' i intelligentsiia: iz istorii vovlechenii staroi intelligentsii v stroitel'stvo sotsializma* (Moscow, 1972), pp. 190–91.

28. Peter F. Krug, "Russian Public Physicians and Revolution: The Pirogov Society, 1917–1920" (Ph.D. diss., University of Wisconsin-Madison, 1979), p. 238.

29. By the mid-1920s, Vsemediksantrud (later Medsantrud), had a membership of 11.4 percent physicians, 7 percent *shkol'nye* feldshers and feldsher-midwives, 2.7 percent *rotnye* feldshers, 2.7 percent midwives, 8.1 percent male and female nurses, and 25.2 percent *mladshii* medical personnel. Overall, medical and dental personnel made up only 60.7 percent of the union; 28.5 percent were workers and service personnel, 7.3 percent were pharmaceutical personnel, and 3.5 percent veterinary personnel (statistics for 1926). A. Aluf, *Spravochnik srednego medpersonala (fel'dshera-tsy, sestry, akusherki)* (Moscow, 1928), pp. 13–14.

30. "Nasha pozitsiia," *Fel'dsherskii vestnik,* 12, nos. 41–44 (November 1–23, 1918), pp. 422–26. N. I. Popov, the editor of *Fel'dsherskii vestnik* who had been so adamant in his opposition to the Soviet regime, was in a minority by late 1918 and resigned.

31. Aluf, *Kratkaia istoriia,* p. 57.

32. Ibid., pp. 46–47.

33. Krug, "Russian Public Physicians," chap. 8.

34. The pioneering, mostly laudatory, studies of early Soviet medicine are Sir Arthur Newsholme and John Adams Kingsbury, *Red Medicine: Socialized Health in Soviet Russia* (Garden City, N. Y. 1934); and Henry E. Sigerist, *Socialized Medicine in the Soviet Union* (New York, 1937). For a more critical scholarly approach to the Soviet medical system see Mark G. Field, *Doctor and Patient in Soviet Russia* (Cambridge, Mass., 1957); and idem., *Soviet Socialized Medicine: An Introduction* (New York, 1967).

35. *Dekrety sovetskoi vlasti* (Moscow, 1964), 3: 141.

36. Krug, "Russian Public Physicians," p. 246. *Shkol'nye* feldshers, it should be noted, immediately objected that "the quick closing of feldsher schools would cause enormous harm to public health and force the population to resort to healers who have nothing in common with medicine." *Dvenadtsatyi delegatskii s"ezd Vserossiiskogo Soiuza soiuzov pomoshchnikov vrachei (8–14 maia n. st. 1918 g.),* p. 14.

37. L. F. Raukhvarger, "Fel'dsherskie shkoly," in L. F. Raukhvarger, ed., *Pervyi Vserossiiskii s'ezd po meditsinskomu obrazovaniiu* (Moscow, 1920), pp. 36, 71.

38. L. F. Raukhvarger, "Zavershenie medobrazovaniia fel'dsherov," in ibid., pp. 27–28.

39. E. K. Sepp, "Opyt uskorennogo prokhozhdeniia meditsinskogo fakul'teta okonchivshimi normal'nye fel'dsherskie shkoly," *1-aia Vserossiiskaia konferentsiia po srednemu meditsinskomu obrazovaniiu* (Moscow, 1922), pp. 25–26.

40. Two-thirds of the graduates of this accelerated program were between the ages of 26 and 35. Just over forty percent were of peasant origin, and about a quarter were of proletarian origin. *Revoliutsionnym putem—k znaniiu. Sbornik, posviashchennyi pervomu vypusku vrachei uskorennogo kursa meditsinskogo fakul'teta v Moskve* (Moscow, 1925).

41. Z. Chernyshev, "O prieme fel'dsherov na medfaki," *Meditsina,* no. 4 (April 1927), p. 9.

42. In 1930, when the First Five-Year Plan placed a renewed emphasis on the importance of trained cadres, numerous *shkol'nye* feldshers complained that they had not been able to take advantage of the various programs through which feldshers could become physicians. They urged the government to provide new and better opportunities for them to complete medical school. See *Meditsina,* no. 14 (July 1930), p. 16.

43. Narkomzdrav, *Tezisy i rezoliutsii tret'ego vserossiiskogo s"ezda zdravotdelov* (Moscow, 1921), p. 22.

44. By 1922 the training of auxiliary medical personnel had been transferred from Narkomzdrav to Narkompros, of which Glavprofobr (*Glavnyi komitet professional'no-tekhnicheskogo obrazovaniia*) was a subordinate department. The 1922 conference on auxiliary medical education was sponsored by Narkompros.

45. *1-aia Vserossiiskaia konferentsiia po srednemu meditsinskomu obrazovaniiu* (Moscow, 1922), p. 11.

46. Narkomzdrav RSFSR, *Statisticheskie materialy,* p. xxii.

47. *1-aia Vserossiiskaia konferentsiia po srednemu meditsinskomu obrazovaniiu,* p. 11.

48. Ibid.

49. Ibid.

50. Ibid.

51. Ibid.

52. Ibid., p. 17.

53. Ibid.

54. Ibid., pp. 13–14.

55. Ibid., p. 14.

56. Ibid., p. 16.

57. V. M. Banshchikov and N. I. Propper, *Srednee meditsinskoe obrazovanie* (Moscow, 1928), p. 119.

58. *1-aia Vserossiiskaia konferentsiia po srednemu meditsinskomu obrazovaniiu*, pp. 36–37.

59. Banshchikov and Propper, *Srednee meditsinskoe obrazovanie*, pp. 117–19.

60. Reports that the introduction of fees for services led to a rise in *znakharstvo* were widespread. See A. Vernyi, "Plenum pravleniia Tverskogo Gubotdela [Vsemediksantrud]," *Meditsinskii rabotnik*, no. 7 (September 10, 1922), pp. 5–6; and "Pskov," *Meditsinskii rabotnik*, no. 8 (October 15, 1922), p. 15.

61. P. S. Pozdniakov, quoted in A. Aluf, "K polozheniiu v uezdakh," *Meditsinskii rabotnik*, no. 7 (September 10, 1922), pp. 1–2.

62. A. Aluf, "K polozheniiu v uezdakh," *Meditsinskii rabotnik*, no. 7 (September 10, 1922), pp. 1–2.

63. Ibid.

64. D. V. Gorfin, "Lechebnaia pomoshch' rabochim, sluzhashchim i chlenam ikh semeistv na mestakh," *Meditsinskii rabotnik*, no. 10 (December 22, 1922), p. 5.

65. For a thorough analysis of the impact of the transfer of health care to local budgets see Christopher Davis, "Economic Problems of the Soviet Health Service: 1917–1930," *Soviet Studies*, 35, no. 3 (July 1983), pp. 343–61.

66. Ibid., p. 345.

67. Lekpom D. [Lekarskii pomoshchnik] "Likvidatsiia fel'dsherizma dybom," *Meditsina*, no. 1 (January 1927), p. 17.

68. A. Aluf, *Itogi shestogo vsesoiuznogo s"ezda Soiuza Medsantrud* (Moscow, 1926), p. 18; idem., *Itogi sed'mogo vsesoiuznogo s"ezda Soiuza Medsantrud* (Moscow, 1928), pp. 31–32.

69. *Biulleten' Narodnogo komissariata zdravookhraneniia*, no. 21 (November 5, 1923), p. 3.

70. Ibid.; also, Shestoi vsesoiuznyi s"ezd Medsantrud (3–12 iiunia 1926 g.), *Rezoliutsii i postanovleniia*, 2d ed. (Moscow, 1926), p. 69.

71. Davis, "Economic Problems," p. 352.

72. Banshchikov and Propper, *Srednee meditsinskoe obrazovanie*, p. 139.

73. Ibid., pp. 139–40.

74. Ibid.

75. Ibid., p. 141.

76. Quoted in ibid.

77. Quoted in ibid., p. 142. For similar proposals in the prerevolutionary period, see G. E. Rein, *Rodovspomozhenie v Rosii (Sbornik dokladov na IX Pirogovskom s"ezde)* (St. Petersburg, 1906).

78. V. P. Lebedeva, "Okhrana materinstva i mladenchestva," *Shestoi vserossiiskii s"ezd zdravotdelov. Sputnik delegata s"ezda* (Moscow, 1927), p. 267.

79. S. Erman, "Okhrana materinstva i zadachi akusherki," *Meditsina*, nos. 17–18 (September 1930), pp. 11–13.

80. Ibid.

81. These schools for feldsher-midwives were sanctioned as temporary expedients in provincial capitals such as Arkhangel'sk, Vladivostok, and Krasnoiarsk.

82. Banshchikov and Propper, *Srednee meditsinskoe obrazovanie*, appendix 2, pp. 33–46. Since 57 of the 137 auxiliary medical institutes reporting in 1928 did not list their programs of study specifically, these figures can only give a general impression.

83. On the establishment of auxiliary medical polytechnical institutes see ibid., pp. 155–71.

84. Vsesoiuznyi professional'nyi soiuz Medsantrud, *Statisticheskii sbornik*, 1st ed. (Moscow, 1928), pp. 124–27.

85. Vsesoiuznyi professional'nyi soiuz Medsantrud, *Statisticheskii sbornik,* 3d ed. (Moscow, 1930), p. 24.

86. Vsesoiuznyi professional'nyi soiuz Medsantrud, *Statisticheskii sbornik,* 1st ed. (Moscow, 1928), pp. 124–25. The available statistics lump *shkol'nye* feldshers and feldsher-midwives together, making it impossible to judge the proportion between them. This is unfortunate, since it gives no indication of how many female feldsher-midwives were engaged in rural practice.

87. Vsesoiuznyi professional'nyi soiuz Medsantrud, *Statisticheskii sbornik,* 3d ed. (Moscow, 1930), p. 24.

88. M. Vladimirskii, *Ocherednye zadachi zdravookhraneniia* (Moscow, 1930), p. 20.

89. Aluf, *Itogi sed'mogo vsesoiuznogo s"ezda,* p. 21.

90. For a report reflecting these kinds of conditions in 1920 see the short entry "Irkutsk," *Meditsinskii rabotnik,* 2, nos. 5–8 (September 1, 1920), pp. 31–32.

91. Certainly this was not entirely new, given the tension between local governments and the medical personnel they hired in the prerevolutionary period. See Nancy M. Frieden, *Russian Physicians in an Era of Reform and Revolution, 1856–1905* (Princeton, N. J., 1981).

92. N. A. Semashko, "Sostoianie dela zdravookhraneniia i ego zadachi," *Trudy shestogo vserossiiskogo s"ezda zdravotdelov* (3–9 maia 1927) (Moscow, 1927), pp. 22, 27, 30.

93. Vladimirov, "Obespechenie strany medpersonalom," *Trudy shestogo vserossiiskogo s"ezda zdravotdelov,* p. 161.

94. Ibid, pp. 161–62.

95. For a full discussion of "specialist-baiting" see Kendall E. Bailes, *Technology and Society under Lenin and Stalin: Origins of the Soviet Technical Intelligentsia, 1917–1941* (Princeton, N. J., 1978), pp. 69–156.

96. A. Aluf, "Itogi vsesoiuznogo s"ezda Medsantrud (3–12 iiunia, 1926)," *Shestoi vsesoiuznyi s"ezd Medsantrud (3–12 iiunia 1926: Rezoliutsiia i postanovleniia,* 2d ed (Moscow, 1926), p. 17.

97. Aluf, *Kratkaia istoriia,* p. 115.

98. Ibid.

99. Shestoi vsesoiuznyi s"ezd Medsantrud (3–12 iiunia 1926 g.), *Rezoliutsiia i postanovleniia,* 2d ed. (Moscow 1926), p. 70.

100. P. I. Kal'iu and N. N. Morozov, eds., *Postanovleniia KPSS i Sovietskogo pravitel'stva ob okhrane zdorov'ia naroda* (Moscow, 1958), pp. 112–13.

101. Ibid.

102. Aluf, *Itogi sed'mogo vsesoiuznogo s"ezda,* p. 40.

103. "Preniia po dokladam t.t. Vladimirova i Proppera," *Trudy shestogo vserossiiskogo s"ezda zdravotdelov,* p. 171.

104. Mark Field suggests that refusal to go the countryside may have been a sign of protest against the Soviet regime. This does not seem to have been a major factor in the 1920s. Field, *Doctor and Patient in Soviet Russia,* p. 80.

105. Ibid., p. 40.

106. This was true of feldshers as well as physicians. See Vasily Grossman, *Forever Flowing,* tr. Thomas P. Whitney (New York, 1972), p. 154. Quoted in Robert Conquest, *The Harvest of Sorrow: Soviet Collectivization and the Terror-Famine* (New York, 1986), p. 246.

107. V. Shishakov, "Antipaskhal'naia kampaniia i medrabotniki," *Meditsina,* no. 7 (April 1930), p. 2.

108. "Pis'ma chitatelei," *Meditsina,* no. 1 (January 1930), p. 14.

109. "Pis'ma chitatelei," *Meditsina,* no. 4 (February 1930), p. 14.

110. Sigerist, *Socialized Medicine in the Soviet Union,* p. 144.

111. "O podgotovke srednikh meditsinskikh, zubovrachebnykh i farmatsevticheskikh kadrov." (Postanovlenie SNK SSSR ot 8 sentiabria 1936 g.), in Kal'iu and Morozov, *Postanovleniia KPSS,* p. 273.

112. On the continuing difficulties which the Soviet regime experienced in getting phy-

sicians to go to the countryside and the persistence of independent feldsher practice see Field, *Doctor and Patient in Soviet Russia,* pp. 95–101. On the importance of the contemporary rural feldsher see Lillian Liu, ''Rural Feldshers and the Public Health in the Soviet Union,'' unpublished paper delivered at the Southern Conference on Slavic Studies, October 19–20, 1979.

113. D. V. Gorfin, *Ocherki istorii razvitiia sel'skogo zdravookhraneniia SSSR (1917–1959 gg.)* (Moscow, 1961), p. 76.

CHRISTOPHER M. DAVIS

Economics of Soviet Public Health, 1928–1932

Development Strategy, Resource Constraints, and Health Plans

In the late 1920s the Soviet Union was an underdeveloped nation trying to solve or ameliorate a wide range of serious problems with scarce domestic resources and little outside assistance. In this context the health sector was under particular stress. The already poor state of national health was aggravated by the low average standard of living of the population, inadequate public sanitation and water supply, and illiteracy. Disease rates were high by European standards and there was a substantial backlog of untreated illness. During the twenties there had been some expansion of the facilities, personnel, and services of the state-financed, territorial-based medical system, as well as improvements in its management. Nevertheless, the general quality and effectiveness of curative medical services remained low; medical facilities experienced chronic shortages of all types of inputs (labor, capital, pharmaceuticals); and the medical system was unable to supply sufficient preventive or curative medicine to satisfy demand. Furthermore, as a result of inertia and of conscious decisions by health administrators, there was significant social and geographic inequality in the distribution of medical care.

The policy of rapid industrialization adopted by the Bolshevik party in 1928 posed new challenges for the health service. That policy resulted in large-scale population movements to cities and industrial regions, growing threats to public sanitation, increased demands for medical care from workers covered by social insurance, and rising opportunity costs of illness. The party and government demanded that health administrators develop an appropriate strategy to cope with this situation. Yet, the Stalinist leadership also made it clear that in the immediate future priority would be given to investment over consumption and to heavy industry over welfare services. Thus the task facing decisionmakers in health was to obtain the best performance from the medical system and the most equitable distribution of services given severe constraints on anticipated resources.

As the Soviet economy shifted from the market-oriented system that prevailed under the New Economic Policy (NEP) to a centrally planned one, the leading organization in the health field, the Commissariat of Public Health RSFSR (Narkomzdrav), was asked to express its strategy in a five-year plan. Two alternative strategies were proposed to guide the development of the Soviet medical system during the first five-year plan period. Initially, in 1928–29, Narkomzdrav, with the support of the RSFSR State Planning Committee (Gosplan RSFSR), prepared a plan that called for a modest expansion of the health service consistent with the anticipated levels of resources and for the maintenance of a territorial health system that distributed medical care primarily on the basis of need. In 1929, as it became increasingly clear that the optimal variant of the general plan for the national economy would be adopted, the first health plan was strongly criticized. The critics advocated a different strategy: it called for the rapid growth of a medical system oriented to providing care at the place of work, with preference given to patients in those socioeconomic groups deemed most important by political authorities. The institutions associated with this second approach included the Council of People's Commissars RSFSR (Sovnarkom), Gosplan USSR, the trade unions, and social insurance agencies.

Given the political climate of that time, sharp conflicts between these two opposing groups of actors came to the fore in the debate over the formulation of the health plan. In the end, some party leaders intervened to end the dispute in favor of supporters of the second plan variant. The intervention resulted in a purge of Narkomzdrav, the adoption of an ambitious five-year plan for health, and a restructuring of the medical system.

This essay analyzes the reasons for the "great turnabout"(*velikii povorot*) in the Soviet health service in 1929–30 and traces its consequences. Two sets of questions are addressed. The first concerns the conditions in the health care sector and the challenges of health planning. How severe were the problems confronting the medical system by the end of the 1920s? To what extent did the first plan drawn up by Narkomzdrav reflect an awareness of the severity of the problems? Is it possible to argue that the second variant of the plan of 1930 was more realistic than the first? The second set of questions relates to the politics of the economic planning process itself, a subject very much on the research agenda since E. H. Carr and R. W. Davies's authoritative study of Soviet economic planning in the 1920s.[1] Why did Narkomzdrav propose and defend a five-year health plan that appeared inconsistent with the announced objectives of some of the most powerful party leaders? Did Gosplan as a supracommissariat have a better understanding of political requirements, social needs, and resource availability than did the more narrowly oriented Narkomzdrav RSFSR? Finally, what does this case study of institutional conflict over the health plan reveal about the broader phenomenon of bureaucratic politics in the Soviet Union in this period?

THE STATE OF THE MEDICAL SYSTEM IN 1927–28

In the period 1923/27 the Soviet health sector recovered from the damage and disruption caused by war, economic collapse, and political upheaval.[2] As S. G. Wheatcroft has shown, improvements in the agricultural sector resulted in a rapid increase in per capita consumption of food.[3] This combined with better public hygiene, health education, and preventive medicine to lower the rates of virtually all infectious diseases. For example, from 1923 to 1927 the number of reported cases of smallpox in the USSR dropped from 46 to 15 thousand and of malaria from 5.7 to 3.7 million.

As Neil Weissman points out in his essay in this volume, during the 1920s there were substantial developments in the organization of medical care in the USSR, but no central authority was charged with planning and managing the national health service.[4] Instead, most medical facilities were controlled by the republican-level commissariats of public health. Of these, Narkomzdrav RSFSR was the oldest, having been created in July 1918. It was headed by N. A. Semashko, a doctor and long-standing Bolshevik party member.[5] By 1928, Narkomzdrav RSFSR had a large and experienced staff, a well-developed structure, and a clear strategy.[6] This agency played a leading role in the health area and tried to carry out objective analyses of the health situation and to defend the public medical system while adhering to socialist principles. Nevertheless, health care in the 1920s was still a low priority and its bureaucracy was weak relative to other commissariats. As a result Narkomzdrav was sometimes forced to adopt measures and programs that ran counter to its desires.[7] Below the republican level were the *oblast*, city, and rural district health departments. Some of these, such as the Moscow Oblast Health Department, were staffed by competent medical specialists committed to the ideals of a national, territorial-based health service and a preventive approach to medicine.[8] But many other lower administrative units were ill-equipped to fulfill their growing responsibilities and tended to follow the path of least resistance.

While expenditures on the Soviet medical system increased significantly during the NEP period (from 140.2 million rubles in 1923–24 to 384.9 million rubles in 1926/27,[9] resulting in improvements in virtually all medically related input and output indicators[10]), the medical system remained seriously deficient in many respects. In an effort to improve the situation Narkomzdrav RSFSR attempted to obtain additional resources and launched several major campaigns to promote cost-effective public sanitation based on prevention, upgrade rural medical care, and raise economic efficiency in medical institutions.

Throughout the 1920s there was much discussion in the USSR of the need for preventive medicine (for example, immunization, health education) as well as for broader programs to improve public health (for example, those that improved housing, sanitation, and water supply).[11] According to a Soviet medical analyst of the 1920s, D. Gorfin, the Fifth Congress of Health Departments in the summer of 1924 was a "turning point" in the activities of the medical system, after which strenuous attempts were made to give all aspects of health service work a preventive orientation.[12] This appears to be an exaggeration. The preventive medicine campaign was gradually undermined by the resistance of traditional curatively oriented doctors, as well as that of social insurance and trade union officials who defended their closed medical facilities and the privileged treatment of industrial workers.[13] Furthermore, medical staff did not have spare time to devote to retraining in preventive medicine and there were insufficient capital funds to finance the conversion of existing facilities into dispensaries. Consequently, by 1927/28 public sanitation and preventive medicine were still underdeveloped branches of the health service.

A second campaign was devoted to improving rural medicine. Throughout 1924/25 there was much discussion of the backward state of medical care in the countryside and exhortations were made by Narkomzdrav to local authorities to increase expenditure on the construction of rural medical facilities, to attract more doctors to the countryside, and to reduce urban-rural inequalities.[14] The convocation in December 1925 of the First All-Union Congress of Microdistrict Doctors and the publication of decrees concerning rural medicine indicated high-level support for this remedial campaign.[15] Nevertheless, in the mid-1920s few resources were available to correct the widespread deficiencies in rural medical care, and, in any event, both the state apparatus and the infrastructure that supported it in the countryside were underdeveloped. Thus this campaign, too, was unsuccessful.

The third campaign was the "regime of economy" in the health service.[16] In February 1926 a national economy-wide drive was initiated to cut costs, rationalize production, and increase labor productivity. An attempt was made in June to introduce a similar campaign in the medical system. Most medical staff opposed this program because they were aware that the main problem was lack of resources, not inefficiency in their utilization.[17] Some administrators did respond energetically to the call for economies, usually to the detriment of staff and patients:

> One administrator, with the objective of economizing in mind, decided to heat water for the baths of medical personnel once a month, and not each week as it had been before the regime; another started to administer less medicine to patients; a third hit upon the idea of using milk instead of serum; a fourth proposed in his budget that the horse of the district doctor, used for home visits, be cut and that the health department statistician be eliminated, etc.[18]

The failure of these campaigns meant that by 1928 Narkomzdrav was confronting many of the same problems that had plagued it five years earlier. Meanwhile, in the 1927/28 budget year, Narkomzdrav received less funding from social insurance authorities than had been projected. In the RSFSR an allocation from the social insurance Fund of Medical Assistance (FMA) of 208 million rubles would have been required to maintain real per capita spending on medical care for the insured. Instead, only 175.5 million rubles were spent.[19] The three other sources of health finance (state budget, local budget, and special means) did increase sufficiently to ensure that total health spending in the RSFSR rose from 384.9 million rubles in 1926/27 to 410.5 in 1927/28. But this represented a decline in real terms and an insignificant rise in per capita health spending from 3.82 to 3.94 rubles. According to a July 1928 assessment by the Collegium of Narkomzdrav RSFSR, the health service in 1927/28 was in a "strained" general financial position and the situation in industrial regions was "especially debilitating."[20]

The financial crisis in 1927/28 had both short- and long-term consequences for the national medical system. Its immediate effects were evident in the deterioration of medical care in Moscow and other industrial regions.[21] In a critical report on the health situation in 1927–28 the commissar of health RSFSR, Semashko, noted that the medical system was woefully inadequate: hospitals refused assistance on a mass scale, outpatient clinics were plagued by queues and overcrowding, patient food norms in hospitals were insufficient, and there were chronic shortages of all medical supplies.[22] In addition, the wages paid to medical staff were low relative to other sectors and to prerevolutionary levels.[23] This adversely affected motivation and the quality of services provided.

The long-term effects of the financial situation were two-fold. First, it undermined the program of capital repair and new construction, which had been receiving a disproportionately high share of support from social insurance medical funds. In the Moscow region, for example, expenditures on new construction fell from 7.4 million rubles in 1926/27 to 5.2 million rubles in 1927/28.[24] Second, it intensified the dissatisfaction of trade unions and the Central Social Insurance Administration of the People's Commissariat of Labor (Narkomtrud) with the procedures used by Narkomzdrav to allocate medical services to insured workers on a privileged basis. Throughout the twenties, as Sally Ewing argues in her essay in this volume, Narkomzdrav and social insurance authorities were in conflict.[25] But by 1928 the complaints of the latter may have convinced decisionmakers in state bureaucracies such as Gosplan USSR that in the future special measures would have to be implemented to protect the medical care of the industrial proletariat from the adverse consequences of economic disruptions.

The impact of the financial constraints on the Soviet medical system in 1927/28 did not fall equally across all sectors and groups. At that time there existed several "closed" subsystems which provided medical care for the Bolshevik party elite, the Red Army, and railway workers. Within the public territorial health service substantially more was spent on the city inhabitants than on peasants, on insured workers (and their families) than on the uninsured, and on the regions of European Russia than on more remote ones. Table 1 provides an estimate of the inequality of health spending in the RSFSR in 1927/28.

Unequal spending, of course, resulted directly in inequality in medical care provision. The insured also received most of their treatment in better endowed urban facilities (91.5 per cent of their hospitalization was in cities) and "in scientific and central establishments the insured obtain 89 percent of bed-days and 90.6 percent of outpatient visits."[26]

When considered in concert, all these indicators show that the Soviet medical system in 1928 was, in fact, in better shape than it had been in 1923. The numbers of facilities and medical staff had grown, financial support was at higher levels, and the output of medical services had increased substantially. Nevertheless, health conditions remained poor, the quantity of medical care supplied to the population was insufficient, its quality was low, and distribution of medical services was unequal. The campaign for the "regime of economy" revealed that there were few untapped internal reserves and that the instability of external sources of finance, such as the social insurance funds, impeded development of the medical system. In sum, this was not a health service that was in a good position to respond to major new challenges.

TABLE 1
Inequality in Health Spending in the RSFSR, 1927–28

Population Group	Distribution of Population		Total Health Expenditures		Per Capita Health Expenditures
	Thousands	%	Millions of Rubles	%	Rubles
Total Population	104,188	100.0	410.5	100.0	3.94
Insured	17,395	16.7	320.8	78.2	18.44
Uninsured	86,793	83.3	89.7	21.8	1.03
Urban Insured	14,786	14.2	292.6	71.3	19.79
Rural Insured	2,609	2.5	28.2	6.9	10.81
Urban Uninsured	3,030	2.9	29.4	7.1	9.70
Rural Uninsured	83,763	80.4	60.3	14.7	0.72

Sources: See Appendix A

THE FIRST VARIANT OF THE FIVE-YEAR PLAN FOR HEALTH

Prior to 1928/29 the Soviet medical system did not operate in accordance with a plan, although some work on health planning was carried out during the 1920s. In December 1925 the Planning Commission of Narkomzdrav RSFSR prepared a rough ten-year "general plan" covering the years 1926–1936 for several medical branches and regions of the RSFSR.[27] The first control figures for the health service were prepared by the Socio-Cultural Section of Gosplan RSFSR for 1926/27 and 1927/28 fiscal years, but these were imperfect documents.[28] Despite the instructions of May 1927 from Narkomzdrav RSFSR to local departments to prepare draft five-year plans, little progress was made over the next year.[29]

During the course of 1928 this situation began to change. At the First Narkomzdrav Planning Conference in early April, deficiencies in past plans were criticized and a first draft of a financial plan for the medical system covering the years 1927/28 through 1931/32 was presented.[30] This plan did not remain in effect for long. On April 26 Narkomzdrav changed the five-year plan period to 1928/29–1932/33 and ordered an acceleration of preparations of the medium-term plan and the 1928/29 control figures.

In its subsequent attempts to prepare the draft of the five-year plan, the Planning Commission of Narkomzdrav RSFSR worked closely and compatibly with the Socio-Cultural Section of Gosplan RSFSR. But the work was hindered by several immediate problems. First, declining standards of living in urban areas apparently generated dissatisfaction among workers and increased pressure on welfare service organizations to safeguard existing levels of social consumption.[31] In 1928 the trade unions and the social insurance authorities criticized Narkomzdrav for neglecting the medical needs of insured workers. This forced health administrators to maintain per capita expenditures on the insured, despite the cut in the fund of medical assistance, and to safeguard their head-of-queue privileges.[32] Second, uncertainty remained over future spending on health by local government and social insurance agencies. Third, the five-year national economic plan was undergoing substantial revisions, which made it difficult to provide a firm foundation for health sector planning.

The 1928/29 Gosplan RSFSR control figures for the health service were published in January 1929.[33] They projected a 16 percent increase in total health expenditure, to 477.9 million rubles. The anticipated increments of most health indicators were fairly modest. Hospital bed provision was to rise by 5.6 percent and the number of doctors by 6.9 percent. But respective per capita indicators were to go up by less than 2 percent. These targets were consistent with those of the health plan that was being prepared by Narkomzdrav.

The Second Narkomzdrav Planning Conference in February 1929 discussed the first variant of the five-year plan for the medical system.[34] This draft plan was subsequently published in the document *Tezisy po piatiletnemu perspektivnomu planu zdravookhraneniia RSFSR*, which included an introductory essay by Commissar Semashko, entitled "Health Policy during the Five-Year Plan.[35] Although Semashko claimed that the plan targets were realistic and the plan correctly formulated, he was clearly unhappy about the inadequate level of medical care in the RSFSR in 1927/28 and considered the targets too low to alter the situation radically by 1932/33.

The financial section of the plan projected a growth in total RSFSR health expenditure from 410.5 million rubles in 1927/28 to 850.9 million rubles in 1932/33 (see Table 2). But concern was expressed about the likelihood of obtaining this financing given continuing uncertainty over social insurance funds and local budgets. From the *Tezisy* and the Gosplan RSFSR control figures it is clear that major obstacles to plan fulfillment were also envisaged in the area of capital construction.[36]

Problems of labor were anticipated as well. The average wage of doctors was to increase from 114 rubles in 1927/28 to 220 in 1932/33. But this would only bring it up to prerevolutionary levels in real terms, whereas the wages of qualified labor in industry would be 150 percent of the 1913 standard.[37] Furthermore, the growth of positions for doctors in the medical system was expected to increase substantially more than the supply. To cover this gap, doctors would have to hold multiple positions in medical establishments. The plan assumed that each doctor in 1932/33 would simultaneously occupy 1.33 positions, which implies that his or her work load would be 33 percent above normal.

THE MEDICAL SYSTEM IN 1929

In 1929, developments in the economy contributed to a worsening of health conditions, increased pressure on the medical system, and financial constraints on the

TABLE 2

Projected RSFSR Health Expenditure in the First and Second Variants of the First Five-Year Health Plan, 1928/29–1932/33

Millions of Rubles

Source of Finance	1927/28		1928/29		1929/30	1930/31	1932/33	1931/32		TOTAL (1928/29–1932/33)		
	First Variant (actual)	Second Variant (actual)	First Variant (actual)	Second Variant (actual)	Second Variant (target)	Second Variant (target)	Second Variant (target)	First Variant (target)	Second Variant (target)	First Variant	Second Variant	Second as % of First
State Budget	45.6	40.2	48.7	35.7	35.4	65.1	88.8	85.8	119.2	325.4	344.2	106
Local Budget	167.4	168.4	198.6	213.0	278.5	400.0	583.6	388.0	864.3	1,460.0	2,339.4	160
Fund of Medical Assistance	175.5	178.5	207.0	188.7	228.7	340.0	492.5	336.6	742.7	1,322.9	1,992.6	151
Special Means	22.0	17.0	23.6	18.8	20.8	23.5	26.0	28.5	29.0	168.7	118.1	70
Subtotal	410.5	404.1	477.9	456.2	563.4	828.6	1,190.9	838.9	1,755.2	3,277.0	4,794.3	146
Other Expenditures[1]	—	14.2	—	19.2	54.6	162.0	238.5	12.0	338.1	100.0	812.4	812
TOTAL	410.5	418.3	477.9	475.4	618.0	990.6	1,429.4	850.9	2,093.3	3,377.0	5,606.7	166

Note: (1) Includes (a) industry, (b) state farms, (c) collective farms,
(d) local communities, (e) wage funds, (f) resort funds,
(g) pharmacies, (h) cooperatives, (i) Commissariat of Railways,
(j) other sources.

Sources: First Variant: Narkomzdrav RSFSR, *Tezisy po Piatiletnemu Perspektivnomu Planu Zdravookhraneniya RSFSR,* Moscow-Leningrad, 1929.
Second Variant: Narkomzdrav RSFSR, *Materialy k Piatiletnemu Planu Zdravookhraneniya RSFSR,* Moscow-Leningrad, 1930

provision of health care. The mediocre 1929 harvest led to a disruption of food supply and light industry production, substantial rises of agricultural prices in private markets, food rationing, and a decline in real wages.[38] Rapid migration to the cities and a 38 percent underfulfillment of the 1928/29 housing construction plan severely strained housing supply and adversely affected urban areas and worker settlements.

In April 1928 the projected total RSFSR expenditure on health in 1928/29 had been 490.5 million rubles. Owing to reduced expectations about social insurance contributions, the January 1929 control figures had a lower target of 477.9 million rubles. The new target for the territorial FMA fell from 177.7 to 169.8. In March 1929, however, the government decided to allocate only 151 million rubles to health from the FMA.[39] Subsequent reports indicate that actual expenditure from the territorial funds was 153.3 million rubles and from transport FMA 35.4, for an FMA total of 188.7 million rubles. This was 9 percent below control figures.

Final health expenditure from the state budget in 1928/29 was 35.7 million rubles, or 27 percent below the control figure, while special means spending was 18.8 million rubles or 20 percent lower. These reductions meant that considerable pressure was put on local government to make compensatory increases in health finance. Although the health share of local budgets remained constant at 13.4 percent in 1928/29, the rapid growth in the total budget generated expenditure of 213 million rubles on the medical system. In consequence, total health finance in 1928/29 was 456.2 million rubles, or 95.5 percent of the control figure. In real terms, this was equivalent to the 1927/28 level.

During 1929, work on the Five-Year Plan for health intensified. At the Sixteenth Bolshevik Party Conference, the first variant prepared by Narkomzdrav RSFSR and Gosplan RSFSR was severely criticized for two main defects: its projected slow rate of growth and its failure to incorporate a "proletarian class line" in distributional plans. It is likely that a major figure behind this criticism was M. F. Vladimirskii, who was then chairman of the Central Revision Commission VKP(b) and in 1930 became commissar of health RSFSR.[40]

In response to the dissatisfaction expressed at the party conference, the Planning Commission of Narkomzdrav passed a resolution in May 1929 calling for "significant correctives and supplements in all plans."[41] At the Third Planning Conference of Narkomzdrav in September a decision was made to raise the targets of the 1929/30 control figures above equivalent levels of the Five-Year Plan.[42] In October Narkomzdrav RSFSR was reorganized and a new powerful Planning Administration was created.[43]

One of the most contentious issues in the health planning debate was the extent to which insured workers should be given preferential treatment. In early 1929 social insurance agency and trade union authorities attacked Narkomzdrav for not utilizing all FMA resources exclusively for the care of the insured. A Narkomzdrav study disputed this and argued that "the insurance resources are fully spent on the insured and that in addition a supplement of 30 percent of this sum is spent on medical assistance for the insured from budget sources."[44] Nevertheless, the deterioration of medical care in industrial regions kept up the pressure on Narkomzdrav to adopt measures which would ensure that the urban proletariat and peasants in socialized agriculture would continue to enjoy priority in the health care system.

In June 1929 the Collegium of Narkomzdrav stated that in the "second stage" of planning care was being taken to concentrate most of the projected increases in medical services on the insured. They were to obtain 93.3 percent of the anticipated 16.1 million additional hospital bed-days during the Five-Year Plan period. To some even this scale of inequality was insufficient. In July Sovnarkom RSFSR criticized Narkomzdrav's plans and ordered it to prepare within five months a revised plan which would demonstrate a commitment to "broadening and improving medical assistance to the insured."[45] This particular intervention may have been the result of the fact that in May 1929 A. I. Rykov, who was associated with the right-opposition, was replaced as the head of Sovnarkom RSFSR by S. I. Syrtsov.[46]

Over the next several months additional criticisms were made of the inadequate "proletarian class orientation" of the plan. The situation was complicated in November at the All-Russian Conference on Medical Assistance for the Socialist Sector of the Village hosted by Narkomzdrav RSFSR. Delegates criticized medical care in the countryside, called for a shift in rural health strategy toward one of preferential treatment of members of the socialized sector of agriculture, and demanded appropriate adjustments in the five-year health plan and the 1929/30 capital construction program.[47]

The 1929/30 control figures for the national economy were ratified by a plenary session of the Bolshevik party Central Committee in November 1929.[48] A month later Gosplan RSFSR published its health control figures.[49] These targets were marginally more ambitious than the ones of the first variant Five-Year Plan, although continued emphasis was placed on financial difficulties. Expenditure on health from the four main sources was to increase by 20 percent, to 557.2 million rubles, and an additional contribution of 56.5 million rubles from industry was anticipated, bringing total finance of health to 613.7 million rubles, or 42 million more than the Five-Year Plan target.

Although Narkomzdrav RSFSR, Gosplan RSFSR, and subordinate organizations, such as the Moscow Oblast Health Department, attempted to adjust plans and policies in accordance with the directives of higher party and government bodies during 1929, it is evident that they resisted calls both for overly ambitious planning and for the reorientation of medical care from the territorial principle to one based on the socioeconomic importance of patients. This reluctance dissatisfied a range of powerful institutions in the USSR, including Sovnarkom RSFSR, Gosplan USSR, the social insurance authorities, trade union officials, and Vladimirskii himself. Given the political climate of the time, Narkomzdrav's resistance to directives was viewed as an expression of "right" opposition and a challenge to central authority. This interpretation was clearly expressed in an assessment of the situation in 1929 by the head of the Health Sector of Gosplan USSR, M. I. Barsukov, and his assistant, A. P. Zhuk.[50]

This ideological criticism, coupled with the growing urgency of health problems, the continuing complaints by trade unions and social insurance bodies, and the prevailing political environment, made it almost inevitable that the central authorities would intervene to bring the medical system under firmer control. The first target was the Moscow Oblast Health Department. As mentioned above, its leaders favored territorial-based preventive medicine and were critical of closed, occupational health services and of inequality in medical care provision.[51] For failing to introduce a firm proletarian class line in medicine, and perhaps for supporting too enthusiastically the "united dispensaries," the top staff of the Moscow Oblast Health Department was purged in October 1929. Obukh was removed from his positions of chief of the Health Department and editor of the *Biulleten' organov zdravookhraneniia Moskovskogo soveta*.[52] He was replaced by N. F. Popov, an official without medical training whose previous experience lay in the construction industry.

Attention was then turned to the republican-level health authorities. On December 18, 1929, the Central Committee of the Bolshevik party issued a resolution entitled "About the Medical Service of Workers and Peasants," which marked the *velikii povorot* in the medical system.[53] The resolution criticized a number of defects in health administration and called for a radical restructuring of the work of the republican health commissariats. It also demanded a speedy resolution of medical labor supply problems, the introduction of an appropriate class line, and fundamental revisions in the five-year health plan to bring it in line with those of other sectors.

Even this criticism, however, did not immediately change the line of Narkomzdrav RSFSR. To the very issue of *Voprosy zdravookhraneniia* which contained the party decree, Semashko contributed an article in which he agreed that some of the complaints were justified but pointed out that financial constraints nevertheless existed. He claimed that the drop in state budget and FMA health finance, coupled with unchanging levels of local budgetary allocations, made it unlikely that the desired goals could be attained.[54] This skepticism was not appreciated by party authorities. In January and February of 1930, Semashko was relieved of his responsibilities as commissar and as editor of the Narkomzdrav journal. Colleagues of Semashko who had written about health planning and finance in the 1920s, such as M. Ginzburg, K. Konovalov, V. Goriushin, and G. Dreisin, also lost their jobs at this time. Semashko's replacement as commissar of health RSFSR was M. F. Vladimirskii. Although Vladimirskii had medical qualifications, his postrevolutionary career had included service in the RSFSR NKVD, Sovnarkom and Gosplan in the Ukraine, Gosplan USSR, and the Central Revision Commission VKP(b).[55] We therefore can assume that he was assigned to Narkomzdrav to implement the policies called for in the December decree.

THE SECOND VARIANT OF THE FIVE-YEAR HEALTH PLAN

After Vladimirskii assumed control of Narkomzdrav RSFSR, remedial work on the five-year health plan intensified. The faster pace of plan preparation manifested itself in the publication in July of the 1930/31 control figures; this was the first time the figures were ready before the financial year commenced.[56] A month later, in August 1930, the second variant of the plan was published in the document entitled *Materiali k piatiletnemu planu zdravookhraneniia RSFSR.*[57]

In an introductory essay to this document, Vladimirskii criticized the past administration of the health service for developing an unambitious first draft of the Five-Year Plan that caused health to become a "retarding sector" of the economy. He claimed that the new variant of the health plan incorporated more ambitious rates of development and took into account the demands for "the differentiated medical treatment of various groups of the population in accordance with their role in the socialist construction of the republic."[58]

The 152-page plan document was divided into two sections: finance and medical system development. The section entitled "The Budget and Capital Investment" made it clear that few of the long-standing financial problems of the health service (severe lack of capital investment and the "acute backwardness" of medical wages) had been solved by the summer of 1930.[59] The solution to these problems was to be achieved through large increases in health expenditure in the final three years of the plan period. Total expenditure was to increase from 418.3 million rubles in 1927/28 to 618.0 million rubles in 1929/30. Expenditures were then supposed to accelerate so that by 1932/33 annual spending would be 2,093.3 million rubles. To support increases of this magnitude, allocations from the four major sources (state budget, local budget, FMA, and special means) were to rise from 456.2 million rubles in 1928/29 to 1,755.2 in 1932/33. In addition, "other contributions" from ten sources were expected to go up from 19.2 to 338.1 million rubles over the same period.

The ambitious nature of the second variant plan becomes evident when its financial targets are compared with those of the first variant. Table 2 shows that in 1928/29 the four-source subtotal of the first variant exceeded that of the second, but with "other contributions" taken into account they are roughly equivalent. In 1932/33, however, all second variant targets, except for special means, were significantly higher than those of the first variant. Over the whole five years the projected expenditure of the second variant plan (5,606.7 million rubles) exceeded that of the first (3,377.0 million rubles) by 66 percent.

The five-year health plan for the whole Soviet Union, summarized in Table 3, was less ambitious than the RSFSR second variant health plan.[60] This can be explained by the fact that the national plan was compiled in spring 1929 by aggregating the existing republican plans. Since the RSFSR was the largest republic, its contribution had great weight. At that time Narkomzdrav RSFSR had only prepared its first variant plan. As a result, even the optimal variant targets for the medical system in the *Piatiletnii plan* document of Gosplan USSR appear modest relative to second variant standards.[61]

In the 1930 third edition of the *Piatiletnii plan* there are a number of indications that Gosplan was aware of the modest nature of the health plan and had tried to make some adjustments—principally in socio-cultural items. But this still did not bring the official national health plan up to the ambitious level of the revised 1930 one for the RSFSR.

TABLE 3
USSR Five-Year Health Plan, 1928/29–1932/33

Plan Indicator	1927/28	1928/29	1929/30	1930/31	1931/32	1932/33	1932/33 as % of 1927/28
A: Medical Facilities							
Total Hospital Beds (optimal)	210,000	221,000	276,000	301,000	338,000	365,000	174
Total Hospital Beds (minimum)	210,000	221,000	233,000	245,000	262,000	280,000	133
Urban	138,000	143,000	149,000	156,000	166,000	176,000	127
Rural	57,000	61,000	66,000	71,000	76,000	82,000	144
Transport	15,000	17,000	18,000	19,000	20,000	22,000	147
Urban Hospital Beds per 1,000	4.9	--	--	--	--	5.8	118
Rural Hospital Beds per 1,000	0.5	--	--	--	--	1.1	220
Rural Doctor Microdistricts	7,102	7,529	7,871	8,238	8,633	9,069	128
B: Medical Personnel							
Doctors	45,095	47,696	51,439	54,867	58,297	61,479	136
Middle Medical	95,966	101,913	110,498	118,053	125,486	132,523	138
Junior Medical/Service	193,728	203,673	213,618	223,563	233,508	243,457	126
Total (minimum)	334,789	353,282	375,555	396,483	417,483	437,459	131
Total (optimal)	335,000	353,000	401,000	434,000	478,000	505,000	151
Doctors per 10,000	2.9					3.5	121
Health as % Total Labor Force	3.4	3.4	3.4	3.3	3.3	3.3	97

C: Medical Wages

Doctors	(rubles)	1,476	--	--	--	--	2,280	154
Middle Medical	''	607	--	--	--	--	876	144
Junior/Service	''	480	--	--	--	--	660	138
Total (optimal)	''	608	663	721	779	841	912	150
Health as % of Economy Ave. Wage		88	89	90	90	91	92	105

D: Health Finance (optimal)

State Budget	(million rubles)	50.0	56.0	62.0	75.0	87.0	100.0	200
Local Budget	''	230.0	248.0	303.0	366.0	453.0	530.0	230
FMA	''	240.6	252.0	298.0	350.0	390.0	430.0	179
Special Means	''	87.0	109.2	132.4	150.9	175.0	198.0	228
Total	''	607.6	665.2	795.4	941.9	1,105.0	1,258.0	207
Health Spending per capita (rubles)		4.04	4.32				6.50	163
Health Investment (million rubles)		89	93	122	150	186	227	258

Source: *Piatiletnii plan narodno-khoziaistvennogo stroitel' stva SSSR*, 3rd ed. (Moscow, 1930), vol. 2, pt. 2, pp. 171, 206–8, 239, 241, 268–70.

THE DEVELOPMENT OF THE
SOVIET MEDICAL SYSTEM IN 1930-32

The period 1930-32 was one of great turbulence in political and economic life in the Soviet Union.[62] The intensification of collectivization and disequilibrium in industry led to a marked decline in living standards and affected adversely health conditions and the performance of the medical system.

By 1930 sanitation and housing standards were low and deteriorating. Only 218 of 508 RSFSR cities had water supply systems and 23 had sewerage.[63] Housing was in short supply and seriously overcrowded. According to Barber, in 1930 the norms of per capita housing provision were exceptionally low in industrial regions and cities (2.7 square meters in the Kuzbas and 3.85 in Sverdlovsk).[64] The ranks of people on central food rations swelled from 26 million in 1930 to 40 million in 1932.[65] In the countryside the poorly planned and brutally implemented collectivization and "dekulakization" campaigns resulted in mass deportations of peasant families, severe disruption of agricultural production, and a drastic drop in food consumption by the rural population. By 1932 the policies of the Stalinist regime had caused a severe famine in large regions of the country, especially in the Ukraine.

The decline in health conditions in the USSR produced an increase in the number of cases and rates of most illnesses. With the onset of the famine in rural areas after the 1932 harvest, illness and death rates soared among the peasantry,[66] while throughout this period the Soviet population as a whole suffered numerous premature deaths as the result of repressive actions by the state such as the large-scale deportations of peasant families.

Following the December 1929 Resolution of the Central Committee, one of the primary tasks of the new leadership of Narkomzdrav RSFSR was to prevent the health of the population from deteriorating so markedly that it interfered with the fulfillment of economic plans. With these objectives in mind, a number of steps were taken to reorient the medical system so that it could better serve the economy. First, attempts were made to shift medical resources to economically and politically important regions.[67] Second, by the end of 1930 it was decided to provide workers with medical care directly at the place of employment through a new institution, the industrial health point (*punkt*). Narkomzdrav was ordered to reassign doctors from territorial facilities to these new closed units immediately.[68] A third policy initiative was to formalize socioeconomic group priorities and rationing procedures in the public medical system. On January 31, 1930, Sovnarkom RSFSR passed a resolution "About the Order of Service of the Rural Population with Medical Assistance," which repealed an existing law that guaranteed all peasants equal access to medical facilities. Instead, the rural population was to be divided into three carefully designated groups, defined by political and economic criteria, which would determine treatment priorities.

Finally, steps were taken to abolish the private medical sector. The significance of this sector was underscored in a *Rabkrin* (People's Commissariat of Workers' and Peasants' Inspection) survey which found in 1930 that about 5 percent of hospitals, 0.5 percent of hospital beds, and 6.4 percent of outpatient clinics were in private hands.[69] Many doctors practiced privately on the side, and those working in the public system made use of state facilities in their private work. It was estimated that 1,500 doctors in Moscow alone, or 17.5 percent of the total number, were engaged in private practice and that they wrote 2,700,000 prescriptions for medicines for private patients per year.[70] Contrary to expectations, most of its patients (82.9 percent of those requiring abortions and about 70 percent of those making outpatient visits) were insured workers or members of their families, who were willing to pay for medical treatment because of dissatisfaction with the state system:

> The reasons which force the insured to visit private practitioners are: (1) one must wait a long time in queues [in state establishments]—it is better to pay but not lose time; (2) it is difficult to wait in a crowd, in uncomfortable conditions; (3) state doctors are exceedingly overworked and give patients little attention; (4) after a long wait it is possible all the same that one will not be admitted (refusals); (5) the attitude of the medical personnel is insufficiently courteous, and sometimes rude; (6) "doctors write longer than they examine"; (7) there are too many demands for various documents.[71]

Despite the fact that the private sector primarily served the proletariat, Narkomzdrav administrators ordered the responsible authorities in January 1930 to liquidate private medical care. Their opposition to fee-for-service medicine was not a principled one. Indeed they had just reintroduced fees in state facilities for certain categories of the population. Predictably, the campaign to eliminate private practice met with considerable opposition and was later moderated on orders from above. At a medical congress in March 1930, M. I. Kalinin condemned the attempt to eliminate private medicine as a left-wing deviation and called for greater tolerance on this issue.[72]

Another concern of health administrators was the medical labor force. The second variant of the five-year health plan called for increases in the number of doctors from 43,792 in 1928/29 to 93,143 in 1932/33 and of middle medical personnel from 83,949 to 217,813. The existing medical education system could not produce these numbers: deficits of 37,349 doctors and 89,511 middle medical personnel for the end of the plan period were projected. In June 1930, Sovnarkom RSFSR issued a decree "About the Reorganization of the System of Preparation of Medical Personnel," ordering a large increase in the number of places in medical schools, a corresponding increase in admissions without regard to qualifications, a reduction in training time (to four years for doctors), and a revised curriculum which would reduce the emphasis on formal study and put students to work immediately in the health system.[73] Students in medical schools were to spend their first year working as junior medical staff (for example, as orderlies) and to progress in successive years to assistant middle medical staff, middle medical staff, and probationary doctor. This policy, reinforced by a June 1931 Central Committee decree, enabled the Soviet Union to increase dramatically the number of places and students in

medical schools. But these quantitative advances were achieved at the cost of reducing drastically the quality of medical education and, ultimately, of the staff
working in the medical system.

A final major problem which attracted the attention of the party, the state apparatus, and health policymakers was that of public sanitation and the control of
epidemic disease. The worsening of public health contributed to absenteeism, job
turnover, and low labor productivity, all of which threatened the industrialization
program. In an effort to resolve this problem Sovnarkom RSFSR passed a resolution
in May 1930 "About the Sanitary Minimum," which had as its objective to stimulate
economic and social institutions to invest time and money (above the level specified
by the plan) in projects such as water supply, sewerage, housing amenities, and
cleanliness of living and working areas.[74] In August, *Sovnarkom* passed another
decree "About the Battle with Epidemics." In that same month Vladimirskii wrote
an article in *Na fronte zdravookhraneniia* entitled "The Battle with Illness Gives
Industry New Resources."[75] He argued that over the remaining three years of the
plan the cost of illness to the economy would be "no less than two to two and one-
half billion rubles" and that more than 50 percent of diseases (infectious, digestive,
and dermatological) were caused by poor public health.

Substantial inputs of finance, material, and labor would be required to implement
these ambitious plans. In the period 1928–32 the increase in total USSR health
expenditure substantially exceeded the optimal target implied in Table 3. However,
the reported health expenditures contain a significant inflationary bias. One can best
appreciate the effects of inflation at this time by assessing real trends in health
investment and wages.

Actual investment in health rose from 99 to 148 million rubles from 1928 to
1932, as shown in Table 4. This was lower than the optimal USSR target (growth
from 89 to 227) and substantially below the RSFSR second variant (68 to 610
million rubles). Over this period the health share of total investment for the whole
economy declined significantly from 2.4 percent to 0.8 percent. The final row of
Table 4, derived from calculations by Zaleski, indicates that real investment in
health increasingly fell below target, and by 1932 its plan fulfillment rate of 35.4
percent was the lowest of any branch in the national economy.[76]

From 1928 to 1932 average wages in the health sector rose from 638 to 1,248
rubles. This was more than had been called for in the USSR plan (Table 3), which
had a 1932/33 goal of 912 rubles. Nevertheless, the average wage in the health
sector fell from 91 percent of the national average in 1928 to a low of 83 percent
in 1931 and then climbed back up to 87 percent in 1932 (the original plan had the
share rising from 88 to 92 per cent). If one applies Zaleski's real wage index to
the health sector we find that the average earnings of medical staff in real terms
fell from 638 rubles to 278 rubles.[77]

The actual increase in the medical labor force considerably exceeded the plan
targets shown in Table 3. Despite this, the growth rate of employment in the medical
system was lower than the average for the whole economy, with the consequence
that the health share of the total labor force fell from 3.4 to 2.8 percent. The number
of doctors in the USSR is reported to have risen from 63,219 in 1928 to 76,377 in

1932. Much of the increment in medical staff was generated by the recruitment of women. The female share of health sector employment rose from 64.6 percent in 1929 to 70.2 percent in 1932.

Table 4 also suggests that there was some reduction in urban-rural disparities. Presumably these trends can be explained by the greater attention given in the revised health plan to the socialized agriculture sector and the desire of the party and state to provide medical care to the expanding numbers of their representatives in rural areas. The growth of medical facilities rose substantially, exceeding the plan target of the optimal variant. There were substantial increases in outpatient clinics, industrial health *punkty,* and rural doctors' microdistricts. Most likely, however, quantitative advances were achieved at the expense of quality. For example, the growth in the numbers of beds probably was accomplished by crowding them into existing ward space. Many of the new "outpatient clinics" and "industrial health points" were crude conversions of existing buildings not designed for medical purposes.

The goals of the second variant health plan for differentiated distribution of medical care may well have been fulfilled. After the *velikii perelom,* Soviet medical authorities introduced new rationing schemes that distributed medical services between social groups on the basis of priority rankings. In addition, medical resources were reallocated to the benefit of the new "health points" in factories and of industrial regions. In sum, it is possible that inequality in medical care distribution was greater by the end of the first five-year plan period than it had been at the beginning.

CONCLUSION

Planning for health required a choice between two conflicting strategies. The first strategy involved retaining the territorial structure and preventive orientation of the medical system, upholding the principle of distribution in accordance with need, and raising levels of provision across the board at the modest pace dictated by projecting into the future resources currently available. The alternative was to break through resource constraints by using aggressive policies to expand the medical system at a rapid pace, reorganize it so that facilities were located at places of work, and distribute services in accordance with the politico-economic importance of population groups.

In the initial phase of plan preparation it appears that Narkomzdrav RSFSR favored the first strategy, as did other bodies such as the Socio-Cultural Section of Gosplan RSFSR. The first variant of the health plan prepared by Narkomzdrav in early 1929 proposed the retention of the existing medical organization, modest increases in the quantities of medical staff, facilities, and medical services, maintenance of quality standards, and some reduction in distributional inequalities.

But Narkomzdrav was not working in a vacuum. During 1928/29 health conditions in the USSR were worsening, illness rates were rising, and economic plans were becoming more ambitious. Many influential individuals and institutions believed that the projected low growth rates and relatively egalitarian distributional

TABLE 4
USSR Medical System Development 1928–32

	1928	1929	1930	1931	1932	1932 as % of 1928
A: Medical Facilities						
Hospital Beds	246,100				405,800	165
Somatic/Childbirth	143,600				230,000	160
Urban	60,000				107,000	178
Rural						
Urban per 1,000	4.47				5.38	120
Rural per 1,000	0.77				1.23	160
Urban Outpatient Clinics	5,673				7,340	129
Urban Outpatient Visits	190,144,000				318,522,000	168
Industrial Health Points	1,942				6,532	336
Rural Doctor Microdistricts	7,531				9,883	131
Rural Outpatient Visits	99,832,000				159,165,000	159
B: Medical Labor						
Total Health Workers	399,000	438,200	476,500	562,200	647,200	162
Health as % Total Workers	3.4	3.6	3.3	3.0	2.8	82
Women as % Health Workers		64.6	67.1			--
Doctors	63,219		68,516		76,377	121
Average Health Wage (rubles)	638	727	799	938	1,248	196
Health Wage as % of Economy Average	91	91	85	83	87	96

C: Health Finance

Total Health Expenditure (million rubles)	660.8				2,105.8	319
State Budget Health	48.5[1]	42.2[2]	58.9[3]	68.0	91.7	189
Local Budget Health	211.8[1]	266.5[2]	450.7[3]	470.3	635.0	300
FMA	246.5		442.8	478.9	759.3	308
Health Capital Investment[4]	99	116	128	141	148	149
Health as % Total Capital Investment	2.4	2.0	1.3	0.9	0.8	33
% Fulfillment Real Health Investment Plan	90.2		81.0	43.8	35.4	---

Notes: (1) 1927/28, (2) 1928/29, (3) 1929/30 plus final quarter 1930, (4) includes investment in social insurance objects

Sources: Gosplan, *Itogi vypolneniia pervogo piatiletnego plana razvitiia narodnogo khoziaistva soiuza SSR* (Moscow, 1933), p. 185; *Sotsialisticheskoe stroitel' stvo SSR: Ezhegodnik* (Moscow, 1935), pp. 464–65, 474, 484–85, 544–55, 647, 654, 661, 668–69, 675; Gosplan, *Trud v SSSR* (Moscow, 1936), pp. 14–15, 25; Gosplan, *Zdorov' e i i zdravookhranenie Trudiashchikhsia SSSR* (Moscow, 1937), pp. 54, 60; Narkomzdrav SSSR, *Narodnoe zdravookhranenie za 25 let sovetskoi vlasti* (Moscow, 1942); E. Zaleski, *Planning for Economic Growth in the Soviet Union, 1918–1932* (Chapel Hill, N.C., 1971), p. 374; and *Sotsialisticheskoe stroitel' stvo SSSR: Statisticheskii ezhegodnik* (Moscow, 1934), pp. 314–19, 322, 424–33, 443, 446–64.

policy of the first variant health plan were ill-suited to the times. The critics of Narkomzdrav came from organizations representing privileged industrial workers— the trade unions and Central Social Insurance Administration of Narkomtrud. Complaints about Narkomzdrav's policies and plan proposals led to investigations by *Rabkrin* of the provision of medical care to workers and drew the attention of higher level state and party bodies to problems in the health sector. During 1929 Gosplan USSR became concerned about the growing discrepancies between the requirements of the optimal variant economic plans for medical services and the supplies projected by Narkomzdrav. By that summer, Sovnarkom RSFSR, under the new leadership of Syrtsov, became more critical of the work of Narkomzdrav and demanded radical revisions in the health plan. The stage was set for institutional conflict.

The Bolshevik party apparatus became enmeshed in this bureaucratic dispute. Earlier in the twenties, a variety of orientations existed in the party and thus an important Old Bolshevik such as Semashko could find high-level support for his policies, especially when they seemed consistent with revolutionary principles and the ideas of Lenin. By 1928, however, Stalin had eliminated the left, had promoted his own people, and was moving strongly against the right opposition. It appears that Semashko had good connections with leading right-opposition figures, which placed him at a disadvantage by 1929. Ranged against Semashko were other Old Bolshevik doctors affiliated with the Stalinist faction, such as Vladimirskii and M. I. Barsukov, who favored the second health strategy. These changes in the balance of power and personnel in the Bolshevik party help explain the strong criticisms of the first variant health plan at the Sixteenth Party Conference and the subsequent intervention by the Central Committee in December 1929 to force a *velikii perelom* in the work of Narkomzdrav RSFSR.

The study of the debate on the health plan illustrates some intriguing features of bureaucratic conflict in 1928/29. First, one cannot assume a priori that organizations functioned consistently as units in bureaucratic struggles. In the dispute over the health plan at least eight party, state, and social institutions participated. Within a single organization there were often differing positions on an issue. For example, it is likely that the Socio-Cultural Section of Gosplan RSFSR was considerably more sympathetic to its client commissariat, Narkomzdrav, than was the Presidium of Gosplan RSFSR, which had close links to Sovnarkom RSFSR and Gosplan USSR.

Second, the documents produced may have played a role in political conflict. Following the replacement of Semashko by Vladimirskii in January 1930, intensive work began on the revision of the five-year health plan so that it would reflect a strategy of rapid growth, occupationally based medical delivery, and differentiated distribution. The newly created Health Department of Gosplan USSR, headed by M. I. Barsukov, played an important role in this process. By August 1930 an ambitious second variant health plan that expressed the "class proletarian line" was ready. But this elaborate draft was not incorporated into official plans for the whole economy and was later reported never to have been ratified (*utverzhden*). Ironically, the second variant health plan may have had more significance as an instrument in a political struggle than as a guide to medical system development.

Third, although important issues were often involved in a bureaucratic conflict (for example, the insufficiency of planned medical services for industrial workers), individual personalities could exert substantial influence on the pace of conflict resolution, if not the outcome. The weight of those personalities was probably the greater because some of the relations between commissariats were not yet routinized. It is probable that the high status of Semashko protected Narkomzdrav from political interference for a long time, although in the end he could not prevent the "great turnaround."

In evaluating the welfare orientation of a state or its achievements in a given period, attention should be focused on final results rather than intermediate processes. In the case of the health sector, this means that studies of trends in the population's health status, illness, and mortality are probably more informative than are assessments of changes in the relatively ineffectual medical system. If this approach is adopted, then the movements of final output indicators all suggest that the welfare of the population worsened during 1928–32. Illness rates rose significantly because of rapid urbanization, decline in public hygiene, deterioration in urban housing and food supply, famine in the countryside, and the effects of mass deportations of peasants. The medical system was unable to cope with this situation, so mortality rates rose and life expectancy declined. This provides eloquent testimony to the low priority which the Stalinist regime attached to the welfare of the Soviet people.

APPENDIX A

ESTIMATED INEQUALITY IN
1927/28 RSFSR HEALTH SPENDING

The sources and estimation procedures used in preparing Table 1 are summarized in this appendix.

COLUMN 1: DISTRIBUTION OF POPULATION (THOUSANDS)

Row 1: The 1927/28 RSFSR population of 104,188 thousand was estimated by dividing officially reported total RSFSR health expenditure of 410.5 million rubles (Donskoi, "Kontrol'nye tsifry, 1928/1929," p. 9 [see note 21]) by per capita RSFSR health spending of 3.94 rubles ("Finansovoe polozhenie," p. 61 [see note 20]). This population estimate falls appropriately within the range of the December 17, 1926, census figure of 100,921 thousand and the January 1, 1929, estimate of 105,989 thousand shown in *Sotsialisticheskoe stroitel'stvo SSSR: Statisticheskii ezhegodnik* (Moscow, 1934), p. 354.

Row 2: The insured consist of eligible workers and family members receiving benefits from both territorial and transport social insurance funds. The number of insured workers in the territorial scheme in 1927/28 was 5,846 thousand (*Tezisy po piatiletnemu*, p. 10 [see note 22]). The average size of an insured family is assumed to be 2.3 members (M. Ginzburg, "Vozmozhno li bez ukhudsheniia medpomoshchi zastrakhovannym iz'iat' kakie-libo summy iz fonda medpomoshchi," *BNKZ*, no. 22 [1927], p. 32) so the number of territorial insured is 13,446 thousand. To this must be added transport workers and family members. An estimate of their numbers (3,949 thousand) can be obtained by dividing the number of RSFSR transport hospital beds (12,242) by the transport beds per 1,000 (3.1/1,000) and multiplying by 1,000 (*Tezisy po piatiletnemu*, p. 25 [see note 20] and *Materiali k piatiletnemu*, p. 96 [see note 57]). Thus, the total of insured plus families is 17,395.

Row 3: Row 1 minus row 2.

Rows 4 and 5: Ginzburg reported that 15 percent of the insured lived in rural areas (Ginzburg, "Vozmozhno," p. 32), so 85 percent lived in urban areas. Multiply the row 2 numbers of insured by these percentages to obtain estimates of urban and rural insured.

Row 6: The urban share of the RSFSR population rose from 16.6 percent in 1926 to 17.6 percent in 1929 (*Sotsialisticheskoe stroitel'stvo 1934*, p. 354). It is assumed that it was 17.1 percent in 1927–28, or 17,816 thousand. Subtract from this the urban insured to obtain the residual urban uninsured.

Row 7: Subtract rural insured from total rural population of 86,372 thousand (104,188 thousand minus 17,816 thousand) to obtain 83,763.

COLUMN 2: DISTRIBUTION OF POPULATION (%)

Divide column 1 row entries by 104,188 and multiply by 100.

COLUMN 3: TOTAL HEALTH EXPENDITURES (rubles)

Row 1: Donskoi ("Kontrol'nye tsifry 1928/1929," p. 9), gives a total 1927/28 expenditure of 410.5 million rubles.

Row 2: The insured benefited from 1927/28 FMA spending of 175.5 million. In addition 145.3 million was spent on them from state budget, local budget, and special means funds. This supplemental spending was estimated by multiplying reported per capita amounts for the population in general by relevant insured populations: urban (9.70 rubles x 14,786), plus rural (0.72 rubles x 2,609) (Donskoi, "Kontrol'nye tsifry 1928/1929," p. 12; *Tezisy po piatiletnemu*, p. 10; Ginzburg, "Vozmozhno," p. 32).

Row 3: Spending on the uninsured from the state budget, local budget, and special means was calculated by multiplying appropriate per capita expenditures for urban (9.70 rubles) and rural populations (0.72 rubles) given in Donskoi, "Kontrol'nye tsifry 1928/1929," p. 11, by population numbers. Total (89.7) = urban (29.4) plus rural (60.3).

Row 4: Calculated as 85 percent of both territorial and transport FMA = 119.4 + 29.8 = 149.2. In addition there was supplemental spending of 143.4 million rubles on the urban insured (9.70 rubles x 14,786 thousand).

Row 5: Calculated as 15 percent of total FMA (26.3 million rubles) plus a supplement estimated at 1.9 million rubles from other rural health finance sources (0.72 rubles x 2,609 rural insured).

Row 6: According to Donskoi in 1927/28 the RSFSR spent 9.70 rubles per urban resident out of state budget, local budget, and special means, or a total of 172.8 million rubles on the urban population. Of this, 143.4 was spent on the urban insured. This leaves a residual of 29.4 million rubles.

Row 7: Donskoi reported that 0.72 rubles was spent out of general funds per rural inhabitant of the RSFSR. So total spending was 83,763 thousand x 0.72 rubles = 60.3 million rubles.

COLUMN 4: TOTAL HEALTH EXPENDITURES (%)

Divide column 3 entries by 410.5 million rubles and multiply by 100.

COLUMN 5: PER CAPITA HEALTH EXPENDITURES

For each row divide the column 3 entry by that of column 1.

NOTES

The author would like to thank IREX for its sponsorship of his exchange visit to Moscow State University in 1976–77, the Centre for Russian and East European Studies, University of Birmingham, for support of work in economic history during 1978–87, Professor R. W. Davies and Dr. Stephen Wheatcroft for comments on the initial draft, and Professor Susan Gross Solomon for her assistance in revising the chapter.

1. E. H. Carr and R. W. Davies, *Foundations of a Planned Economy 1926–29*, Vol. I (Harmondsworth, England, 1974).

2. Among the good sources of background information about the economic and political developments in the 1920s are: Carr and Davies, *Foundations*; A. Nove, *An Economic History of the USSR* (Harmondsworth, England, 1972); E. Zaleski, *Planning for Economic Growth in the Soviet Union, 1928–32* (Chapel Hill, N.C., 1971); M. McAuley, *Politics and the Soviet Union* (Harmondsworth, England, 1977); J. F. Hough and M. Fainsod, *How the Soviet Union Is Governed* (Cambridge, Mass., 1979); and E. H. Carr, *Foundations of a Planned Economy 1926–1929*, vol. 2 (Harmondsworth, England, 1976).

3. S. G. Wheatcroft, "Population Dynamic and Factors Affecting It in the Soviet Union in the 1920s and 1930s" CREES Discussion Papers, SIPS no. 2 (Birmingham, England, 1976).

4. The historical development of the Soviet health service bureaucracy has been covered in the English-language literature by M. Field, *Soviet Socialized Medicine: An Introduction* (New York, 1967); G. Hyde, *The Soviet Health Service: An Historical and Comparative Study* (London, 1974); and M. Kaser, *Health Care in the Soviet Union and Eastern Europe* (London, 1976). Appropriate Soviet sources include M. I. Barsukov, ed., *Ocherki istorii zdravookhraneniia SSSR* (Moscow, 1957); *Zdravookhranenie v gody vosstanovleniia i sotsialisticheskoi rekonstruktsii narodnogo khoziaistva SSSR: 1925–1940 (Sbornik dokumentov i materialov)* (Moscow, 1973); and N. A. Vinogradov, ed., *Organizatsiia zdravookhraneniia v SSSR*, 2d ed. (Moscow, 1962).

5. Biographies of N. A. Semashko can be found in S. A. Blinkin, *N. A. Semashko* (Moscow, 1976), and B. M. Potulov, *N. A. Semashko—vrach i revoliutsioner* (Moscow, 1986).

6. See Neil B. Weissman, "Origins of Soviet Health Administration: Narkomzdrav, 1918–1928," in this volume.

7. See C. Davis, "Economic Problems of the R.S.F.S.R. Health System, 1921–1930," CREES Discussion Paper, SIPS no. 19 (Birmingham, England, 1978); and C. Davis, "Economic Problems of the Soviet Health Service: 1917–1930," *Soviet Studies*, 35, no. 3 (July 1983), pp. 343–61, for a discussion of the low priority of the health service and policy compromises that it was forced to make.

8. Information about the work of the Moscow Health Department can be found in the journals *Biulleten' organov zdravookhraneniia Moskovskogo soveta* [henceforth, *BOZMS*] and *Moskovskii meditsinskii zhurnal* [henceforth, *MMZ*].

9. Davis, "Economic Problems of the Soviet Health Service," p. 348.

10. Ibid., p. 352.

11. I. V. Vengrova and Iu. A. Shilinis, *Sotsial'naia gigiena v SSSR* (Moscow, 1976). Certain health departments were energetic and innovative in developing preventive programs. For example, the Moscow *oblast* health department under the leadership of V. A. Obukh and Ia. Iu. Kats devised the concept of the "united dispensaries" and introduced it on a local basis with some success. See Ia. Iu. Kats, "Revoliutsiia v obshchestvennoi meditsine," *MMZ*, no. 1 (1925), pp. 63–74; and Ia. Iu. Kats, "Osnovy piatiletnego plana sanitarnoi deiatel'nosti v Moskovskoi oblasti," *BOZMS*, no. 16–17 (1929), pp. 230–36.

12. D. Gorfin, "Okhrana zdoroviia proletariata za 10 let," *Biulleten' Narodnogo komissariata zdravookhraneniia RSFSR* [hereafter, *BNKZ*], no. 20 (1927), pp. 25–38.

13. Kats, "Osnovy"; "Sostoianie zdravookhraneniia v Moskve v 1927/28 g. i perspektivy

Moszdrava na 1929 g.,'' *BOZMS*, no. 1 (1929), pp. 2–8; and I. A. Liberman, ''Doktor Kats i Moskovskaia Blagodat,'' *Profilakticheskaia meditsina*, no. 12 (1926), pp. 117–25.

14. For example, see M. Ginzburg, ''Mestnyi biudzhet i zdravookhraneniia,'' *Izvestiia Narodnogo komissariata zdravookhraneniia RSFSR*, no. 1 (1924), pp. 66–69; and N. A. Vinogradov, *Zdravookhraneniia v period perekhoda na mirnuiu rabotu po vosstanovlenniiu narodnogo khoziaistva (1921–1925 gg.)* (Moscow, 1954).

15. S. Cherniak, ''Rol' s''ezdov zdravotdelov v organizatsii dela zdravookhranenie,'' *BNKZ*, no. 20 (1927), pp. 21–25; and Vingradov, *Zdravookhranenie (1921–1925 gg.)*, p. 15.

16. The ''regime of economy'' campaign is discussed in more detail in Davis, ''Economic Problems of the R.S.F.S.R. Health System,'' pp. 43–46. See also Samuel C. Ramer, ''Feldshers and Rural Health Care during the Early Soviet Period,'' in this volume.

17. See, for example, D. Rostotskii, ''O rezhime ekonomii,'' *BNKZ*, no. 2 (1927), pp. 23–27.

18. K. Konovalov, ''Dva goda rezhima ekonomii v dele zdravookhraneniia,'' *Voprosy zdravookhraneniia* [hereafter cited as *VZ*], no. 10 (1928), pp. 3–9.

19. Davis, ''Economic Problems of the R.S.F.S.R. Health System,'' pp. 21–25.

20. ''Finansovoe polozhenie dela zdravookhraneniia,'' *VZ*, no. 14 (1928), pp. 61–62; and ''Zasedanie 26 avgusta: Finansovo-kal'kuliatsionnyi otchet za 1927/28 god,'' *VZ*, nos. 16–17 (1929), pp. 127–29.

21. M. Donskoi, ''Kontrol'nye tsifry zdravookhraneniia RSFSR na 1928/29 g.,'' *VZ*, no. 2 (1929), p. 13.

22. N. Semashko, ''Politika zdravookhraneniia v piatiletnem plane,'' in Narkomzdrav RSFSR, *Tezisy po piatiletnemu perspektivnomu planu zdravookhraneniia RSFSR* (Moscow-Leningrad, 1929).

23. M. Ginzburg, ''Voprosy zdravookhraneniia v predstoiashchem biudzhete,'' *Izvestiia Narkomzdrava*, nos. 2–3 (1925), pp. 9–22; and A. Rozova, ''Finansirovanie dela zdravookhraneniia v RSFSR,'' *VZ*, no. 8 (1928), pp. 9–16.

24. ''Zasedanie 26 avgusta,'' pp. 128–29.

25. See Sally Ewing, ''The Science and Politics of Soviet Insurance Medicine,'' in this volume. The conflict between Narkomzdrav RSFSR and social insurance authorities is also discussed in Davis, ''Economic Problems of the R.S.F.S.R. Health System'' and Davis, ''Economic Problems of the Soviet Health Service.''

26. ''Zasedanie 26 avgusta,'' p. 129.

27. S. M. Daniushevskii, ''Vvedenie,'' in A. P. Zhuk, *Planirovanie zdravookhraneniia v SSSR* (Moscow, 1968).

28. M. Donskoi, ''Kontrol'nye tsifry po zdravookhraneniiu na 1926–27 g.,'' *BNKZ*, no. 19 (1926), pp. 3–7; and K. Konovalov, ''K voprosu o perspektivnom planirovanii zdravookhraneniia,'' *VZ*, no. 7 (1928), pp. 3–17.

29. ''Instruktsiia: Mestnym organam zdravookhraneniia k sostavleniiu 5-letnego perspektivnogo plana,'' *BNKZ*, no. 10 (1927), pp. 56–59.

30. Konovalov, ''K voprosu''; and Konovalov, ''K itogam.''

31. Gorfin, ''Okhrana zdoroviia''; ''Finansovoe polozhenie''; Carr and Davies, *Foundations;* and N. A. Vinogradov, *Zdravookhranenie v gody bor'by za sotsialisticheskuiu industrializatsiiu strany (1926–1929)* (Moscow, 1955).

32. ''Vrachebnaia ekspertiza invalidnosti,'' *BOZMS*, nos. 4–5 (1929), pp. 31–55; and ''Pechataemye nizhe tezisy po sostavleniiu 5-letnego plana po zdravookhraneniiu utverzhdeny planovoi komissiei NKZdrava,'' *VZ*, no. 12 (1928), pp. 48–52.

33. Donskoi, ''Kontrol'nye tsifry, 1928/1929.''

34. E. Neishtat, ''2-e planovoe soveshchanie zdravotdelov,'' *VZ*, no. 6 (1929), pp. 32–39.

35. Narkomzdrav RSFSR, *Tezisy po piatiletnemu perspektivnomu planu zdravookhraneniia RSFSR* (Moscow-Leningrad, 1929).

36. Donskoi, ''Kontrol'nye tsifry, 1928/1929,'' p. 12.

37. Neishtat, "2-e planovoe soveshchanie zdravotdelov," p. 36.

38. Zaleski, *Planning,* pp. 83–91.

39. K. Konovalov, "K voprosu ob ispol'zovanii FMP," *VZ,* no. 5 (1929), pp. 3–7.

40. For information on the career of Vladimirskii see S. Ia. Chikin, "M. F. Vladimirskii— Vydaiushchisiia organizator sovetskogo zdravookhraneniia," *Sovetskoe zdravookhranenie,* no. 9 (1977), pp. 60–64.

41. "V planovoi komissii NKZ," *VZ,* no. 9 (1929), p. 77.

42. K. Konovalov, "K itogam 3-go planovogo soveshchaniia," *VZ,* no. 20 (1929), pp. 54–61.

43. "Reorganizatsiia Narkomzdrava," *VZ,* no. 20 (1929), pp. 17–19.

44. Konovalov, "K voprosu," p. 3.

45. K. Konovalov, "Dal'neishee utochnenie piatiletki zdravookhraneniia," *VZ,* nos. 16– 17 (1929), pp. 5–7.

46. Carr, *Foundations,* pp. 203–4.

47. Vinogradov, *Zdravookhranenie (1926–1929),* p. 15.

48. Zaleski, *Planning,* pp. 90–98.

49. Donskoi, "Kontrol'nye tsifry, 1929–30."

50. In 1932 Barsukov and Zhuk wrote that "In the recovery period a whole series of opportunistic distortions arose in the theory and practice of medicine. . . . These were re- flected in the influence exerted on the weakest links of leading personnel in the health field by hostile class elements, who used the positions they occupied in the Soviet apparatus and medical facilities to confuse party members who did not display sufficient class vigilance and to force through their counterrevolutionary and bourgeois objectives under the flag of the socialist health service. These opportunistic distortions caused the lagging behind of the health service from the pace of development of the economy and of the requirements of workers and peasants, and reduced the health service to one of the bottlenecks of socialist building in the reconstruction period. . . . Overall, it is necessary to classify these deficiencies as right-opportunistic deviations" (M. Barsukov and A. Zhuk, *Za sotsialisticheskuiu rekon- struktsiiu zdravookhraneniia: Osnovye polozheniia vtorogo piatiletnego plana zdravookh- raneniia v SSSR* [Moscow, 1932], pp. 14–16). It is worth noting that Mikhail Ivanovich Barsukov played an important role in organizing the Soviet health service after the 1917 revolution. Before becoming head of the Health Sector of Gosplan USSR in April 1930 he occupied numerous top health positions, including commissar of public health of the Belo- russian republic. He probably had close connections with M. F. Vladimirskii and was an active participant in debates on health strategy in the late 1920s. He later worked as a historian of the Soviet health service and was editor of *Ocherki istorii zdravookhraneniia SSSR (1917– 1956 gg.)* (Moscow, 1957). For information on his life see *Bol'shaia meditsinskaia entsik- lopediia* (Moscow, 1929), vol. 3, and also the essay in this volume by Neil Weissman, "Origins of Soviet Health Administration: Narkomzdrav, 1918–1928." A. P. Zhuk went on to become a leading specialist on health planning and was the author of *Planirovanie zdra- vookhraneniia v SSSR* (Moscow, 1968).

51. Kats, "Osnovy."

52. "Novyi zaveduiushchii Mosoblzdravotdelom," *BOZMS,* nos. 23–24 (1929), title page.

53. *Zdravookhranenie v gody 1925–40,* pp. 131–33.

54. N. A. Semashko, "Na novye rel'sy," *VZ,* no. 1 (1930), pp. 2–4.

55. "Novyi narkom zdravookhraneniia—M. F. Vladimirskii," *Sovetskii vrach,* no. 4 (1930) p. 80; and Chikin, "M. F. Vladimirskii."

56. G. Karanovich, "Kontrol'nye tsifry zdravookhraneniia na 1930/31 g.," *Na fronte zdravookhraneniia* [hereafter, *NFZ*], nos. 13–14 (1930), pp. 27–43.

57. Narkomzdrav RSFSR, *Materialy k piatiletnemu planu zdravookhraneniia v RSFSR* (Moscow-Leningrad, 1930).

58. Ibid., pp. 5–6.

59. Ibid., p. 86.

60. The USSR five-year health plan for 1928/29–1932/33 can be pieced together from material presented in *Piatiletnii plan narodno-khoziaistvennogo stroitel'stva SSSR*, 3d ed. (Moscow, 1930), vol. 2, pt. 2.

61. For example, the USSR plan called for an increase in national health capital investment from 89 million rubles in 1927–28 to 227 million rubles in 1932–33, whereas respective RSFSR second variant figures for the RSFSR alone were 68.3 and 610.0 million rubles. Ibid., pp. 58–59, and Narkomzdrav, *Materialy*, p. 135.

62. Information about political and economic developments in the 1930–32 period can be found in: Hough and Fainsod, *How the Soviet Union Is Governed*, chap. 5; M. Heller and A. M. Nekrich, *Utopia in Power* (New York, 1986), chap. 5; S. Fitzpatrick, ed., *Cultural Revolution in Russia 1928–31* (Bloomington, Ind., 1978); Zaleski, *Planning;* and R. W. Davies, *The Socialist Offensive: The Collectivisation of Soviet Agriculture, 1929–1930* (London, 1980), chaps. 4 and 5.

63. Narkomzdrav, *Materialy*.

64. J. Barber, "The Standard of Living of Soviet Industrial Workers, 1928–1941," SIPS Seminar Paper (Birmingham, England, December 1980). See also T. Sosnovy, *The Housing Problem in the USSR* (New York, 1954), for an analysis of housing conditions, construction, and policy in this period.

65. R. W. Davies, "The Soviet Economic Crisis of 1932: The Crisis in the Towns," SIPS Seminar Paper (Birmingham, England, January 1985).

66. Assessments of the famine in the USSR in the early 1930s and its effects on the population's health are provided in Wheatcroft, "Population Dynamic"; in S. G. Wheatcroft, "Famine and Factors Affecting Mortality in the USSR: The Demographic Crises of 1914–1922 and 1930–1933," CREES discussion paper, SIPS nos. 20–21 (Birmingham, England, 1981); and in R. Conquest, *The Harvest of Sorrow: Soviet Collectivization and the Terror-Famine* (London, 1986).

67. This regional redistribution policy is expressed in a December 26, 1929, SNK USSR resolution, "About Hospital Construction in Industrial Regions," and a February 20, 1930, directive of Narkomzdrav RSFSR, "About the Mobilization of Qualified Medical Workers in Regions of Mass Collectivization." See *Zdravookhranenie v gody 1925–40*.

68. N. A. Vinogradov, *Zdravookhranenie v period bor'by za kollektivizatsiiu sel'skogo khoziaistva: 1930–1934* (Moscow, 1955), pp. 9–11.

69. V. Korneev, "K voprosu o chastnom sektore v dele zdravookhraneniia," *VZ*, no. 2 (1930), pp. 4–11.

70. The private sector tended to specialize in certain services—for example, it provided 40 percent of all abortions in Moscow.

71. Korneev, "K voprosu o chastnom sektore," p. 7.

72. Vinogradov, *Zdravookhranenie 1930–1934*, p. 7.

73. Ibid., pp. 27–36.

74. Ibid., pp. 17–23.

75. M. Vladimirskii, "Bor'ba s zabolevaemosti dast promyshlennosti novye resursy," *NFZ*, nos. 13–14 (1930), pp. 1–3.

76. Zaleski, *Planning*, p. 374.

77. Ibid., p. 392.

Part Three

Varieties of
Soviet Social Medicine

SUSAN GROSS SOLOMON

Social Hygiene and Soviet Public Health, 1921–1930

The first decade and a half after the Bolshevik Revolution brought to Russia a number of American physicians—travelers and fellow-travelers. Fortunately for the comparative historian of public health, some of those doctors left detailed descriptions of the "revolution" in public health that was sweeping the Soviet Union: the commitment to provide universal health care that was free and of high quality, health care that was directed as much at the prevention as at the cure of disease.[1]

In fact, this "revolution" in Soviet public health was more far-reaching than any of the American visitors appreciated at the time. The American physicians focused on the changes in the delivery of health care, but there were equally important reforms in the teaching of and research on Soviet public health. Indeed, according to the architects of the changes, the success of the "revolution" in health care delivery depended on the emergence of a new type of physician, one "who would be as much at home in sociology as biology, as much interested in preventing illness as in curing it."[2] In the training of such a physician-researcher, the pivotal discipline was to be social hygiene—*sotsial'naia gigiena*—a public health specialty with a distinctive philosophy of health and disease.

Soviet social hygienists defined their field as the science which studied the influence of the economic and social conditions of life on the health of the population and the means to improve that health.[3] Disease, they insisted, was not primarily a biological phenomenon; it was first and foremost a social phenomenon, best understood in its societal context. Health was not simply the absence of disease; it was the active promotion of the well-being of the population at large. The aim of social hygiene as a science was both to describe and to prescribe: its practitioners were to examine the social conditions within which disease occurred and spread and to propose social measures which would contribute to the all-important goal of preventing disease.

Within Russian public health, social hygiene was a relatively late arrival. Although some of its roots could be traced to the tsarist period, the field did not find institutional expression in Russian medical schools and research institutions until five years after the Bolsheviks took power. The emergence of social hygiene as a distinctive teaching and research enterprise in the 1920s is the subject of this essay.

As we shall see, the fact that a field which played such a prominent role in the "new" Soviet public health was still in the process of securing its own legitimacy had important implications both for the content of the emerging field and for those aspects of public health that the field was attempting to reshape.

SOCIAL HYGIENE IN PUBLIC HEALTH

The institutionalization of social hygiene in Soviet public health required the introduction of a new specialty into a well-defined intellectual terrain. The core of the Russian public health curriculum on the eve of the Revolution—and indeed for the half-century that preceded it—was "general hygiene." General hygiene had a venerable history in Russian public health. The first *kafedry* ("departments") in this subject were established in the medical schools as early as the end of the 1860s. Not surprisingly, by 1917, general hygienists had clearly delineated their subject and methodology. Theirs was the study of the impact on health of such environmental factors as air, water, and climate; theirs were the methods of physics, chemistry, and biology.[4] But the forging of that identity had not come easily: in the twenty years before the Revolution, the content of general hygiene was challenged several times by spokesmen for a variety of intellectual disciplines.

At the end of the nineteenth century, speaking as the advocates of the purely biological approach to public health, a group of bacteriologists led by Mechnikov made a bid to displace the field of general hygiene in Russia. While they accepted the importance of the laboratory for the study and solution of public health problems, general hygienists argued the merits of a broader approach which included sanitary statistics and engineering. General hygienists staved off the challenge from bacteriologists; within the next decade, bacteriology was established as a separate field in the medical schools and in specialized research institutes.[5]

In the first decade of the twentieth century, the scope of general hygiene was challenged by proponents of "community medicine." Speaking on behalf of a social approach to problems of public health that had been gaining ground among zemstvo physicians since the late 1880s,[6] those who represented community medicine urged that the concept of the environment—so central to general hygiene—be broadened to include social as well as biological factors. In part because of the onset of the First World War, the efforts of these spokesmen came to little: some courses in community medicine were introduced into economic and technical institutes but not into medical faculties.[7] As a consequence, on the eve of the Revolution, general hygiene looked much the way it had a decade earlier.[8]

Soon after 1917, the claim of environmentally oriented general hygienists to speak on behalf of public health as a whole was contested by spokesmen for the field of social hygiene. This time the challenge to the hegemony of general hygiene was successful. Capitalizing on both the widespread enthusiasm for new fields that followed the Revolution and on the unassailable Marxist, if not Bolshevik, credentials of many of their leading members, social hygienists gained the support of a highly visible patron, the commissar of public health. With the encouragement and protection of this patron, social hygiene broke away from general hygiene and was established as a distinctive specialty within Soviet public health. The recognition of their distinctiveness opened new challenges for social hygienists: they had to justify their separation and secure the legitimacy of their enterprise.

At least in a formal sense, social hygiene was institutionalized in the Soviet Union in a remarkably short time. In 1922 the first *kafedra* of social hygiene was opened for the medical faculties of the two Moscow state universities. Within six years there were fifteen such *kafedry* throughout the RSFSR.[9] In 1923, with social hygiene still emerging as a distinctive discipline, a new research institution, the State Institute for Social Hygiene (GISG) was founded to conduct and coordinate research on problems in social hygiene.[10] Even before GISG opened its doors, there was created under the aegis of the *kafedra* of social hygiene of I Moscow University a special journal, *Sotsial' naia gigiena*, whose mandate was to publish important works on social hygiene written by researchers from all over the country.[11] By the end of the 1920s, teaching and research in public health looked substantially different from the way it had at the outset of the decade.

SEMASHKO AND SOCIAL HYGIENE

The rapid pace at which social hygiene was institutionalized was a function of the fact that the new field was established by government fiat. The field emerged under the umbrella of the Commissariat of Public Health (Narkomzdrav). Its chief patron was the commissar himself, N. A. Semashko. In deference to his prerevolutionary friendship with Lenin, Semashko was (and still is) referred to in official Soviet literature as Lenin's comrade-in-arms.[12] During Lenin's lifetime, Semashko enjoyed access to those who made decisions for public health, and even after Lenin's death in 1924, the commissar continued for more than half a decade to carry with him the charisma of an Old Bolshevik.

Semashko's personal stature, however, was not matched by the prestige of the ministry over which he presided. As Neil Weissman has shown, public health was one of those ministries which was given a fundamentally new structure after the Revolution.[13] As a result, its administrators could not reap any of the benefits which flow from long-standing procedures or arrangements. Even more important, official pronouncements notwithstanding, the delivery of health care was a fairly low priority for the new leadership. Throughout the 1920s, investment in health care was, at best, modest, and at the end of the decade, when resources were needed for industrial development, the delivery of health care was cut back severely.[14]

In his role as chief patron of the fledgling field of social hygiene, Semashko was constrained by factors other than the relatively weak position of his ministry. For one thing, the Commissariat of Public Health had to share jurisdiction over public health with other ministries. For example, between 1922 and 1930, the Commissariat of Enlightenment (Narkompros) had jurisdiction over medical education, as it did over all of higher learning;[15] to Narkomzdrav fell the task of regulating physicians after they graduated. In a similar vein, research on public health problems was often conducted under the combined aegis of a number of commissariats. For example, some of the most important research on industrial hygiene was jointly sponsored by the Commissariats of Health and Labor.[16] Even within his own commissariat, Semashko was constrained in his support of social hygiene because Narkomzdrav was home to a wide array of intellectual disciplines, some of which were based on philosophical principles diametrically opposed to those underlying other disciplines. In the 1920s, for example, Narkomzdrav supported both social hygiene with its nurturist principles and eugenics with its naturist foundations.[17] To make the commissariat home to such a variety of disciplines required restraint in championing the cause of any single discipline.

Nowhere was this restraint more evident than in the definition of social hygiene which Semashko used to argue for the legitimacy of the fledgling field. That definition emerged piecemeal. In 1921, Semashko wrote a small brochure entitled "Nauka o zdorovye obshchestva," which was notable for its traditional approach to public health. In this brochure, social hygiene appeared as "the science of the health of society," but the list of subjects included under the rubric of this science scarcely differed from that conventionally included in the field of general hygiene: soil and water, clothing, living space, nutrition, labor and sexual hygiene. Semashko did say that disease should be seen as a social phenomenon because it affected various segments of the population differently, but he made only minor allusions to the ways in which the important indicators of public health might vary with social class.[18]

A year later, Semashko wrote an article (whose core was later enshrined in the Bol'shaia Sovetskaia Entsiklopediia) that differentiated social hygiene more sharply from general hygiene.[19] He began not with the subject matter of the field, but with its philosophy of disease. Semashko insisted that the old formula "microbe + organism + (physical) environment = disease" was outmoded; he argued that it ought to be replaced by an analysis of the social factors involved in disease. The carrier of this new philosophy of disease must be a new and separate field, social hygiene. In support of this proposal, Semashko cited such German pioneers in social medicine as A. Grotjahn, B. Chajes, and A. Kisskalt, but in making the case for social hygiene, Semashko was much less bold than those he claimed had inspired him. To argue for the utility of the new field, he used two noncontroversial problems: living space and nutrition. As Semashko laid it out, whereas general hygiene focused on the suitability (space, air, location) of a particular dwelling, social hygiene would concentrate on the relationship between living conditions and social structure. Similarly, whereas general hygiene studied the quality and sanitation of food, it would fall to social hygiene to examine the nutrition of the various classes.

Semashko's use of the examples of nutrition and living space sent a clear message to spokesmen for social hygiene that the commissar was prepared to argue for the legitimacy of the field simply on the grounds that it had a distinctive approach to familiar problems; the field did not need to display substantive novelty. In making this point, Semashko inadvertently signaled opponents of social hygiene that the field did not have a specific content. For many, as we shall see, this was to be the Achilles heel of social hygiene.

Among those who challenged the legitimacy of social hygiene, one of the most powerful was G. V. Khlopin, the one-time Social Democrat who was the doyen of general hygiene at Leningrad's prestigious Military Medical Academy.[20] Khlopin's authoritative textbook on general hygiene, *Osnovy gigieny,* appeared in print in 1921—at the very time Semashko was working toward a definition of social hygiene.[21] In his text, Khlopin demarcated the terrain of his field broadly: general hygiene embraced the study of ways to make the environment healthy, of ways to prevent professional illness, and of the etiology of and most effective means to prevent infectious disease. At Khlopin's hands, general hygiene was broader than bacteriology and epidemiology; it built on chemistry, physics, specific bacteriology, and physiology.

Nor was Khlopin content to stop here. He insisted that Russian general hygiene had always been concerned with social conditions and reminded the reader that both the general hygienists A. P. Dobroslavin, who taught the subject in the Military Medical Academy in St. Petersburg from 1871 to 1889, and F. F. Erisman, who taught the subject at Moscow University from 1882 to 1896, stressed the importance of social factors.[22] To rip away these social concerns now would deprive general hygienists of the right to cover such important topics as the protection of labor, community nutrition, reform of housing, and sanitary legislation. Bluntly put, this would drive general hygiene back into the laboratory.[23] Khlopin's polemic was pointed: his targets were unnamed German proponents of social medicine who were trying to separate social hygiene from "scientific" (read laboratory) hygiene and whose example Soviet social hygienists seemed determined to emulate.

The sources do not tell us the precise source of Semashko's conception of social hygiene. It may well be that before the Revolution he had been inspired by reading German works in social medicine; alternatively, the commissar may have taken his ideas of social hygiene from Russian colleagues such as Z. G. Frenkel and V. Ia. Kanel who were familiar with the German work.[24] Whatever the case, Soviet social hygienists openly acknowledged their debt to German social medicine of the first two decades of the twentieth century: they translated into Russian many of the leading German textbooks in social medicine.[25] Moreover, throughout the 1920s Soviet social hygienists made every effort to maintain the link with the Germans: they inserted articles in the leading German journals of public health[26] and publicized their research in a joint German-Russian periodical.[27] (Close relations between German and Russian physicians of the type evident among specialists in social medicine were found in many branches of medicine. The German-Russian links may have been close because in the interwar period both Russia and Germany were treated as pariahs in the international arena.)

Among those most active in maintaining the Russian-German connection in social medicine was Semashko himself. A reading of Semashko's references to German work suggests that, in his view, its debt to German social medicine did not adversely affect the stature of Soviet social hygiene. On the contrary, Semashko behaved as though the German lineage added luster to the field he championed. In doffing his hat to the Germans, Semashko was sending a clear signal that, for him, the legitimacy of Soviet social hygiene did not depend on its being original on the world stage; it was enough that the field was "new" to Russia after the Revolution.

In delineating the roots of social hygiene in Russia, Semashko omitted any mention of the contribution of prerevolutionary Russian community medicine (*ob-shchestvennaia meditsina*). In this, he was virtually alone among Soviet social hygienists. The self-appointed historian of Soviet social hygiene, Z. G. Frenkel, devoted half of his best-known work to a careful delineation of the intellectual and personal connections between the prerevolutionary community medicine and the postrevolutionary field of social hygiene.[28] How extensive was the debt of social hygiene to community medicine? There was a substantial overlap in personnel: a number of the prime movers in Soviet social hygiene had tried before the Revolution to mount courses on social aspects of hygiene in the medical schools.[29] Moreover, the research agenda of social hygiene overlapped partially with that of some spokesmen for "community medicine." But the resemblance was far from perfect: most of the Russian pioneers in community medicine do not appear to have had a clear definition of their field of research. As a result they included in their agenda not only everything that had a vaguely social cast but also that which did not fit into the field of general hygiene (for example, questions of health care delivery and organization).[30] The Soviets, by contrast, used their categorical statement about the primarily social nature of health and disease as a strict principle of inclusion and exclusion of subject matter in their field. Therefore while there were several specific points of similarity between "community medicine" and social hygiene, the amalgam that was social hygiene was distinctive: in the main it was an adaptation of German *soziale Medizin* to the Soviet context, with the addition of some concerns of prerevolutionary Russian community medicine—all overlaid with a strong critical thrust that derived from the notion of health and disease as fundamentally social in nature.

Semashko's selective approach to the roots of social hygiene was probably deliberate: in any case, it afforded the commissar considerable room for maneuver. He was able to answer critics who challenged the legitimacy of social hygiene by pointing to the German roots of the field; he was able to answer opponents who challenged the novelty of the field by arguing that as such the field of social hygiene did not exist in prerevolutionary Russia. Semashko made it clear that in his view the legitimacy of social hygiene was beyond dispute. He contended that the differentiation of fields was the natural course of knowledge and that the splitting up of general hygiene into different fields was completely in keeping with the progress of science. Semashko went even further: social hygiene was legitimate not simply because it was different from, but because it was better than, general hygiene. "Social hygiene stands on the shoulders of general experimental hygiene."[31]

There was a streak of realism in this patron. However demonstrable the merits of social hygiene, Semashko predicted that the battle to institutionalize that field would be a pitched one, particularly on the educational front. It would not be easy, he declared, to get a special course devoted to the concerns of social hygiene into the curriculum of the medical faculties, the foremost of which tended to be somewhat hidebound.[32] In fact, the establishment of special courses on social hygiene between 1922 and 1927 was not problematic; what proved exceedingly difficult was securing legitimacy for the new discipline.

TEACHING SOCIAL HYGIENE

Given the prominence of social hygiene's leading patron, Semashko, and the complexity of the task of defining a new field, one might assume that Semashko's definition of social hygiene would be replicated in all Russian medical faculties. But the attentive reader of social hygiene textbooks and course outlines in the second half of the 1920s will discern intriguing variations in the definition of the "new" field.

As a rule, social hygiene was defined in opposition to general hygiene but, as we shall see, the boundaries of general hygiene itself varied from place to place, and therefore in every instance social hygiene had to adapt to a different ecology of fields in public health. Not only was the current shape of teaching general hygiene significant; it turned out that the history of that teaching also had an impact. Finally, in each region the intellectual interests and strengths of the regional spokesmen for social hygiene strongly influenced the way in which the field was conceived and transmitted to students.

The heart of the Moscow approach to social hygiene was the commitment to study a wide range of diseases in their societal contexts. And yet, while the Moscow "school" stressed social factors, it never neglected their biological substrate. This balanced approach was patent in the lectures on social hygiene delivered at the *kafedry* of social hygiene of I Moscow University (headed by A. V. Molkov, a sanitary doctor active in the Pirogov Society who became a member of the Communist party in 1919[33]) and II Moscow University (headed by Z. P. Soloviev, the long-time Bolshevik who was Semashko's deputy commissar of public health[34]). For example, the first course on the subject, offered in 1922, opened with a section on the concept of social hygiene which gave play to the role of natural and sanitary science in the development of that concept.[35] The same evenhandedness was patent in the first original textbook on social hygiene published in 1927 under the editorship of A. V. Molkov. In this text, discussions of the "problems of collective life" (dwelling, nutrition, work, sexual life) were peppered with references to the works of general hygienists.[36]

The Moscow approach to social hygiene owed much to the fact that the field's alter-ego, general hygiene, was taught by individuals (the sanitarian A. N. Sysin in I Moscow University,[37] the bacteriologist P. N. Diatroptov in II Moscow University[38]) who did not have to be persuaded of the salience of social factors for the incidence and spread of disease. Indeed, the sensitivity of Moscow general hygienists to social factors dated back to the work of F. F. Erisman in the 1870s. In the Soviet period, the tempered approach of the Moscow social hygienists was further reinforced by the prominence in the capital of Semashko who, as commissar of public health, was responsible for maintaining as broad as possible a constituency among public health physicians.

In Leningrad, by contrast, social hygiene was characterized by an overriding emphasis on social analysis that was unique among those who taught in the field. For most Soviet social hygienists, social analysis was nothing more than crude class analysis. But in Leningrad, at both the Military Medical Academy and the Leningrad Medical Institute, the head of the *kafedra* of social hygiene was A. F. Nikitin, the social theorist who had been drawn to Marxist circles in his twenties and later studied with Khlopin.[39] Both in the course he taught and in the textbook he wrote, Nikitin defined social hygiene as the "hygiene of the social collective."[40] This broad definition of the field allowed Nikitin to present social hygiene as a field which integrated all studies of man as a bio-social being and then to include under its rubric such subjects as lifestyle and labor, disease and poverty, and social dynamics. With its focus on society and social problems, Nikitin's social hygiene bore an intriguing resemblance to American sociology of the same period.[41]

How can one explain the approach taken by Nikitin? It is important to recall that Leningrad had a long-standing interest in social analysis: well before the Revolution, this city witnessed the development of a burgeoning literature in empirical social research under the direction of such luminaries as Pitirim Sorokin.[42] Although that empirical sociology was forcibly cut off in 1922 when some of the leading sociologists went into exile, the legacy of sociological thinking here proved enduring.

In addition to the existence of an indigenous sociological tradition in Leningrad, Nikitin's approach to social hygiene was doubtless influenced by the commanding presence of G. V. Khlopin in the major medical schools in the northern capital.[43] Even as Khlopin's high profile retarded the opening of *kafedry* of social hygiene in Leningrad,[44] his conservative position vis-à-vis the new field forced social hygienists to the margin and made them define their field in a more profoundly social way than did any other cohort of Soviet social hygienists.

The traditional centers of bacteriology and public health had their distinctive approaches to social hygiene, approaches which differed in important respects from those followed in the old and new capitals. Kharkov, for example, emerged as the center of the psycho-neurological approach to social hygiene. The pivotal figure here was S. A. Tomilin, the wide-ranging intellectual who served as the head of *kafedra* of social hygiene in the I Kharkov Medical Institute from 1925 on.[45] In his many writings on social hygiene, Tomilin acknowledged the importance of biological factors in disease but urged social hygienists to study the psychological factors that were superimposed on biology, factors which he believed profoundly affected human well-being.[46] Curiously, for all the originality of his definition of social hygiene, Tomilin never denied the usefulness of general hygiene; he argued only that this traditional field should be supplemented by social hygiene.

The Kharkov approach to social hygiene owed much to the catholic intelligence of Tomilin. But the success of Kharkov in developing the psycho-neurological approach was partly a function of timing. As one observer explained, the fact that the Kharkov *kafedra* of social hygiene was not opened until 1925 meant that social hygienists there could avoid becoming enmeshed in the debates between Bekhterev and Pavlov that had engulfed psychologists in Leningrad.[47]

Given the considerable support of the Commissariat of Public Health for the establishment of social hygiene, the variations in the teaching of the discipline were understandable: each regional center, confident of the broad endorsement of the patron, developed its own brand of social hygiene. Such variety certainly attests to a high degree of creativity among teachers of social hygiene. It may equally well bespeak the existence of competing visions of the newly emerging discipline.

The absence of agreement on the core of social hygiene was not problematic as long as the field was expanding. Even the most cursory glance at the journal *Sotsial'naia gigiena* in the years 1922–1925, when the number of *kafedry* of social hygiene was increasing dramatically, suggests that the goal at this juncture appeared to be to proselytize—to open new *kafedry* of social hygiene, to mount new courses, to activate new student groups; concern about the content of the field was secondary. This pride in the proliferation of social hygiene was clearly reflected at the First All-Union Meeting of Representatives of Prophylactic Kafedry in the RSFSR held in Moscow in April of 1925.[48]

The 1925 meeting was scheduled to focus on preventive medicine, but, as the published transcript of the meeting makes clear, the meeting developed into a contest for leadership between spokesmen for general and social hygiene. The social hygienists, acting now as a united force despite the existence of significant differences in approach, bent every effort to assert hegemony over the field of public health as a whole. For a fledgling field which had been institutionalized for less than a half decade, this was a Herculean task.

To accomplish it, social hygienists pursued two strategies. First, they argued for the right to include certain subjects in the syllabus of their courses on the grounds that the approach to these same subjects taken by general hygienists was too narrow. In fact, there was little overlap in the content of the two courses,[49] but the social hygienists' argument had a polemical purpose. So assertive were the social hygienists at the 1925 meeting that G. A. Batkis, the young hothead Bolshevik doing his graduate studies at Moscow University, suggested publicly that social hygiene be regarded as the basic course in the "hygiene cycle," the core of the prophylactic curriculum.[50] Even as ardent a supporter of social hygiene as S. A. Tomilin expressed amazement that social hygiene, "the newest guest at the table," aimed at taking a leading role in public health.[51]

Second, the social hygienists laid claim to paternity over the two newest prophylactic *kafedry*—hygiene of education and hygiene of labor. Proponents of general hygiene had a long-standing interest in these two areas: indeed, Khlopin's 1921 text on general hygiene had covered hygiene of labor and education hygiene.[52] But it was the *kafedra* of social hygiene which had applied to the Main Committee of Professional Education (*Glavprofobr*) of the Commissariat of Enlightenment for permission to set up new *kafedry* devoted specifically to the teaching of these subjects.[53] And a 1924 circular of the Commissariat of Public Health enjoined *kafedry* of social hygiene to teach material on hygiene of education and labor whenever separate *kafedry* had yet to be formed.[54] If this were not enough to establish the paternity of social hygiene over the two new fields, S. I. Kaplun, the energetic young Communist party member who headed the new *kafedra* of hygiene of labor at I Moscow University, declared that his *kafedra* had sprung from social hygiene![55]

To be sure, the offensive of the social hygienists at the 1925 meeting did not go unopposed. Khlopin launched a powerful fusillade against the claims of the social hygienists: social hygiene had no specific content, he argued; it was simply an approach (*podkhod*), and not a distinctive approach at that. It was an amalgam of sociology, anthropology, and nonmedical sciences.[56] At the time, Khlopin's critique fell on deaf ears because social hygienists seem to have occupied the high ground in public health—despite the absence of a settled core of the field.

In the wake of the 1925 conference, social hygienists, assuming the role of standardbearers of the preventive emphasis in medicine, attempted to infiltrate the teaching of clinical subjects. As I have shown elsewhere, that attempt was most successful in fields with their own clinics and with established well-check procedures; it was far less successful in such bastions of the biological approach as pathology.[57] Indeed, the efforts of social hygiene to spearhead the "prophylactization" of the clinical subjects engendered considerable resistance. That resistance contrasts sharply with the lack of interest that attended the initial establishment of *kafedry* of social hygiene in the first half of the 1920s. But then, at the outset of the decade, spokesmen for social hygiene had appeared moderate; half a decade later, the ambitions of some of the discipline's leaders had become patent.

In May 1928, the Second Conference of Representatives of Prophylactic Kafedry met in Leningrad to review the results of the preceding three years of teaching prophylactic disciplines in the medical schools. Semashko opened the conference with the statement that "the time had passed when one could have prevention in one pocket and cure in the other."[58] Judging from the content of the discussion that followed, it is clear that the commissar's words should be read not as a sign of satisfaction at the achievements of the preventive *kafedry,* but as a desperate plea for their survival.

What was the source of Semashko's desperation? The stepped-up pace of industrial development was draining resources from all sectors of the economy other than industry. In these conditions of financial stringency, a field like social hygiene, whose contribution lay in its new approach to old problems rather than in its ability to treat problems not handled by other fields, was expendable. Apparently, the Commissariat of Workers-Peasants Inspection (RKI) was threatening to disband many of the prophylactic *kafedry* because they were not functioning in twelve medical schools![59]

But it emerged in discussion that the prophylactic *kafedry* had also failed to win the allegiance of students and faculty. Kedrov, the representative of Narkompros's Main Committee for Professional-Technical Education, asserted that although 5,000 places were available in these *kafedry,* only 1,800 students showed up.[60] Interviews I conducted in 1985 with former Soviet physicians who were trained in the 1920s and early 1930s confirmed these attitudes. Those most drawn to social hygiene were the students who did not come from medical families; students who came from established medical families, who were upwardly mobile, and who were from major urban centers tended to view social hygiene as a diversion whose principles could be assimilated on the job.[61] Indeed some teachers of clinical subjects were apparently saying to students, "We are here to teach you so that you can earn a living, not be sanitary doctors."[62]

Not surprisingly, then, the 1928 meeting of teachers of prophylactic subjects reads like the record of dashed hopes. Although the conference ended with resolutions prohibiting the closure of the prophylactic *kafedry,* the survival of the preventive emphasis in medicine was clearly far from assured. In recognition of the tenuousness of their enterprise, a high proportion of the speakers at the Leningrad meeting, both from the large urban centers and from the provinces, tried to move the battle outside the medical school. They suggested that the survival of the preventive emphasis in medicine depended on tying prevention to curative (in-patient or out-patient) facilities.[63] That is, prophylactic medicine had to demonstrate its utility. Otherwise, as one speaker from the provinces put it, "in two to three years, we can forget the prophylactic *kafedry.*"[64]

SETTING RESEARCH AGENDAS

In the course of the 1920s, the range of topics studied under the rubric of social hygiene was impressive. The research agenda for 1926–27, when the field was at its height, embraced problems of population, (birth, death, migration), consumption (nutrition and alcoholism), sexual life (sex education and prostitution), work (professional selection and women's work), and collective life (housing, education, leisure). The list of topics is deceptive, however. It included three distinct categories of subjects: those which emerged under the protection of social hygiene and remained under its umbrella (for example, problems of sexual life), those which were initially part of social hygiene but subsequently differentiated themselves from that field and were studied as independent areas (for example, hygiene of labor), and those in which other fields had a long-standing interest and into which social hygienists were attempting to make inroads (for example, alcoholism).

The differences among research topics were reflected in the organization of research. Formally, social hygiene research was centered in GISG. That institution, formed in 1923 from the State Museum of Social Hygiene, was created specifically to exercise intellectual and organizational leadership over researchers working in the fledgling field. In practice, the situation proved somewhat more complex. For those areas of research which emerged under the aegis of social hygiene and remained there, GISG performed the task of leadership admirably. In the case of research areas which acquired legitimacy under the umbrella of social hygiene and then developed into independent areas of inquiry, GISG had to cede its hegemony to other research units, some of which were under the jurisdiction of ministries other than public health. For the third group of research areas, those in which disciplines other than social hygiene had a long-standing involvement, GISG was forced to carve a place for itself in an already demarcated institutional terrain. The difficulties of institutionalizing their field of research are most clearly illustrated by social hygienists' experience with this last category of subjects.

ALCOHOLISM AND THE UTILITY
OF SOCIAL HYGIENE RESEARCH

One research area that fell clearly into the third category was the study of alcoholism. Well before the Revolution, the problem of alcoholism had engaged the professional attention of Russian psychiatrists, criminologists, and police.[65] In the mid-1920s, social hygienists were provided with the opportunity to demonstrate the distinctiveness of their approach to this most intractable of social problems. To succeed in this demonstration, they had to show not only descriptive, but prescriptive, novelty.

In 1926, the Council of People's Commissars (Sovnarkom) passed an edict which entrusted to Narkomzdrav the task of studying the problem of alcoholism and leading the prophylactic fight against it.[66] Although the mandate formally sanctioned some "medicalization" of the alcohol problem, it did not specify the type of physician responsible for studying alcoholism. Almost immediately the Commissariat of Public Health made clear its interpretation of the 1926 edict: it commissioned GISG—by then the bastion of the field of social hygiene—to conduct research on alcoholism as a social problem and to coordinate the research on alcoholism being conducted by other research institutes under the ministry's aegis.[67] To accomplish this task, a small *kabinet* (office) was opened in GISG under the directorship of E. I. Deichman.[68]

The nod to GISG should not be seen as unambiguously according authority over alcoholism to social hygienists. For in the original enabling edict of 1926, Sovnarkom targeted the neuro-psychiatric dispensaries as the institutions most appropriate for leading the fight against alcoholism. Moreover, in 1927 Narkomzdrav itself licensed these out-patient dispensaries to collect data on alcoholics—thus requiring GISG to share the research function.[69] The stage was set for the confrontation between social hygienists and psychiatrists over the right to speak authoritatively on this subject.

From the beginning, social hygienists insisted that alcoholism was a "social disease," that is, a disease whose appearance, frequency, and spread were all affected by social factors. In the 1922 curriculum for the course on social hygiene prepared by GISG, alcoholism appeared under the heading "social disease" along with tuberculosis and venereal disease. In the 1925 revised curriculum for the same course, alcoholism was subsumed under the general heading of "social disease" but it now appeared along with narcotics and nervous disease in a subgroup entitled "addiction and nervous disease."[70] By the middle of the 1920s, social hygienists were expressing the view that alcohol consumption was habit-forming and that the habit was socially conditioned.

After GISG received the official mandate to study social aspects of alcoholism, social hygienists began to carve out a specific facet of the alcohol problem which would be theirs alone—the study of the habitual or *bytovoi* (lifestyle) alcoholic, whose numbers were increasing dramatically in the Soviet period.[71] Although this drinker imbibed less than the chronic alcoholic, his consumption interfered with the maintenance of public order, adversely affected the quality and quantity of industrial production, and perverted family and social life.[72]

To lay claim to authority over the *bytovoi* alcoholic, GISG researchers had to differentiate the *bytovoi* alcoholic clearly from the chronic alcoholic and to develop a methodology of research which could be used to ferret out those social conditions most frequently associated with habitual or lifestyle drinking. In 1926, A. V. Molkov, the director of GISG and the leading intellectual spokesman for social hygiene, wrote an article which presented the habitual alcoholic as an individual whose drinking was a function of such social factors as the desire to compensate for insufficient food, exhausting conditions of work, the absence of good living conditions, the lack of elevated interests or the organizational possibilities for intellectual pursuits.[73] Although he did not say so explicitly, Molkov clearly subscribed to the nurturist as opposed to naturist hypotheses about the causes of alcoholism.[74]

Included in the article was a questionnaire which Molkov designed. That questionnaire, which conferred a degree of scientist legitimacy on a field like social hygiene that lacked the paraphernalia of the laboratory, subsequently became the official instrument for all systematic research on the social aspects of alcoholism; it was used by GISG researchers themselves, by field workers *(korrespondenty)* collecting data on the local level, and by researchers from other ministries. Not surprisingly, the questionnaire revealed the importance of habit in the consumption of alcohol by peasants and workers, adults and children alike. From the several studies of drinking patterns among these groups conducted between 1926 and 1929,[75] the *bytovoi* alcoholic emerged not as a vicious deviant, but as a victim of his social circumstances (poor living, poor nutrition, taxing work, isolation, parents who drank).

Significantly, Soviet social hygienists rested their claims to authority over alcoholism on methodological rather than on substantive grounds. They pointed with pride to the comprehensiveness of Molkov's questionnaire and to the ingenious use of field workers to carry out inquiries on the periphery.[76] Only secondarily did the Deichman team tout the value of the research findings in understanding the *bytovoi* alcoholic.

The emphasis GISG researchers placed on methodological originality must be understood in the context of the strong and pervasive commitment of postrevolutionary Soviet culture to "science." Although interest in scientific positivism was evident in many countries of Europe at this time, in the Soviet case commitment to science was part of official ideology. For Soviet social hygienists in the 1920s, a successful claim to being considered "scientific" could not be mounted on the basis of social theory. Almost from the beginning of the decade, Marxism was the only officially sanctioned social theory, and its insights had not been cast into propositions that could be used to direct research on social problems.[77] The focus on methodology as the heart of science was much more promising. Devices like the questionnaire carried with them an aura of science; besides, the use of such devices allowed Semashko and his followers to press their claims to legitimacy while not treading on the toes of historical materialism.

It is also possible that GISG researchers studying alcoholism stressed their methodological novelty because they did not want to draw attention to their substantive contribution. Pushed only slightly further than they took it, social hygienists' research on *bytovoi* alcoholism would have shown that behind the seemingly random social factors which made for habitual drinking lay the patterns of Soviet social structure; this in turn would have given grounds for the argument that, in order to reduce habitual alcoholism, what was needed was profound social change. But the social hygienists declined to push their analysis that far. Acting as mandated experts rather than free-wheeling social critics, they stopped short of formulating an indictment of Soviet social structure. (Ironically, the same social hygienists criticized "bourgeois" researchers on social diseases for producing a factorial rather than a structural account of the conditions leading to illness!)[78]

Apart from the risky political implications of their work, there was the question of its scope. Deichman and his team had staked their claim to authority over alcoholism on their ability to analyze the *bytovoi* alcoholic. But this was a wager on narrowness for, in addition to the "habitual" alcoholic, there was the chronic alcoholic over whom social hygienists claimed no expertise whatever.

And finally, as the self-proclaimed intellectual heirs of the German pioneer in social medicine, Alfred Grotjahn, Soviet social hygienists consistently maintained that theirs was a prescriptive as well as a descriptive science. To achieve recognition as the authorities over alcoholism, Soviet social hygienists would have to demonstrate that their analysis led logically to policies that would be effective in dealing with the intractable problem of the habitual drinker.

Unfortunately their approach to treatment proved to be the great weakness of the social hygienists. Social hygienists invariably put their faith in cultural work (propaganda and resocialization) aimed at softening the attachment of the alcoholic to "the little beaker of vodka."[79] But cultural work was a long-term therapy. What ought to be done with the habitual alcoholic in the short term? As public health physicians-turned-researchers, the social hygienists had little first-hand experience in treating alcoholics. The treatment facility closest to the philosophy of the social hygienists was the *narko-dispanser* (narcotics dispensary), an out-patient unit which approached the habitual drinker as a patient suffering from a social, rather than a mental, problem.[80]

When it came to questions of therapy, however, the social hygienists were easily outclassed by the psychiatrists who had been involved in treating alcoholics since well before the Revolution. Prior to 1917, the psychiatrists had concentrated their attention on chronic alcoholics, leaving to the police the handling of habitual drinkers who did not constitute a threat to themselves or to society. In the course of the 1920s, as I have shown elsewhere, the psychiatric profession began to lay claim to speak authoritatively about the *bytovoi* alcoholic, thus entering into direct rivalry with the social hygienists.[81] In contrast to the social hygienists, the psychiatrists pictured the *bytovoi* alcoholic as a species of mental patient whose drinking was a function of his inability to adapt to the challenges of life rather than a response to his unfavorable social circumstances. Touting the results of their empirical studies of the patients in psychiatric institutions,[82] the psychiatrists maintained that they alone had the knowledge to treat this type of alcoholic effectively.

The psychiatrists' claim of hegemony over the question of treatment easily won the day. In the first place, the *narko-dispansery*—the outpatient units most consistent with the approach of the social hygienists—were not making the kinds of inroads into life style alcoholism that had been predicted for them. In fact, psychiatric hospitals were getting increasing numbers of referrals of patients who had been treated in the dispensaries without success.[83] Equally important, the long-term strategy of resocialization and propaganda urged by social hygienists seemed out of place in the late 1920s. As the decade progressed, the emphasis was increasingly on rapid transformation; where spontaneous transformation had not occurred, force was now considered legitimate. Thus by the end of the decade the general climate favored the short-term solutions of restricted access to liquor[84] and forced treatment[85] which the psychiatrists advocated. In the face of this shift in the climate of opinion, the social hygienists' attempt to demonstrate the utility of their approach fell on deaf ears. Not surprisingly, no new social inquiries on the subject of alcoholism were reported in the review of GISG activities for 1929.[86]

1930: ON THE CUSP

Beginning in 1930, a series of structural changes occurred which fundamentally altered the position of social hygiene within Soviet public health. These changes appear to have been triggered by the removal in January of 1930 of the field's chief patron, N. A. Semashko, as commissar of public health.[87] No specific reasons for Semashko's replacement were ever given. It may well be, as Christopher Davis suggests in his contribution to this volume, that Semashko's failure to endorse what he considered the overambitious pace of development of health care called for in the First Five-Year Plan led to his removal.[88] Alternatively, it may have been that Semashko's credentials as an Old Bolshevik made him appear threatening to Stalin; Lunacharskii, the commissar of enlightenment whose Bolshevik credentials were of the same vintage, was also removed from his post in 1930.[89]

If historians cannot pinpoint the reasons for Semashko's removal, they can infer a good deal from the profile of the man who replaced him. Semashko was succeeded by M. F. Vladimirskii, whose prerevolutionary involvement with the Bolshevik cause brought him into direct contact with Semashko as early as 1911, if not earlier. Though trained as a physician, Vladimirskii appears to have confined his activities after 1917 to administrative positions only tangentially related to health care.[90]

The effects of Semashko's removal were felt first in the area of social hygiene research. In late 1930, GISG was converted into the Institute of Organization of Health Care and Hygiene under the aegis of the Commissariat of Public Health RSFSR. The top priorities of the new institute were administrative: practical health care and organization.[91] To the extent that it endured at all, social research on health and disease was conducted by statisticians. But by the mid-1930s even statistics had dried up. In October 1934, a decree of the Council of People's Commissars officially eliminated thirty-eight research institutes dealing with questions of public health, including the institute that had been created to replace GISG.[92]

With hindsight, it is clear that substantial changes in the limits of permissible social hygiene research had occurred well before 1930. GISG was initially organized along methodological lines (three of the five *kabinety* of the institute were methodological in focus[93]), but by 1929 even the methodologically oriented divisions of the institute were licensed to work on social hygiene problems only insofar as those problems illuminated questions of methodology.[94]

The full impact of Semashko's removal on the teaching of social hygiene occurred somewhat later than it did on research work. Not until May 1941 were *kafedry* of social hygiene formally renamed *kafedry* of the organization of health care, although the preoccupation with health care organization was patent by 1936 if not earlier.[95] In 1930, a series of decrees was passed creating three distinct faculties in the medical schools: the curative-prophylactic faculty, which prepared specialists in surgery, therapy, and stomatology; the sanitary-prophylactic faculty to which medical students interested in social hygiene gravitated; and the faculty of protection-of-mothers-and-children (*okhmatdet*), which prepared specialists in maternity and infant care.[96] The division of the medical school into three distinct faculties was effectively the death-knell of the experiment to integrate social hygiene into the medical school curriculum. Equally important, it introduced into the medical schools a system of educational streaming, for the curative-prophylactic and *okhmatdet* faculties were more demanding and took longer to complete than did the sanitary-prophylactic faculty.[97] As might be expected, the best-prepared and most able students did not flock to the sanitary-prophylactic faculties. Thus, at the very time when, according to Christopher Davis, almost all the health care indicators reflected a deepening crisis, those responsible for medical education made a series of decisions which could only contribute to rather than alleviate the problems.

CONCLUSION

The rise and fall of social hygiene in Soviet public health raises a series of interesting issues. Traditionally, scholarly treatments of the relationship of government and science have examined well-established scientific disciplines for indications of resistance or receptivity of science to government direction.[98] In these treatments, government almost invariably emerges as an intrusive force seeking, through the use of positive or negative incentives, to limit scientific autonomy. In Soviet social hygiene we have a discipline which was formed through government fiat. In this instance, government acted not as an intruder, but as a patron which facilitated the emergence of a new discipline. Prior to the Revolution, specialists in "community medicine" had tried in vain to create a niche for their field in the medical schools and in research institutes. The Bolsheviks' accession to power provided a window of opportunity for social hygienists. Secure in the support of their patron, they defined an intellectual enterprise and presided over its establishment in teaching and research institutions. Without the support of the Commissariat of Public Health, it is highly unlikely that social hygiene would have come into being as a distinctive intellectual enterprise in the 1920s. Left to the tender mercies of more traditional medical men, social hygiene might well have remained, as did Russian "community medicine" before it, a would-be discipline.

In a setting where government is both sole patron and client of science, one might think that the institutionalization of any field by government fiat would ensure the success of that field. Our story suggests that such success is far from axiomatic. Although government fiat can establish a field, it cannot secure its legitimacy. Legitimacy comes from the acceptance of an intellectual enterprise by professionals working in the field itself and in allied fields. In this instance, there were serious obstacles to the new field's securing of legitimacy.

To begin with, a large proportion of professors in the medical school—particularly those teaching clinical medicine, were unwilling to endorse the new field. As Semashko was to reflect in 1947, nearly two decades after the demise of social hygiene, suspicion of the new *kafedra* at the time of its formation was fueled by the fact that its leaders, A. V. Molkov, A. N. Sysin, S. I. Kaplun, and Semashko himself, were not "diplomaed scholars."[99] By mid-decade, that suspicion had become opposition because to many teachers of clinical medicine the ambitions of social hygienists for a leading role in public health appeared to threaten their emphasis on cure.

Wariness of social hygiene was not confined to the professoriate; students, too, were reserved in their enthusiasm. As Batkis explained it, the students of 1922/23 were receptive to the approach of social hygiene: having just been through the Revolution and civil war, they were eager to put their faith in the new curriculum. The students of 1927/28, however, were the product of more normal times: upwardly mobile, they were more interested in specialized education and had little time for diversions.[100]

The final obstacle to the social hygienists' securing legitimacy for their enterprise stemmed from the increasing use of the yardstick of practical utility to judge the worth of intellectual fields. In any setting, the acceptance of a field depends in part on its success in addressing the problems to which its spokesmen have committed themselves. But as the 1920s wore on, the criterion of practical utility came to surpass all other yardsticks for evaluating the worth of Soviet fields. Though many social hygienists began as "men of practice" (to use Semashko's phrase), the 1920s saw them devoting their time to teaching social hygiene or to charting directions for research. When some social hygienists were provided with the opportunity to apply their findings to concrete social problems, they were not always able to demonstrate the usefulness of their approach in solving the pressing problems of public health (for example, alcoholism).

The obstacles confronting social hygiene in its quest for legitimacy could not be surmounted by the patronage of Semashko. For Semashko himself was operating under palpable constraints: for much of his tenure, he had to share jurisdiction over social hygiene with other commissariats (such as Narkompros) which were not as committed as he was to the fledgling field. More important, social hygiene did not secure the allegiance of those ministries responsible for its funding (Sovnarkom) or regulation (Workers-Peasants Inspection). Having hitched their star to a single patron, social hygienists found themselves, when Semashko was replaced, without bureaucratic support; not surprisingly, their field foundered.

Apart from the reliance of its leaders on a single patron, was there something about Soviet social hygiene which made the field particularly vulnerable at the end of the 1920s? This essay has suggested that the Soviets adapted a good deal of German social medicine—particularly its research agenda and methods—to their own context. And they did not trouble to hide that adaptation: in fact, for a variety of reasons Soviet social hygienists underscored the extent to which they were following the German lead. But there was one crucial difference between the two which the Soviets studiously avoided mentioning. The German pioneers in social medicine had been engaged in a protracted struggle to institutionalize their field. In the early 1920s, in order to secure acceptance and an institutional niche for their field—so argues a recent study—the leading figures in German social medicine abandoned the critical posture that had characterized their work since the turn of the century and conducted research that did not threaten the state.[101] By contrast, for most of the 1920s, the thrust of the Soviet work was critical. Relying on the patronage of the top leadership of the Commissariat of Public Health and on the unassailability of their credentials as Bolshevik supporters, social hygienists carried out research on a range of sensitive issues and produced results that were social dynamite. Soviet social hygienists thus attempted the highly dangerous practice of biting the hand that feeds.

For some time, one suspects, the vaunted novelty of social hygiene, in the name of which so many disciplines were brought into being in the 1920s, protected the discipline. Toward the end of the 1920s, there was a discernible shift in cultural policy: the Cultural Revolution of 1928–31, which accompanied the policy of forced industrialization, brought with it a selective enthusiasm for originality. Radical ideas were entertained, even encouraged, as long as they did not conflict with or undermine the official version of truth. The arbiter of acceptability in all fields became the party.[102] In this climate, venerable Bolshevik credentials proved an impediment, rather than an asset, to those who claimed authority in fields of learning.

The field of social hygiene did not survive the Cultural Revolution intact. The achievement of rapid industrial development, to which the regime had committed itself in 1928, was perceived as requiring a high degree of social stability. Studies conducted by social hygienists of the influence of social factors on disease revealed disturbing social realities. The tension between what was desired and what was found to be the case was resolved by truncating almost every area of social research on health and disease.

Although the field of social hygiene as such did not survive the Cultural Revolution, in striking contrast to Bolshevik scholars in other fields of learning, a significant number of the individuals who figured prominently in the development of social hygiene did manage to continue doing public health work into the 1930s. Some of those individuals made lateral moves into other areas of public health. From 1928 to 1938, Nikitin was head of the *kafedra* of hygiene of labor at Leningrad Medical Institute.[103] In 1931, Z. G. Frenkel became head of the *kafedra* of communal hygiene in the State Institute of Medical Sciences (GIMZ), a post he continued to occupy until 1953.[104] Other social hygienists stayed in what remained of the *kafedry* of social hygiene through the early 1930s[105] and then took refuge during the hard years (1934–38) in departments of sanitary statistics (G. A. Batkis,[106] S. A. Tomilin[107]). Still other social hygienists (in fact, the leading figures) assumed top positions in the institutions that replaced the *kafedry* of social hygiene. Molkov, who had a talent for surviving political change, in 1934 became director of the Institute of Hygiene, an informal umbrella organization for ten hygiene *kafedry* in I Kharkov Institute.[108] Semashko, after being removed as commissar of public health, served as head of the *kafedra* of health care organization in I Kharkov

Institute, a post from which he pressed actively for the revival of social hygiene throughout the 1940s.[109]

In the demise of social hygiene as a distinctive field, there is a bitter lesson to be learned about fields of learning created by government fiat. Soviet social hygiene owed its existence to its ability to appeal to a patron in what was undeniably a crowded intellectual terrain. Throughout the 1920s, the field continued to enjoy, indeed to bask in, the endorsement of that patron. The strength of that support encouraged social hygienists to claim for themselves a leading position in both the teaching of and research on public health. The audacious claims of the spokesmen for social hygiene goaded their critics to attack. The replacement of Semashko as commissar of public health in early 1930 brought home harsh realities. The patronage of the Commissariat of Public Health, which had been the envy of those who criticized social hygiene, had become its weakness.

NOTES

1. For example, see Horsley Gantt, *A Medical Review of Soviet Russia* (London, 1928); Arthur Newsholme and John Kingsbury, *Red Medicine: Socialized Health in Soviet Russia* (London, 1934).

2. N. A. Semashko, "Sotsial'naia gigiena, ee sushchnost', metod, i znachenie," *Sotsial'naia gigiena* (1923), 1:8.

3. Ibid., pp. 8–9.

4. Z. G. Frenkel, *Obshchestvennaia meditsina i sotsial'naia gigiena* (Leningrad, 1926), pp. 43–46; "Gigiena," *Bolsh'aia Sovetskaia Entsiklopediia*, 1st ed (Moscow, 1929), 16: 619–23.

5. L. Ia. Shkorokhodov, *Materialy po istorii meditsinskoi mikrobiologii v dorevoliutsionnoi Rossii* (Moscow, 1948), pp. 200ff.; I. D. Strashun, *Russkaia obshchestvennaia meditsina v period mezhdu dvumia revoliutsiiami, 1907–1917 gg.* (Moscow, 1964). For an English-language discussion of the bacteriological revolution, see John F. Hutchinson, "Tsarist Russia and the Bacteriological Revolution," *Journal of the History of Medicine and Allied Sciences*, 40, no. 4 (October 1985), pp. 420–39.

6. For the increasing importance of "community medicine" in the 1880s and 1890s, see Frenkel, *Obshchestvennaia meditsina*, p. 52.

7. Ibid., pp. 19–21.

8. The leading spokesman for social hygiene—hardly a disinterested observer—argued that teaching in the *kafedry* of hygiene did not advance beyond the "gloomy 1890s." A. V. Molkov, "K voprosu o peresmotre obshchego plana prepodavaniia gigienicheskikh ditsiplin v vysshe medshkole," *Sotsial'naia gigiena* (1923), 2: 20. Significantly, the same point was made by the doyen of general hygiene, G. V. Khlopin, at the 1925 meeting of the representatives of prophylactic *kafedry* described below.

9. Between 1922 and 1923, *kafedry* of social hygiene were opened in Leningrad, Kharkov, Kiev, Minsk, Voronezh, Smolensk, and Odessa. See I. V. Vengrova and Iu. A. Shilinis, *Sotsial'naia gigiena v SSSR (Ocherk istorii)* (Moscow, 1976), pp. 115, 122–23.

10. The institute had its origins in the State Museum for Social Hygiene founded in 1919, which had evolved from the Pirogov Society's Commission on the Spread of Sanitary Education. The first director of the institute was A. V. Molkov, who had been director of the

museum and head of the commission. The institute's yearly research plans and reports of its activities were published in the journal *Sotsial'naia gigiena.*

11. The journal, which appeared between 1922 and 1930, was under the general editorship of A. V. Molkov.

12. N. A. Semashko (b. 1874), one of the most prominent Bolshevik physicians, began his involvement with Marxism in 1893. Arrested for Marxist activities, he emigrated to Switzerland in 1906, where he developed a close friendship with Lenin. In April of 1917, Semashko returned with Lenin to Russia. In July of 1918, he was named first commissar of public health. See the entry on Semashko in *Bol'shaia Sovetskaia Entsiklopediia* Vol. 50 (1944), p. 738.

13. See Neil B. Weissman, "Origins of Soviet Health Administration: Narkomzdrav, 1918–1928," in this volume.

14. Between 1923 and 1926, investment in medical services increased by two and a half times, but in 1926 the Soviet government instituted a regime of economy which severely hampered the delivery of health care. See Christopher Davis, "Economics of Soviet Public Health, 1928–1932: Development Strategy, Resource Constraints, and Health Plans," in this volume.

15. See Susan Gross Solomon, "Social Hygiene in Soviet Medical Education, 1922–1930" (forthcoming).

16. For example, the State Institute for the Protection of Labor, founded in 1925, was under the aegis of the Commissariat of Labor, the Commissariat of Health, and the Supreme Council of the National Economy (*Vesenkha*).

17. See Mark B. Adams, "Eugenics as Social Medicine in Revolutionary Russia: Prophets, Patrons, and the Dialectics of Discipline-Building," in this volume.

18. N. A. Semashko, *Nauka o zdorovye obshchestva: Sotsial'naia gigiena* (Moscow, 1921).

19. Semashko, "Sotsial'naia gigiena, ee sushchnost'."

20. Grigorii Vitalevich Khlopin (1863–1929) taught general hygiene well before the Revolution. A critic of the tsarist regime, his political sympathies are listed as "social democratic." See A. A. Rachkov, *Grigorii Vitalevich Khlopin* (Moscow, 1965); "Professor G. V. Khlopin," *Gigiena i epidemiologiia*, 8, no. 7 (1929), pp. 127–30; O. V. Perov, "G. V. Khlopin—uchenyi vysokogo obshchestvennogo dolga i gumanizm," *Sovetskoe zdravookhranenie*, no. 80 (1963), pp. 84–87.

21. G. B. Khlopin, *Osnovy gigieny* 1, in three parts (Moscow, 1921); 2, in one part (Moscow, 1922).

22. Khlopin, *Osnovy gigieny*, 1:12–17.

23. This is the celebrated tension between "laboratory and pen" referred to in Russian histories of medicine. Strashun, *Russkaia obshchestvennaia meditsina.*

24. V. Ia. Kanel, "Sotsial'naia meditsina, eia sushnost' i znachenie," *Obshchestvennyi vrach*, no. 4 (1913), pp. 423–53; Frenkel, *Obshchestvennaia meditsina.* V. Ia Kanel is listed as a member of a Moscow-based "literary-physicians" group organized by the RSDLP (Bolshevik). E. I. Lotova and B. D. Petrova, *Vrachi-Bolsheviki—Stroiteli sovetskogo zdravookhraneniia* (Moscow, 1970), p. 16.

25. See Alfred Grotjahn, *Sotsial'naia patologiia,* translated from the German by Drs. L. A. Syrkin, M. Ia. Mirskii, and A. L. Rossels (Moscow, 1925). The original was Alfred Grotjahn, *Soziale Pathologie*, 3d ed. (Berlin, 1923). See also B. Khaes, *Kratkii kurs sotsial'noi gigieny,* trans. from the German by A. A. Letavet (Moscow-Leningrad, 1923). The original was Benno Chajes, *Kompendium der sozialen Hygiene* (Berlin, 1921). Finally, see A. Fisher, *Osnovy sotsial'noi gigieny,* trans. from the German by N. A. Zimilova (Moscow, 1929). The original was Alfons Fischer, *Grundrisse der sozialen Hygiene* (Berlin, 1913).

26. Semashko contributed articles describing the activities of Soviet physicians to more than half of the issues of *Deutsche medizinische Wochenschrift* published between 1923 and 1925.

27. In 1925 there appeared three issues of *Russko-nemetskii meditsinskii zhurnal,* a journal

published by the Russian-German (or, as it was known in Germany, the German-Russian) Medical Society. The editorial board was drawn from both countries. The senior Soviet editor was Semashko.

28. Frenkel, *Obshchestvennaia meditsina*. This was the premier work on community medicine.

29. The only figure to succeed in teaching community medicine before 1917 and social hygiene after the Revolution was Z. G. Frenkel, who became professor of social hygiene at the State Institute of Medical Science and at the Institute for the Up-Grading of Doctors in Leningrad in 1917. L. A. Alekseeva and V. M. Merashbili, *Z. G. Frenkel* (Moscow, 1971).

30. See the research agenda for the institute proposed by Gamaleia. N. F. Gamaleia, "K voprosu o Ministerstve Narodnago Zdraviia," *Gigiena i sanitariia* (1910), 1:1–32.

31. Semashko, "Sotsial'naia gigiena, ee sushchnost'." Curiously, the general hygienist A. N. Sysin made the same argument.

32. Ibid.

33. A. V. Molkov (1870–1947) was director of GISG, head of the *kafedra* of social hygiene of I Moscow University (1924–29), and editor of *Sotsial'naia gigiena* (1922–30). A. P. Shishkin, "A. V. Molkov—organizator i rukovoditel instituta sotsial'noi gigieny narkomzdrava RSFSR," *Sovetskoe zdravookhranenie*, no. 10 (1970), pp. 64–68.

34. Zinovii Petrovich Soloviev (1876–1928) was the first deputy commissar of public health and an editor of the medical section of the *Bolsh'aia Sovetskaia Entsiklopediia*. See L. G. Veber, "Z. G. Solov'ev i sovremennyi etap Sovetskogo zdravookhraneniia," *Sovetskoe zdravookhranenie*, no. 1 (1952), pp. 8–14; "Z. P. Solov'ev—vydaiushchiisia sotsial-gigienist i organizator sovetskogo zdravookhraneniia," Z. P. Solov'ev, *Voprosy sotsial'noi gigieny i zdravookhraneniia. Izbrannye proizvedeniia* (Moscow, 1970), pp. 5–14; B. D. Petrov, "Z. P. Solov'ev—Professor sotsial-gigienist," *Sovetskoe zdravookhranenie*, no. 1 (1976), pp. 62–75.

35. "Programma kursa sotsial'noi gigieny, utverzhdennaia Gosudarstvennym Uchenym Soveta, priniataia v nastoiashchee vremia," Frenkel, *Obshchestvennaia meditsina*, pp. 169–73.

36. A. V. Molkov and N. A. Semashko, *Sotsial'naia gigiena. Rukovodstvo dlia studentov-medikov*, vol. 1 (Moscow, 1927).

37. Aleksei Nikolaevich Sysin (b. 1879) was head of the sanitary-epidemiological section of the Commissariat of Health RSFSR from 1918 to 1931. From 1924 on, he was professor of experimental hygiene at I Moscow University. See the entry on Sysin in *Bol'shaia meditsinskaia entsiklopediia*, 5 (1935), pp. 239–40.

38. P. N. Diatroptov was the director of the Sanitary-Hygiene Institute of the State Institute of Public Health (GIMZ) from 1919 to 1920. See "Professor P. N. Diatroptov," *Gigiena i epidemiologiia*, 8, nos. 3–4 (1929), pp. 7–9.

39. Alexander Fedorovich Nikitin (1873–1965) studied general hygiene with G. V. Khlopin, who apparently marked this student as brilliant. E. Ia. Belitskaia, "Sotsial-gigienist Professor A. F. Nikitin," *Sovetskoe zdravookhranenie*, no. 5 (1972), pp. 85–88.

40. A. F. Nikitin, *Ocherki sotsial'noi gigieny. Sotsial'nyi kollektiv i ego moshchnost'* (Moscow, 1925).

41. For a discussion of Chicago sociology of that period, see Robert E. L. Faris, *Chicago Sociology, 1920–1932* (San Francisco, 1967); Jerzy Szacki, *History of Sociological Thought* (Westport, Conn., 1979), pp. 437–64.

42. For an overview of this nascent tradition, see Elizabeth Ann Weinberg, *The Development of Sociology in the Soviet Union* (London, 1974), chap. 1.

43. From 1906 to 1918, Khlopin taught general hygiene at the Clinical Institute of the Grand Duchess Elena Pavlovna (later the Clinical Institute for the Up-Grading of Doctors); between 1904 and 1929, he taught the same subject at the Petersburg Women's Medical Institute (later the Leningrad Institute of Medical Sciences); from 1918 until 1929, he headed the *kafedra* of general hygiene at the Military Medical Academy. Rachkov, *Khlopin*.

44. In GIMZ (the State Institute of Medical Sciences), where Khlopin declined to teach,

Z. G. Frenkel gave a course on community medicine and social hygiene as early as 1919. In Khlopin's stronghold, the Military Medical Academy, no lectures in social hygiene were delivered until April 1925. Similarly, at the Leningrad Medical Institute, the *kafedra* of social hygiene was not opened until the academic year 1923/24. A. F. Nikitin, "Kafedra sotsial'noi gigieny," *Voenno-Meditsinskaia Akademiia: Nauchno-issledovatelskaia deiatelnost s 1918 po 1928* (Moscow, 1929), p. 358; Vengrova and Shilinis, *Sotsial'naia gigiena*, pp. 122–33.

45. Sergei Arkadevich Tomilin (b. 1877) was one of the few leading social hygienists with no evident Bolshevik or even Marxist connection. See V. P. Piskunov and V. S. Steshenko, "O zhizni i nauchno deiatelnosti S. A. Tomilina (kratkii ocherk)," in S. A. Tomilin, *Demografiia i sotsial'naia gigiena* (Moscow, 1973), pp. 5–21.

46. See S. A. Tomilin, "Sotsial'naia gigiena i ego mesto v sisteme meditsinskogo znaniia"; S. A. Tomilin, "Osnovnye voprosy sotsial'noi gigieny"; S. A. Tomilin, "Biologicheskie elementy v sotsial'noi gigiene." These articles all appeared in the journal *Profilakticheskaia meditsina* between 1922 and 1925. They have been reprinted in Tomilin, *Demografiia.*

47. B. P. Aleksandrovskii, "Opyt psikhonevrologicheskii kharakteristiki ukrainskogo selianstva," *Profilakticheskaia meditsina*, no. 4 (1927), p. 48.

48. The whole of volume 5 (1925) of the journal *Sotsial'naia gigiena* was devoted to a full transcript of the meeting.

49. Social disease was treated by general hygiene as a problem of epidemiology and was covered in one lecture, whereas social hygiene devoted four lectures to the subject, treating it as a problem caused by socioeconomic conditions. Living conditions consumed six sessions in the course in general hygiene, while social hygiene treated it as one of the many "problems of collective life" to which a total of thirteen sessions were devoted. Compare: "Programmy kursov i plany rabot profilakticheskikh kafedr. 1. Eksperimental'naia gigiena," ibid., pp. 91–95; "Programmy kursov i plany rabot profilakticheskikh kafedr. 2. Sotsial'naia gigiena," ibid., pp. 95–102.

50. G. Batkis, "Itogi i dal'neishie tendentsii v razvitii prepodavanii sotsial'noi gigieny," *Sotsial'naia gigiena*, 5 (1925), p. 40. Grigorii Abramovich Batkis (b. 1895) was one of the Young Turks of the social hygiene movement. Batkis was commissar of Public Health of Kiev *guberniia* (1917–20), head of a division of the Ukranian Commissariat of Health (1920–23), and a senior assistant at the *kafedra* of social hygiene of I Moscow University (1925–1930). In 1931, he headed the *kafedra* of social hygiene at II Moscow University. O. Grinin, "G. A. Batkis," *Sovetskoe zdravookhranenie*, no. 2 (1965), pp. 88–89.

51. Tomilin, "Sotsial'naia gigiena i ee mesto."

52. Khlopin, *Osnovy gigieny.*

53. "Rezoliutsii soveshchaniia predstavitelei profilakticheskikh kafedr medvuzov," *Sotsial'naia gigiena*, 5 (1925), p. 11.

54. See *Biulleten' Narkomzdrava*, no. 16 (1924), circular 194. Mention was made of this circular in T. Ia. Tkachev, "Sviaz' gigienicheskikh kafedr s organami i uchrezhdeniiami," *Sotsial'naia gigiena*, 5 (1925), p. 59.

55. S. Kaplun, "Gigiena truda, kak predmet prepodavaniia medvuzov," *Sotsial'naia gigiena*, 5 (1925), pp. 41–42.

56. G. V. Khlopin, "Ustanovlenie i soglasovanie programm obshchei (eksperimental'noi) gigieny mezhdu soboi i so spetsial'nymi kursami gigieny," *Sotsial'naia gigiena*, 5 (1925), pp. 27–29.

57. Solomon, "Social Hygiene in Soviet Medical Education."

58. N. A. Semashko, "O razvitie profilakticheskikh form meditsinskoi deiatel'nosti v strane," *Sotsial'naia gigiena*, 12–13 (1928), p. 215. The transcript of the entire meeting appeared as "Trudy vtorogo soveshchaniia predstavitelei profilakticheskikh kafedr," ibid., pp. 167–265.

59. "Izbrannye stenogram zasedanii," ibid., p. 222. The speaker was Dr. Kedrov, who represented the Commissariat of Enlightenment's Main Committee on Professional-Technical Education (*Glavprofobr*).

60. Ibid., p. 246. Again, the speaker was Dr. Kedrov, who claimed to have obtained these facts from A. V. Molkov himself.

61. Interviews conducted in the spring of 1985 in Israel with three dozen former Soviet physicians who had been trained in the 1920s and early 1930s.

62. "Izbrannye stenogrammy zasedanii," p. 239. The speaker was Professor Danilov from Smolensk.

63. Semashko, in his opening address, suggested a link between preventive medicine and the dispensaries. Semashko, "O razvitie," p. 215. Z. G. Frenkel, the real comparativist in the group, suggested that medical faculties should be organized like the good major hospitals in America and Europe with their *service social*. This would promote recordkeeping and research in a curative setting. "Izbrannye stenogrammy," p. 226.

64. Ibid., p. 223. The speaker was Professor Tarasenko of Tomsk.

65. For a discussion of the study of alcoholism in the prerevolutionary period, see John F. Hutchinson, "Science, Politics and the Alcohol Problem in Post-1905 Russia," *Slavonic and East European Review*, 58, no. 2 (1980), pp. 233–54.

66. See "O blizhaiushikh meropriatiakh po bor'be s alkogolizmom," in R. Vlassak, *Alkogolizm* (Moscow, 1928), p. 257. This book was a translation by S. Iu. Veinberg of Rudolf Wlassak, *Die Alkoholfrage* (Vienna, 1923). The Veinberg translation included a series of Soviet articles on the alcoholism problem in the USSR.

67. See *Biulleten' Narkomzdrava*, no. 5 (1927), pp. 56–58. The entire mandate, which was entitled "O borbe s alkogolizmom," was reprinted in Vlassak, *Alkogolizm*, pp. 258–61. For the mandating to GISG of social analyisis and the allocation to other institutes of research on physiological and neurological aspects of alcoholism, see V. Beliaev, "Bor'ba s alkogolizmom," *Na fronte zdravookhraneniia*, 11 (1927), p. 11.

68. The *kabinet* was small: Deichman had one assistant and two graduate students. Four statisticians were assigned to the *kabinet*.

69. Apart from GISG, the neuro-psychiatric dispensary was the only other institution authorized to conduct social research on alcoholism. Beliaev, "Bor'ba," p. 11.

70. Compare the 1922 curriculum, "Programmy sotsial'noi gigieny," *Sotsial'naia gigiena*, 5 (1925), p. 171, and the 1925 curriculum, "Programmy kursov i plany rabot profilakticheskikh kafedr. 2. Sotsial'naia gigiena," ibid., p. 97.

71. Initially, official sources blamed the high incidence of alcoholism in the 1920s on the easier access to grain and on the persistence of a bourgeois mentality. I. D. Strashun, "Bor'ba s alkogolizmom," in Vlassak, *Alkogolizm*, pp. 171–72. But by the mid-1920s it was clear that alcoholism had risen above prerevolutionary levels and was continuing to rise.

72. E. Deichman, "Problema, zasluzhivaiushchaia vnimaniia," *Bol'shevik*, no. 19–20 (1927), pp. 132–33.

73. A. V. Molkov, "Alkogolizm, kak problema izucheniia," *Gigiena i epidemiologiia*, nos. 7–8 (1926), p. 42.

74. It was easier for social hygienists to ignore the question of the constitutional predisposition to drink because they had been charged with the study of the social factors which strengthened the drink habit.

75. For example, see G. Sinkevich, "Bytovoi alkogolizm vologodskoi gubernii," *Sotsial'naia gigiena*, 7 (1926), pp. 20–24; N. I. Chuchelov, "Opyt izucheniia potrebleniia alkogolia v fabrichno-zavodskom raione sredi muzhskoi molodezhi," *Sotsial'naia gigiena*, 10 (1927), p. 38; Deichman, "Opyt izucheniia alkogolizma."

76. Present-day Soviet historians of medicine also stress the originality of GISG methodology. A. P. Shishkin, "Institut sotsial'noi gigieny i izuchenie problemy alkogolizma," *Sovetskoe zdravookhranenie*, no. 5 (1971), p. 64.

77. In the absence of a social theory which could interrelate macro-theory and empirical data, the discussions of "methodology" were often discussions of methods.

78. D. Gorfin, "Sotsial'nye bolezny," *Bol'shaia Meditsinskaia Entsikolpediia*, 31 (1928), pp. 214–18.

79. The phrase is that of the iconoclastic Moscow psychiatrist A. S. Sholomovich. See

A. S. Sholomovich, "Printsipy, metody, rabota po bor'be s alkogolizmom," *Voprosy zdra-vookhraneniia*, no. 9 (1928), p. 9.

80. See ibid., pp. 7–9. In treating the habitual alcoholic, the *narko-dispanser* did not segregate him from society: the drinker was treated together with his family and was encouraged to retain his customary job throughout the course of treatment.

81. See Susan Gross Solomon, "David and Goliath in Soviet Public Health: The Rivalry of Social Hygienists and Psychiatrists for Authority over the *Bytovoi* Alcoholic," *Soviet Studies* (April 1989).

82. See I. I. Rozenblium, "Kharakteristike alkogolizma rabochikh," *Sotsialisticheskoe zdravookhranenie*, no. 7 (1928), pp. 68–86; P. P. Brukhanskii, "Opyt lecheniia alkogolikov v psikhiatricheskikh bol'nitsakh," *Moskovskii meditsinskii zhurnal*, no. 7 (1927), pp. 15–26; B. F. Didrikhson, "Alkogolizm Leningrada v 1927 godu," *Gigiena truda*, no. 6 (1927), pp. 59ff; K. V. Tseraskii, "Alkogolizm v psikhiatricheskikh bol'nitsakh," *Moskovskii meditsinskii zhurnal*, no. 2 (1928), pp. 73–82.

83. Tseraskii, "Alkogolizm."

84. Almost all physicians, whether social hygienists or psychiatrists, favored some form of restricted access to liquor. Most chronic drinkers who were questioned expressed the same view. The state was slow to implement restrictions because of its perceived need for the revenues from the state monopoly on liquor sales.

85. In April 1927 the Council of People's Commissars passed the "Instruction on the Forced Treatment of Alcoholics Who Consititute a Social Danger." This instruction was modeled on the forced treatment of the mentally ill. See "Instruktsiia NKIu, NKZdrava, i NKVD po primeneniiu prinuditel'nogo lecheniia alkogolikov predstavliaiushchikh sotsial'nuiu opasnost', ot aprelia 1927g, No.94/mv," *Biulleten' NKZ* ot 9 aprelia 1927, as cited in A. I. Elistratov, *Administrativnoe pravo* (Moscow-Leningrad, 1929), p. 341.

86. "Iz deiatel'nosti sotsial'no-gigienicheskikh uchrezhdenii i organizatsii," *Sotsial'naia gigiena*, 3–4 (1929), pp. 178–79.

87. "Ob osvobozhdenii N. A. Semashko ot obiazanosti Narkomzdrav RSFSR," *Voprosy zdravookhranenie*, no. 5 (1930), p. 85.

88. Davis, "Soviet Economic System, 1928–1932."

89. See Sheila Fitzpatrick, *The Commissariat of Enlightenment* (Cambridge, 1970).

90. Mikhail Fedorovich Vladimirskii (b. 1894) was commissar of public health from 1930 to 1934. M. F. Vladimirskii, *Voprosy Sovetskogo zdravookhraneniia: stat'i i rechi* (Moscow, 1960), especially the appreciation by G. A. Batkis, ibid., pp. 5–37. Vladimirskii served in the NKVD RSFSR, as well as in Sovnarkom and Gosplan in the Ukraine. Davis, "Soviet Medical System, 1928–1932." For his prerevolutionary involvement with the Bolsheviks, see *Vrachi-Bol'sheviki*, p. 26.

91. Vengrova and Shilinis, *Sotsial'naia gigiena*, p. 170.

92. Ibid., p. 170–71.

93. Of the institute's five *kabinety*—biometric, statistical, psycho-physiological, medical research, and sanitary hygiene—the first three were methodological in focus. "Iz godovogo ucheta," *Sotsial'naia gigiena*, 7 (1926), p. 114. In addition, GISG created the Council of the Commissariat of Public Health on Social Hygiene Research Methodology.

94. "Iz otcheta GISG NKZ za 1928/1929," *Sotsial'naia gigiena*, 2 (1929), pp. 174–76.

95. Vengrova and Shilinis, *Sotsial'naia gigiena*, p. 171. Describing the content of the 1936 course on social hygiene in an article written in 1947, Semashko underscored the focus on organization. What he did not allude to was the disappearance of social analysis from that course. N. A. Semashko, "Sotsial'naia gigiena v SSSR," *Izbrannye proizvedeniia* (Moscow, 1967), pp. 145–55.

96. "Meditsinskoe obrazovanie v SSSR," *Bol'shaia Sovetskaia Entsiklopediia*, 2d ed., 26:638–39.

97. In 1930, the sanitary-prophylactic faculty required three and a half years to complete, whereas the other two faculties required four years. In 1933, a reform was instituted: the

sanitary prophylactic faculty was upgraded to a four-and-one-half-year course of study, but the other two faculties became five-year courses of study.

98. For example, see Wolfgang van der Daele and Peter Weingart, "Resistance and Receptivity of Science to External Direction: The Emergence of a New Discipline under the Impact of Science Policy," in Gerard Lemaine, et al., *Perspectives on the Emergence of Scientific Disciplines* (The Hague, 1976), pp. 242–77.

99. N. A. Semashko, "K istorii kafedry sotsial'noi gigieny I Moskovskogo ordena Lenina meditsinskogo instituta," *Gigiena i sanitariia*, no. 1 (1947), p. 5.

100. "Izbrannye stennogrammy zasedanii," *Sotsial'naia gigiena*, 13 (1928), p. 226. Batkis made this statement at the Second Meeting of Representatives of Prophylactic *Kafedry* in 1928.

101. Daniel S. Nadav, "Politics of Social Hygiene in Germany" (Ph.D. diss., Tel Aviv University, 1981).

102. For an excellent volume on the Soviet cultural revolution, see Sheila Fitzpatrick, ed., *Cutural Revolution in Russia, 1928–1931* (Bloomington, Ind., 1979).

103. Nikitin retained this post until 1938. Beliskaia, "Sotsial-gigienist Professor A. F. Nikitina."

104. Frenkel retained this post until 1953. Alekseeva and Merashbili, *Z. G. Frenkel*, p. 62.

105. There are indications that social hygiene survived longer in the Ukraine than it did in the RSFSR.

106. Until he died in 1965, G. A. Batkis headed the *kafedra* of the organization of health care at II Moscow Medical Institute. In the hard years, he taught a course on the history of medicine (1932), was "scientific consultant" to the division of sanitary statistics of the Erisman Institute (1935–38), and ran the division of sanitary statistics of NKZ SSSR (1938–41). Grinin, "G. A. Batkis," pp. 88–89.

107. S. A. Tomilin headed the social hygiene sector at the Ukrainian Institute of Nutrition from 1930 to 1934; from 1932 to 1934 he was head of the *kafedra* of social hygiene at the I Kharkov Medical Institute. In the hard years he headed the sector of disease at the All-Ukrainian Institute of Socialist Protection of Health in Kiev (1934–36) and became senior research assistant at the Institute for Demography and Sanitary Statistics at the Ukrainian Academy of Sciences (1934–38). Piskunov and Steshenko, "O zhizni i nauchnoi deiatelnosti S. A. Tomilina," pp. 16–18.

108. Molkov remained at the sanitary-prophylactic faculty of the I Moscow Medical Institute, 1930–34. *200 let I Moskovskogo ordena Lenina meditsinskogo instituta imeni I.M. Sechenova* (Moscow, 1959), p. 630.

109. Semashko received the order of Lenin in 1944. Semashko, "Sotsial'naia gigiena v SSSR," pp. 149–50.

MARK B. ADAMS

Eugenics as Social Medicine in Revolutionary Russia

Prophets, Patrons, and the Dialectics of Discipline-Building

Eugenics and Soviet social medicine? The very juxtaposition may well seem improbable. We are used to thinking of eugenics as a rightwing, stridently hereditarian view of human nature associated with fascist politics, the sterilization of "defectives," and the horrors of Auschwitz. But the Bolsheviks were leftwing in their ideology and stridently "environmentalist," asserting that human nature is a social product. This was most evident in their emphasis on the social determinants of health and disease and their commitment to free and universal health care. What, then, could eugenics have to do with Soviet social medicine?

Yet, officially at least, the Russian Eugenics Society was a creature of the new Bolshevik state. It was organized in 1920 under the auspices of the Commissariat of Public Health—Narkomzdrav—and its progressive commissar, Nikolai Semashko; and it was disbanded in 1930, during the Cultural Revolution, when Semashko was dismissed. This relationship between eugenics and Bolshevik public health takes on added interest because Russian eugenics is the sole example of a eugenics movement in a communist state. These facts invite us to rethink familiar stereotypes. Have we misconceived eugenics, or Soviet public health? The answer, I think, is "Both."

In concentrating on the ways post-revolutionary Soviet social medicine was unique or distinct, we may have overlooked the many features it shared with its European neighbors. In many continental settings, and especially in Germany, a close relationship between state medicine and eugenics was the norm. In creating their own system, Soviet health reformers may well have been more influenced by the German model than we yet understand. Of course, as Susan Solomon demonstrates, in the 1920s Narkomzdrav supported not only "hereditarian" eugenics, but also stridently "environmentalist" forms of social hygiene. This appears anomalous only if we think of Narkomzdrav as having been created "from the top down" in order to develop a single line or to serve a single, coherent policy objective; in fact, for much of the 1920s, its character was shaped by the many enterprises that came under its aegis. Official histories notwithstanding, Narkomzdrav came into being not as a state instrument but as a professional network encompassing divergent agendas.

We may profit in several ways, then, by exploring the way Russian eugenics developed within Narkomzdrav. As a field imported into the Russian context from abroad, eugenics illustrates the ways various intellectual entrepreneurs sought to adapt foreign ideas and models to the Soviet context. As a new field, Soviet eugenics allows us to study the process of self-definition and discipline-building in the Soviet Union in the postrevolutionary decade. Finally, as a field organized and funded under the auspices of Narkomzdrav, Soviet eugenics may afford us a new view of that administrative enterprise, not from the usual perspective of its policymakers and their rhetoric but, rather, from the viewpoint of one group of scientists, researchers, and visionaries who found themselves within its sprawling domain and had to rely on it as a patron.

PROPHETS AND PATRONS

The word *eugenics* was coined by the Englishman Francis Galton in 1883 to denote the ''science'' of the biological improvement of the human kind. Galton was convinced that a wide range of human physical, mental, and moral traits were inherited. If this were so, he reasoned, human progress depended on improving the human stock, and social measures were likely to be truly progressive only by virtue of their effects on the selective transmission of the population's hereditary endowments to future generations. In keeping with his meritocratic, middle-class British values, he did not favor bringing this about by government intervention or coercion; rather, he believed that eventually, through appropriate popular moral and scientific education, a time would come when all people would voluntarily adjust their reproductive behavior to suit the long-range interests of society.

In the decades between 1890 and 1930, eugenics movements developed in more than thirty countries, each adapting the international Galtonian gospel to suit local scientific, cultural, institutional, and political conditions. In some places, eugenics was dominated by experimental biologists, in others by animal breeders, physicians, pediatricians, psychiatrists, anthropologists, demographers, or public health officials. In some places it was predominantly Lamarckian (for example, in France and Brazil); in others Mendelian (in the United States). In some places, eugenicists opposed interracial marriage (for example, in Germany); in others, they advocated it (in Mexico).[1] Patterns of patronage also varied from place to place. In the United States and Britain, eugenics institutions were supported principally through private funding, often by philanthropic contributions or endowments.[2] In Germany, funding for race hygiene involved a mix of private endowments and state support.

Although these national movements joined various international eugenic organizations and acknowledged their commonality, each drew heavily on its own native roots in defining its identity and agenda. In the United States, for example, Charles Davenport and his successors built their movement around Mendelian principles popular among animal breeders, and it rapidly expanded from traveling exhibits at state fairs into the politics of progressivism, immigration restriction, and the promulgation of sterilization laws in Indiana, California, and many other states.[3] In Germany, the term *Eugenik* was rejected in favor of *Rassenhygiene* (race hygiene) reflecting a conception of the field derived less from Galton than from Schallmayer and Ploetz.[4] Although the French eugenic society used the term *eugénique,* demographic concerns about underpopulation helped make *puericulture*—the science of childrearing in its broadest sense—a dominant strain.[5] Elsewhere on the continent, traditional concerns with underpopulation, racial or cultural degeneration, class conflict, physical anthropology, Aryanism, and criminology, derived variously from Broca, von Nordau, Morel, Lombroso, and others, flavored local movements.[6]

THE ORIGINS OF RUSSIAN EUGENICS

Galton's *Hereditary Genius* appeared in Russian translation in 1875.[7] Over the next three decades, European ideas filtered into Russia, some through translations, others brought back by the many Russian students for whom continental experience was a standard part of postgraduate training. In writings addressed to both professional audiences and the general public, various Russian psychiatrists, physicians, and intellectuals reported on European developments and expressed their own views on fertility (*rozhdaemost'*), on congenital (*vrozhdennyi*) defects and diseases, and on the general problem of human degeneration (*vyrozhdenie*). By 1910, the word *evgenika* was used occasionally in books and essays. In the period 1905–17, translations of many Western scientific works were published in Russia, and a number of them dealt with experimental biology, genetics, and evolution. In St. Petersburg, the firm ''Obrazovanie'' commissioned many dozens of anthologies for its series on ''new ideas'' in biology, psychology, sociology, physics, philosophy; in Moscow, a comparable role was played by the firm of M. and S. Sabashnikov.

For the new generation of Russian scientists who were beginning their careers in the prerevolutionary decades, these new research fields from abroad had a special appeal. Intellectually, of course, such fields provided some of the most exciting science of the day, but they also served the professional career interests of young Russian scientists. By importing new scientific trends into Russia from abroad and presiding over their development, young scientists could legitimize the new and independent places they were seeking for themselves in the structure of Russian science. The central roles in creating Russian eugenics were played by two entrepreneurial and prolific members of this scientific generation, two zoologists who had been converted to the new experimental biology in Europe and had returned home to cultivate it in their respective cities.

In Moscow, the key figure in creating Russian eugenics was Nikolai Konstantinovich Kol'tsov (1872–1940). He had traveled to Europe and specifically the Naples Station to study invertebrate morphology beginning in the 1890s—before the rediscovery of Mendel's laws in 1900—so the new ''experimental biology'' to which he became converted did not yet include Mendelism, although he became aware of it on subsequent trips. A docent at Moscow University, he was active in liberal politics and resigned in 1909 in protest over the actions of Minister of Education Kasso. He began teaching full-time at the Bestuzhev Courses for Women and at Shaniavskii University, private institutions partially underwritten by the

Moscow city duma. At both places, he developed laboratories where he trained students who specialized in one of the new experimental disciplines: limnology, experimental psychology, biometrics, blood chemistry, hormone research, organ transplantation, physicochemical biology, developmental mechanics, cytology, and genetics.

Beginning in 1914, he joined L. A. Tarasevich, a leading bacteriologist, as coeditor of the new popular science journal, *Priroda,* based in Moscow. As editor, Kol'tsov reviewed Western developments in experimental biology; he also reported on the funding and organization of science in other countries, detailing the emergence of the Kaiser Wilhelm Institutes in Germany and the lavish efforts of the Carnegie and Rockefeller Foundations in the United States. Kol'tsov had close family ties to the Moscow merchantry, which had been so active in charity, education, civic reform, and democratic politics.[8] After years of lobbying the Moscow merchantry for funds to support his various research enterprises, he managed to create the Institute of Experimental Biology in 1916, under the auspices of the privately funded Moscow Scientific Research Institute Society. His institute was endowed with a substantial grant from the will of Russian railway magnate G. M. Mark and was located in a large house in the city's merchant quarter. At that time, genetics was a relatively minor component of its overall program.

As the Russian capital, St. Petersburg, with its ready access to the Baltic, was Russia's "window to the West." Not surprisingly, it had the lion's share of Russia's scientific institutions. There eugenics developed under the auspices of Iurii Aleksandrovich Filipchenko (1882–1930).[9] Filipchenko spent the academic year 1911–12 working with Richard Hertwig in Munich and at the Naples Station, where he became acquainted with the latest biological trends, especially Mendelism. On his return, he opened Russia's first genetics course at St. Petersburg University in 1913 and began working concurrently in the physiological division of the Veterinary Laboratory of the Ministry of Internal Affairs as assistant to I. I. Ivanov (1870–1932), a student of Pavlov and a pioneering researcher in artificial insemination. Under Ivanov's direction, he mastered the various craniometric indices and used them in a study of the inheritance of skull characteristics in hybrid cattle that earned him a doctorate in 1917. The study was awarded the Von Baer Prize of the Russian Academy of Sciences.

Filipchenko's expertise in the new biology and his study of mammalian crania led to connections with Bekhterev's Psychoneurological Institute. He taught a course there beginning in 1914, was elected its professor of vertebrate anatomy the next year, and served as its academic secretary through 1920. Filipchenko's readings on genetics, craniometry, the inheritance of quantitative characters, and neurology brought him into contact with the eugenics work being developed in the United States and Europe. He began giving popular lectures on eugenics in 1917 and, in 1918, published his first popular article on the subject.[10]

REVOLUTIONARY OPPORTUNITIES

Because of the effects of world war, revolution, and civil war, 1917–22 was a time of both hardship and opportunity for young Russian scientists. On the one hand, scientific work and its financial support were disrupted, there were shortages in food, paper, and equipment, and much scientific talent died or emigrated. On the other hand, for those who remained, the system had opened up and there were new opportunities for professional advancement.

We can observe these effects in the careers of Filipchenko and Kol'tsov. Filipchenko was awarded a doctoral degree in zoology and comparative anatomy from Petrograd University in 1917; on December 18 of that year, he was appointed salaried docent in zoology—and within a year had been promoted to professor. In 1918 he organized the university's Laboratory of Genetics and Experimental Zoology and became its director; in 1919, the laboratory became a university department and Filipchenko became its chairman. Kol'tsov was a decade older and better established than Filipchenko, so the Revolution was a mixed blessing. He became a professor at both the first and second Moscow universities in 1918. On the other hand, the institute he had worked so hard to establish and fund now lost its endowment, and the expensive equipment needed for physicochemical laboratory science became difficult to obtain. Then, too, Kol'tsov had been politically active before the Revolution; in August 1920 he was briefly under arrest as a counterrevolutionary, but his networks of prerevolutionary contacts, including Semashko and Maxim Gorky, were soon able to secure his release.

The special opportunities and constraints of the postrevolutionary years made eugenics an opportune field. We know from his correspondence with Filipchenko that the publisher M. Sabashnikov sought to remain in business by commissioning books that he felt would appeal to political authorities. In keeping with the new materialist approach to man and nature, he tried to assemble many collections dealing with the relationship of the biological and the social, including volumes on the evolutionary origins of human beings, the biological basis of behavior, and sociological works based on biology. One area he found especially promising was eugenics—and no wonder. It fit ideally the new emphasis on science as a way of undermining religion and improving the human condition; it entailed a scientistic, materialist, biosocial concept of human beings; it sought to apply the results of genetics to benefit society; and it emphasized the human power to shape the future.

For its founders, eugenics was not only scientifically intriguing and professionally useful: it also had strong visionary appeal. In characterizing eugenics, both Filipchenko and Kol'tsov initially took their lead from Galton and his concept of a "civic religion"—one that, at a trying time, provided hope for a better future. In his first programmatic statement on eugenics, Kol'tsov echoed Galton's call, making some minor adjustments to the new revolutionary order. Contrasting the ideals of Islam and socialism, Kol'tsov concluded:

> The ideals of socialism are bound up with our earthly life: but the dream of creating a perfect order in the relations between people is also a religious idea, for which people will go to their deaths. Eugenics has before it a high ideal which also gives meaning to life and is worthy of sacrifices: the creation, through conscious work by many generations, of a human being of a higher type, a powerful ruler of nature and creator of life. Eugenics is the religion of the future and it awaits its prophets.[11]

Although Filipchenko never indulged in such effulgent rhetoric, he was even more active than Kol'tsov as an evangelist, writing prolifically on the subject for popular audiences and producing no fewer than four books on eugenics in as many years, including a comparative biography of Galton and Mendel.[12]

Kol'tsov's poetics of 1921 captured something of the early spirit and appeal of eugenics throughout Russia. For readers who had just lived through epidemics, civil war, and famine, it held out the prospect of a better future guaranteed by the authority of science. For biologists, it defined a central role in helping their society. For potential patrons, it offered a reason to fund research at a time of severe shortages. For isolated scientific workers in enclaves throughout the war-torn regions of the former empire, it served to inspire, rally, and recruit. In all, it was a stirring call for the creation of something new. Of course, its creation would entail an important role for the author as well as substantial financial support for his own scientific institute, its programs, and its students. There was nothing contradictory in a religious credo, much less a worldly one, that called for sacrifice from the faithful and at the same time managed to serve the interests of its prophets.

GETTING ORGANIZED

In addition to the ideological utility and visionary appeal of eugenics, important practical reasons made it an opportune field. A mainstay of eugenic research was the collection and analysis of genealogical and anthropometric data from questionnaires and archives. Such work fit the times: all it required was "paper and initiative."[13] More practically, at a time of war, inflation, and famine, it paid and fed students and supported research collectives that were in danger of dissolving. It also helped support other, more theoretical scientific work in laboratory biology and genetics. It is instructive to follow the ways Kol'tsov and Filipchenko used eugenics to obtain social support and funding from public authorities for their broader scientific agendas.

When he became fully aware of the importance of new Western work on genetics in 1918 and 1919, Kol'tsov quickly moved the field to the forefront in his plans, since breeding experiments were relatively cheap and easy to perform. In addition, genetics promised immediate practical benefit in animal breeding at a time of famine. Kol'tsov thus was able to support his student Alexander Serebrovskii through the Commissariat of Agriculture and to obtain funds for a poultry-breeding station linked to his institute. More importantly, with the loss of his institute's endowment, Kol'tsov managed to gain support from the Commissariat of Public Health, headed by his friend Semashko, and his entire institute became part of Narkomzdrav's system of research institutions (GINZ).

By making genetics relevant to human health, eugenics proved useful in solidifying the links between Kol'tsov's institute and its new patron. In the summer of 1920, Kol'tsov created within his institute its new Eugenics Section (*Evgenicheskii otdel*). In September, he wrote to Filipchenko proposing that they combine efforts in developing the field. At a meeting on November 1, however, they agreed that Filipchenko would organize something in Petrograd completely independent of Moscow.[14] Given his location, his contacts, and his research orientation, Filipchenko approached the Russian Academy of Sciences, located in Petrograd. During the prerevolutionary war years, the academy had created the Commission on the Study of Natural Productive Forces (KEPS). On February 14, 1921, the Bureau of Eugenics was established under the auspices of KEPS. Filipchenko was named director, and he in turn appointed to the bureau's staff Jan Janovich Lusis, Denis Karl Lepin, and A. I. Zuitin, three Latvians who were his senior students at the time.[15]

Just how useful eugenics was in supporting the more general research agendas of Filipchenko and Kol'tsov may be seen in the way it functioned in their respective institutions. The Bureau of Eugenics supported Filipchenko's cohort of students in genetics—D'iakonov, Zuitin, Lepin, Lusis, and, after 1924, Dobzhansky, Kerkis, and Medvedev. No matter what kind of genetics they studied, they were all partially funded through the bureau. The utility of the imprimatur "eugenics" for supporting "genetics" may be gauged from the following fact: when the research unit was named the Bureau of Eugenics (1921–25), its bulletin included both eugenic and genetic research; when it was named the Bureau of Genetics and Eugenics (1925–27), it published no eugenic research—only animal and plant genetics. Filipchenko made a point of emphasizing that the bulletin of his bureau published only scientific research carried out by its staff. For Filipchenko, then, eugenics was a "civic religion" and a research interest, but it was also a way of obtaining patronage from the academy for a "socially relevant" field in order to support his research, his students, and his institutional agenda.

For Kol'tsov, eugenics served parallel functions. Work within the Eugenics Section of Kol'tsov's Institute of Experimental Biology had a highly interdisciplinary character: it encompassed not only genealogical research, but also studies of blood chemistry and blood groups, as well as studies of behavioral genetics in mice by Maria Sadovnikova, Kol'tsov's wife and former student.[16] Students trained in animal genetics often worked in eugenics as a matter of course. For example, V. V. Sakharov won a degree at the institute in 1924 for two pieces of research that he carried out in tandem—one on pedigrees of Russian musicians, the other on mutations in fruitflies.[17] In the late 1920s, he served as secretary of the Russian Eugenics Society while continuing his laboratory studies. Thus, although his research agenda was broader and more "physicochemical" than Filipchenko's, Kol'tsov also used eugenics to legitimize his growing research enterprise and the support it was receiving from its patron.

DISCIPLINE-BUILDING

All disciplines are composed of clusters defined by professional and institutional affiliation, theoretical orientation, and problematics.[18] In the case of Russian eugenics, these clusters had more reality than the putative discipline they comprised, for in the early 1920s Russian eugenics was a new imported field that its organizers were seeking to develop in Russia under postrevolutionary conditions. To do so, they sought to tie together appropriate professional, institutional, and regional groups into a unified network and to provide it with a viable and legitimate Russian identity.

The Russian Eugenics Society

In the fall of 1920, weeks after he had created the eugenics section of his institute and at roughly the same time as he was in communication with Filipchenko, Kol'tsov brought up the idea of forming a Russian eugenics society at a meeting of a Nar-komzdrav commission that was working on the creation of a division of race hygiene in its Social Hygiene Museum. A preliminary planning meeting for the society was held on October 15, 1920, at the House of Sanitary Education.[19]

At the founding meeting of the Russian Eugenics Society a month later on November 19, 1920, it was clear that the society's governance would be dominated by Kol'tsov and his students. The gathering was held at the Institute of Experimental Biology. Kol'tsov was elected president. Its bureau was established, consisting of Kol'tsov, psychiatrist T. I. Iudin, and anthropologist V. V. Bunak as regular members, and N. V. Bogoiavlenskii and A. S. Serebrovskii as temporary members (both were promoted to full members the following year). In 1922, M. V. Volotskoi assumed the post of secretary of the society. Bunak, Serebrovskii, and Volotskoi were all young protégés of Kol'tsov who worked in his institute. Like that institute, the Russian Eugenics Society was under the auspices of the State Scientific Institute of the Commissariat of Public Health (GINZ).

During the society's first year it held nineteen meetings at which twenty-six papers were presented, fourteen by workers affiliated with the institute.[20] In subsequent years, except for occasional joint meetings with other professional groups and a few public sessions held at the House of Scientists (*Dom uchenykh*), the society customarily met one or two Fridays a month during the academic year at Kol'tsov's institute and was administered from its Eugenics Section. In late 1920, the Russian Eugenics Society had thirty Muscovite members; by the end of 1921, the number had risen to eighty-three; by the end of 1924, 129. These numbers are significant when we consider that they represent a substantial number of the most distinguished biologists, physicians, psychiatrists, or health officials of Moscow. Beginning in 1922, the society began publishing a journal, *Russkii evgenicheskii zhurnal,* which issued an average of three numbers annually through the beginning of 1930. Especially in its early years, a substantial number of its articles were based on papers presented at society meetings.

Russia had been largely cut off from Western developments since 1916, so there was great interest among society members in genetic and eugenic developments in Germany, France, Scandinavia, Britain, and America. On behalf of the society, Kol'tsov wrote to Davenport and other prominent Western eugenicists to report on Soviet developments and to ask for publications. Kol'tsov was eager to bring the Russian society into the international eugenics organizations. On December 2, 1921, Kol'tsov was elected the official representative of the Russian Eugenics Society to the International Commission of Eugenics, and this was confirmed at its 1922 meeting in Brussels, where Russia became one of its twenty-two cooperating countries and one of only fifteen fulfilling its requirements.[21]

Given the difficulties of travel and communication during and immediately after the Civil War, it was to be expected that a new national society based in Moscow would reflect the work of the Moscow community. Meanwhile, in other cities, eugenics societies were created in the early 1920s through local entrepreneurship; generally, they became affiliated with the central society in Moscow only after several years. Filipchenko's group formed the Leningrad branch of the society in 1924. The Saratov Eugenics Society, formed on December 29, 1923, under the presidency of psychiatrist M. P. Kutanin, soon had a membership of forty-four, dominated by local psychiatrists, gynecologists, and obstetricians; only at the end of 1925 did it become a branch of the Russian Eugenics Society.[22] The Odessa branch of the Russian Eugenics Society was formed in the mid-1920s under the presidency of Nikolai Kostiamin, a professor at the Odessa Institute of Hygiene and a physiological chemist specializing in blood chemistry.[23]

In addition to biologists and physicians, psychiatrists played an important role in Russian eugenics. The most renowned was V. M. Bekhterev, founder and director of the Psychoneurological Institute; its staff helped distribute hundreds of questionnaires for the Eugenics Bureau's study of the Petrograd intelligentsia. In addition, from the outset, psychiatrist T. I. Iudin was one of the society's most active and prolific members, publishing books and numerous articles on eugenics, psychopathology, and constitution, and, beginning in the mid-1920s, psychiatrist P. I. Liublinskii was coeditor of the society's journal. Another link between psychiatry and eugenics was institutionalized in 1927 when the Kozhevnikov Society of Neurologists and Psychiatrists in Moscow created its own genetics bureau at the psychiatric clinic of Moscow University under the direction of the prominent young neurologist and eugenicist S. N. Davidenkov.[24]

Anthropologists were also involved in the 1920s eugenics movement. Following the European tradition, in Russia ethnology (the study of ''ethnos'' or culture) was distinguished from anthropology, a more biological discipline modeled after Broca's school and roughly corresponding to what is called in the United States ''physical anthropology.'' The anthropologist V. V. Bunak became involved in eugenics through his interest in craniometry and his attempt to develop new biometric techniques for measuring skull characteristics. He met Kol'tsov through Moscow University and worked for a time in the Eugenics Section of Kol'tsov's institute. During the 1920s, Bunak edited the leading Russian journal of anthropology and chaired the department of anthropology at Moscow University until 1930.

Professionally, then, Russian eugenics in the 1920s involved a mix of experimental biologists, animal geneticists, hygienists, physicians, psychiatrists, anthropologists, and demographers. Institutionally, it was a loose federation of groups in Moscow associated with the Kol'tsov institute, the university, the medical school clinic, public health, and anthropology; groups in Leningrad associated with the Academy of Sciences, the university, and the Bekhterev institute; and sundry other enclaves in Saratov, Odessa, and elsewhere. How could these disparate workers and interests be harmonized into a coherent Russian field worthy of public support?

RUSSIFYING EUGENICS

In introducing eugenics into Russia, both Filipchenko and Kol'tsov had taken their lead from Galton. As Mandrillon has pointed out, a preoccupation with hereditary talent reflected the central values of the Russian intelligentsia.[25] Yet at times Russian eugenics seemed a distinctly foreign import. When the journal of the Russian Eugenics Society first appeared, for example, on its title page was the society's emblem: a genealogical chart of the linked pedigrees of Charles Darwin and Francis Galton, complete with black and white circles and squares. A larger and more detailed version hung prominently on the wall behind Kol'tsov's desk in the director's office of his institute.

In adapting an imported eugenics to fit postrevolutionary Russian circumstances, the Russian eugenicists, like their counterparts elsewhere, sought a native forerunner. They found one in the person of a certain Florinskii, who had published a book in St. Petersburg in 1866 entitled *The Improvement and Degeneration of the Human Race*.[26] The work did not depart notably from contemporary European literature on degeneration and had been largely ignored in Russia until it was unearthed by Russian eugenicists in the early 1920s. For purposes of establishing the new field's progressive Russian roots, the identity of the author posed something of a problem since the title page of the original listed the author as "F. Florinskii," well known in his day as a religious idealist philosopher. A lengthy footnote to a 1924 article on the subject concluded, however, that this was undoubtedly a mistake, since the clinical examples cited in the work surely made it the product of Vasilii Markovich Florinskii (1833–99), a professor at the Medico-Surgical Academy in St. Petersburg.[27] The 1866 book was republished in 1926 with its authorship corrected.[28]

To be adapted to Soviet conditions in the early 1920s, however, eugenics required more than a legitimate nineteenth-century Russian precursor: it needed a legitimate Soviet identity that assured it a place in the ecology of knowledge in postrevolutionary Russia. If Kol'tsov's characterization of eugenics (and socialism) as an earthly "civic religion" had seemed strategically apt in 1921, it soon became unhelpful. Another way of characterizing eugenics was as an international "movement," and various accounts of the history and state of the eugenics movement (*evgenicheskoe dvizhenie*) appeared in the Soviet Union in the 1920s.[29] But this term too was not without its drawbacks. In particular, why should an international movement be funded by Narkomzdrav's severely strained budget?

Given the character of its Soviet practitioners, institutions, and funding, many eugenicists felt that the legitimacy of eugenics ultimately depended on its recognition as a new scientific discipline in its own right. Among them was Professor T. I. Iudin, who began *Evgenika*, his 240-page textbook for the field, with an opening chapter entitled "Eugenics as an Independent Scientific Discipline: Its Limits, Methods, and Tasks." There he addressed the relation of eugenics to other established disciplines: "Biologists call eugenics 'human genetics', anthropologists call it 'social anthropology', sociologists call it 'political demography', physicians call it 'constitutional pathology', Moll and Forel call it 'sexology', hygienists call it 'part of social hygiene' or 'racial hygiene', Haeckel calls it 'gonionomy.' " Clearly, argued Iudin, a field related to so many existing disciplines but distinct from all of them merited disciplinary status in its own right. He concluded that, although analogous to medicine, eugenics was a union of genetics and sociology and "will become the biology of social types.'"[30]

Iudin's characterization of eugenics as a combination of genetics and sociology went to the heart of its identity problem. In its early years, at least, the field may have allowed geneticists to talk sociology, but few sociologists were talking genetics. A report on the activities of the Russian Eugenics Society during its first year applauded the interest of academics, biologists, and medics in the field but lamented the dearth of sociologists and other social scientists and activists.[31] The call for the involvement of social activists was, however, answered soon enough.

THERAPEUTIC DILEMMAS

Eugenic literature was replete with the rhetoric of human biological improvement and visions of a better, if distant, future. But what of the more immediate future? Whatever its self-image and ideology, Russian eugenics was a field patronized by the public health commissariat because of its actual or potential usefulness, and that body faced immediate and pressing problems in the early 1920s.

Policy Issues

Like discipline-builders elsewhere, the founders of Soviet eugenics felt a tension between reformist zeal and academic and professional caution. For those eugenicists who regarded their research mission as primary, the agenda was relatively clear: learn more. As for educating the public, most eugenicists endorsed the publication of popular works and the establishment of appropriate courses in universities and medical schools, although teaching eugenics to women in secondary schools provoked considerable resistance. For those who sought a guide to immediate practical action, however, it was less clear what eugenics had to offer.

The issue of practical action was especially important for two groups. First, officials of the eugenics society were naturally concerned to legitimate and consolidate their relationship with their singular patron. Kol'tsov may have found a sympathetic friend in Semashko, but the commissar had to balance his friend's agenda against competing interests within his enterprise and justify Narkomzdrav's claims to scarce resources against claims of other commissariats. The Commissariat of Public Health was responsible, after all, for public health; why spend on a new field severely limited resources that might better go to well-established medical specialties or to fields of obvious practical importance—nutrition research, for example, or epidemiology? Eugenicists had sought to legitimate their new field by alluding to its vital practical importance; yet, although they might diagnose human genetic diseases, they could not show how to cure or even treat them. Funded as public health, eugenics could help itself and its patron by demonstrating its practical usefulness.

A second group vitally concerned with action was comprised of Marxist eugenicists. From its earliest years, Soviet eugenics had attracted a number of young Marxist scientific activists who were inspired by its visionary prospects and stimulated by its practical potential. As the government and party consolidated power and began to establish policies and priorities in the mid-1920s, the bourgeois founders of Soviet eugenics retreated from their earlier and somewhat awkward attempts to articulate the relevance of their field to socialist construction, leaving the task to the young Marxist activists they had nurtured. These activists assumed a prominent role in "bolshevizing" eugenics and trying to figure out how it could be made useful.

For those who sought eugenic action, of course, the general policy options were apparent. There were only three ways to improve the hereditary quality of the next generation. First, a human population could be improved by negative selection; a "negative eugenics" approach was aimed at eliminating or limiting the breeding of the "unfit." Second, conceivably a way could be found to control mutation or to induce desirable hereditary traits. Finally, a human population might be improved through positive selection; a "positive eugenics" would seek to increase the number of offspring of people with desirable traits. In charting the dialectics of discipline-building by Soviet eugenicists it is important to keep in mind that these three options defined the limits of the practicable.

OPTION ONE: THE "INDIANA IDEA"

Soviet eugenicists were well informed about the public policies supported by foreign eugenics movements, and in such policies they sought models for social action. Some foreign prescriptions seemed irrelevant: there was hardly a flood of immigrants into Russia, so immigration restriction on the American model was pointless. But one measure seemed more promising: eugenic sterilization. Indeed, in the United States, the legislatures of several states, beginning with Indiana, had passed eugenic sterilization laws, and vasectomies (and to a lesser extent salpingectomies) were being widely used. Even before the Revolution, psychiatrist Liublinskii had reported on the American program of eugenic sterilization, which he called the "Indiana Idea."

One young Marxist activist who found the Indiana Idea especially appealing was M. V. Volotskoi (1893–1944), an officer of the Russian Eugenics Society from 1922 through 1925. In lectures, articles, and a book published in 1923, Volotskoi urged that a sterilization program be undertaken in Russia.[32] He argued that vasectomy was not castration; that it was working well in America; that it could be put to immediate use; and that the success of the U.S. program would undoubtedly improve the biological quality of the American population in the near future. Volotskoi's championing of eugenic sterilization met with considerable opposition: the reviews of his book by Filipchenko and others were hardly enthusiastic, and the discussions of sterilization in eugenic society meetings from Leningrad to Saratov were almost uniformly hostile.

In his text on eugenics published in 1924, Filipchenko opposed the Indiana Idea on moral, programmatic, and scientific grounds. He declared that, morally, "the compulsory sterilization of hundreds of thousands of citizens by some big government" was a purely dystopian notion, a "crude assault on the human person." Moreover, he noted that although "nothing indicates that such measures will have a significant result," programmatically they would undoubtedly be "harmful to the diffusion of eugenic ideas.'' Finally, he argued that, scientifically, the most efficient way of creating a desirable breed is positive, not negative, selection. For Filipchenko, the creation of "especially favorable combinations of traits" was "the chief task of both human reproduction and all eugenics."[33]

Filipchenko's position on sterilization fit his program and its patron. His Bureau of Eugenics was funded by the Academy of Sciences, and, not suprisingly, he regarded the primary task of eugenics to be not social action, but, rather, education and research. Indeed, the research in which his bureau was engaged was an extensive Galtonian genealogical study of talented Leningraders, including members of the Academy itself. Also, according to the testimony of contemporaries, Filipchenko had some disdain for Kol'tsov's transparent attempts to cultivate political authorities—as, for example, Kol'tsov's published suggestion that since Communist party members were hereditarily superior, it was their social duty to have more children. Volotskoi was, of course, one of Kol'tsov's protégés.

It might seem curious that a Marxist like Volotskoi would embrace sterilization. With hindsight, we may associate sterilization of the "defective" or "feebleminded" with extreme right-wing politics and therefore expect to find strong political, moral, and scientific opposition to the idea in any moderately progressive setting. Given a choice between positive and negative eugenics, it may seem that encouraging "gifted" people to breed would be less problematic than compelling "defective" people not to breed; it was certainly so to Filipchenko. In Britain and America, however, it appears that the reverse was the case: as Diane Paul has demonstrated, until the 1940s there was a broad consensus among geneticists from the political right, left, and center that negative eugenics was desirable. If they could not agree on the most desirable human characteristics for which to breed, they could agree on what constituted "unfitness" and shared the conviction that humankind can and should act to eliminate it.[34] In light of the abiding consensus, then, it is natural that Volotskoi would consider sterilization a plausible form of Bolshevik action.

Yet, had Volotskoi not been so preoccupied with the need for action, he would have realized that there was an obvious reason for the widespread Russian opposition to sterilization that had nothing whatever to do with moral, programmatic, or scientific qualms about the procedure. As Gorbunov reported in 1922, Russia was experiencing a population implosion. In the years between 1917 and 1920, Moscow had lost 49.6 percent of its population, Petrograd a staggering 71 percent. And this was not simply the result of migration. In 1910, births had exceeded deaths in Moscow by 101 per 10,000; in 1920, deaths exceeded births by 243. In Petrograd, the comparable figures were even more chilling: in 1910, births had exceeded deaths by 37 per 10,000; in 1920, deaths exceeded births by an awesome 484. Data from the provinces gave comparable figures.[35] It is no wonder, then, that at meetings of the Saratov Eugenics Society most of the discussion concerned the collapse of the local population. Participants urged the elimination of abortion for reasons of both health and demography.[36] Sterilization was simply out of the question: given the social realities, the common perception was that Russia needed not fewer births, but many, many more.

OPTION TWO: LAMARCKISM

What, then, was to be done? By 1925, it appeared to many that a eugenics based on Mendelian genetics had little to say about improving public health in the immediate future. At roughly the same time, biological issues became a subject of controversy in Marxist philosophical circles, where the impression was widespread that genetics itself was incompatible with Marxist revolutionary philosophy and dialectical materialism. One of the chief criticisms of genetics in Marxist circles was that its concept of the immortal germplasm, subject only to rare, random, and generally harmful mutations, was contrary to a materialist view and rendered mankind impotent in directing mutational change. On philosophical grounds, some Marxists preferred Lamarckism: if the Lamarckians were right, then hereditarily desirable traits might be induced deliberately by appropriate environmental or social conditions. The academic geneticists and eugenicists who founded the movement held the facts of science indisputable on the question: for them Lamarckism had no scientific standing. But it became popular among Marxists and social activists who were, after all, equally involved in this "socio-genetic" science.

Interestingly, although this position was hostile to genetics, it was not necessarily hostile to eugenics. Many Marxist Lamarckians followed the lead of the Viennese biologist Paul Kammerer, who enjoyed great popularity in the Soviet Union in the mid-1920s. Lunacharskii had written a scenario for a film entitled *Salamandr,* which lionized Kammerer as a great scientist vilified in the West because of his communist sympathies. Many of Kammerer's books and articles were translated into Russian, and the Communist Academy invited him to Moscow to head a laboratory.[37] In one of his most influential books, Kammerer had claimed that Mendelian genetics makes us "slaves of the past" whereas Lamarckism makes us "captains of the future" and had devoted the last third of his text to a stirring call for a Lamarckian socialist eugenics.[38] Several Soviet Marxist Lamarckians responded to that call. Most notable among them was, once again, Volotskoi. Two years earlier he had published a book urging the creation of a sterilization program; now, in 1925, he published a second book—*Class Interests and Modern Eugenics*—echoing Kammerer's call for the creation of a socialist eugenics based on Lamarckism.[39]

Once again, Filipchenko took on the Moscow Marxist, this time by standing his central claim on its head. In a 1925 pamphlet attacking Lamarckism, he pointed out that "if acquired characters are inherited, then, obviously, all representatives of the proletariat bear in themselves the traces of all the unfavorable influences which their fathers, grandfathers, and a long series of distant ancestors have suffered over many, many years."[40] Thus, it was not genetics but rather Lamarckism that would judge the proletariat inferior and render social action pointless. This argument reportedly caused quite a stir in Marxist circles.[41] Perhaps because of this reaction, Filipchenko, in the words of his biographers, "lost interest" in eugenics shortly after this controversy. Of course, however contrary in their science and their politics, both Volotskoi and Filipchenko shared the biosocial rhetoric so characteristic of the 1920s and so central to their common passion, eugenics.

Volotskoi was not alone in preferring Lamarckism to genetics because of his desire for action. He was joined, among others, by the physician Solomon G. Levit (1884-1938?), a party member since 1919 and a member of the administrative board of Moscow University from 1922 to 1925. Levit was a central figure in Marxist circles: in 1924 he organized a society of materialist physicians and subsequently became vice chairman, and then scientific secretary, of the Natural and Exact Sciences Section of the Communist Academy.[42] In a 1925 pamphlet responding to Filipchenko, Levit made the reason for his support of Lamarckism clear: "Does it make any sense to talk seriously about such undertakings [prophylactic medicine] if we accept the invariability of the genotype? . . . The arguments concerning this issue smack of desperate pessimism and impotence. If, indeed, pathology is determined by the genotype, while the latter develops solely under the influence of 'internal forces', independent of the environment, what will become of human efforts to change pathological forms?"[43] Needless to say, such sentiments heightened the need for non-Lamarckian eugenics to demonstrate that it could be useful and posed a serious problem for those attempting to bolshevize it.

A way out of the problem was provided by another of Kol'tsov's protégés, Aleksandr Serebrovskii (1892-1948).[44] In a paper delivered to the Society of Marxist Biologists on January 26, 1926, he asserted that it was wrong to argue that genetics was "unrevolutionary" or "counterrevolutionary" because it "attempts somehow to assign a value to different groups of the population, to various classes, and that its evaluation of the most revolutionary classes can be unfavorable." Western bourgeois eugenicists had been guilty of this, he agreed, but that did not damn genetics, because "the genetic foundations are an entirely objective field." Only when we "move to the question of what is worse and what is better" do we "inevitably leave the precise ground of science and enter the field of opinions, of sympathies, and as with all sympathies, they inevitably reflect the class position of the author who expresses them. . . . Each class must create its own eugenics."[45] Thus, there could indeed be bourgeois and proletarian eugenics, but neither could be based on Lamarckism—both had to be based on the objective science of genetics.

The matter came up at the Communist Academy again almost a year later, on December 7, 1926, when Volotskoi presented a paper entitled "Issues in Eugenics." Arguments broke out in the discussion period, leading Serebrovskii to restate his distinction in the strongest terms:

> Two entirely different things are constantly getting mixed up. On the one side is anthropogenetics, which is an exact science; on the other side is something constructed on it, something that has only a certain relation to science. Eugenics is not a science. It is an attempt to apply scientific data on human heredity in the discussion of ways of solving the problems the eugenicist chooses to address, and those problems are not biological, scientific problems.[46]

Thus, what a few months before had been the "genetic foundations" of eugenics had become a new scientific field, *antropogenetika*.

In 1927, a scientific event occurred that helped win over a number of young Marxist Lamarckians to Serebrovskii's position. In a piece of research that would subsequently win him the Nobel Prize, the American geneticist H. J. Muller demonstrated that X-rays cause genetic mutations. For some Soviet Marxists, Muller's discovery redeemed Mendelian genetics by demonstrating that, far from being eternally fixed, genetic traits could be changed by environmental influences and might eventually be deliberately manipulated and controlled. Serebrovskii emphasized both the scientific and ideological significance of Muller's discovery in an article in the September 11, 1927, issue of *Pravda* entitled "Four Pages That Shook the Scientific World."[47] That autumn, in his laboratory at the Moscow Zootechnical Institute, he replicated Muller's findings.

As a result of these developments, and under the tutelage of fellow Marxist Serebrovskii, Levit abandoned Lamarckism and soon showed for genetics the enthusiasm of a recent convert. In 1927, Serebrovskii left the Kol'tsov institute and established a genetics laboratory at the Communist Academy's Timiriazev Institute, where he pursued innovative studies of gene structure with a distinguished group of young Marxist biologists, including Levit.[48] Much more research would be needed, however, before techniques could be developed to induce desirable gene mutations in humans: most of the X-ray–induced mutations Muller had found in fruit flies were harmful, and some were lethal. Hence, for Bolshevik geneticists, a second option for therapeutic eugenic action had been ruled out.

THE FINAL OPTION: POSITIVE EUGENICS

In context, Serebrovskii's distinction between anthropogenetics (the science) and eugenics (the social construction) was itself revolutionary. It conflicted with the image of eugenics as a scientific discipline that Iudin and other advocates were laboring to establish. It also conflicted with the popular and widely held views set forth by Bogdanov, Bukharin, and other Marxist luminaries that science itself was class-based and came in two different varieties—bourgeois and proletarian.[49] Nonetheless, Serebrovskii's distinction had critically important implications. First, if it denied eugenics the status of a scientific discipline, it did afford that status to eugenic research, suitably relabeled anthropogenetics. Second, it opened the opportunity for creating a Soviet style of eugenics different from and untainted by foreign eugenics movements.

Yet, however useful, Serebrovskii's distinction left him in a dilemma of his own making. On the one hand, he had defended genetics from Lamarckism by declaring it to be objective, scientific, and utterly neutral on social questions—and thereby free of the unsavory taint of foreign bourgeois eugenic programs. On the other hand, he had defended genetics from the charge that it was counterrevolutionary by declaring that human genetics could be of great practical use as the basis for a distinctly proletarian eugenics—but he had not specified any distinctly proletarian eugenics that could be built on genetics, or any distinctly Bolshevik prescriptions for action that such a proletarian eugenics would make possible. Consider his explicit references to the patron of eugenics, Narkomzdrav, which were intended to show that his ideas were "of more than academic interest." Noting that "almost every act of every commissariat affects in one degree or another the interest of the gene fund," he emphasized the role of Narkomzdrav, "which cures and supports the existence of the sick, which saves defective children, etc., which creates such an improvement of living conditions that infant mortality changes and those who formerly would have died have the possibility of living," thereby "serving as an agent which affects the fate of the gene fund."[50] So far so good; but precisely what did he propose the officials of Narkomzdrav do, and how could anthropogenetics help them do it?

This dilemma may have prompted Serebrovskii to devise a truly Bolshevik eugenics, based on anthropogenetics, that would aid the building of communism. In 1928, Serebrovskii set about creating a new institutional base for anthropogenetics together with Solomon Levit. Previously, Levit had rejected genetics because it left the physician therapeutically impotent; now, convinced of its scientific validity, its philosophical plausibility, and its potential for practical action, he threw himself into the study of anthropogenetics. In late 1928, he left the Moscow University Clinic and, together with Serebrovskii, established the Cabinet of Human Heredity and Constitution at Narkomzdrav's Biomedical Institute. In 1929, Levit's office (kabinet) published its first volume of papers and, in a brief note, he laid out its research program: it would use twin studies, genealogical analysis, and case histories from anthropogenetic stations to elucidate the topography of human chromosomes, human population genetics, and the genetic basis of human pathological forms.[51]

What made the volume memorable, however, was its lead article—a startling piece by Serebrovskii entitled "Anthropogenetics and Eugenics in a Socialist Society."[52] In 1928, the party called for discussions and suggestions for revisions in the new First Five-Year Plan. Long a Bolshevik enthusiast, Serebrovskii had recently become a candidate member of the party, and his article was his enthusiastic response to the party's call. Complaining that the plan's architects had taken into account gas, oil, and mineral resources but had "completely left out the tabulation of the biological quality of the population of the Soviet Union," Serebrovskii commented that it was apparent "what a heavy burden is place on man and his works by the accumulation of harmful genes in his gene fund." "If we calculate how much effort, time, and money would be freed if we succeeded in cleansing our country's population of various forms of hereditary ailments," he commented, "then probably it would be possible to fulfill the Five-Year Plan in two-and-a-half years."[53]

Serebrovskii then proposed a concrete Bolshevik form of eugenics that would fit with centralized planning: "the widespread induction of conception by means of artificial insemination using recommended sperm, and not at all necessarily from a beloved spouse." He spelled out the immediate technical possibilities. Given "the tremendous sperm-making capacity of men," and "with the current state of artificial insemination technology (now widely used in horse and cattle breeding), one talented and valuable producer could have up to 1,000 children. . . . In these conditions, human selection would make gigantic leaps forward. And various women and whole communes would then be proud . . . of their successes and achievements in this undoubtedly most astonishing field—the production of new forms of human beings."[54] He predicted that this time was "not far off."

Like Filipchenko and Kol'tsov before him, of course, Serebrovskii also used his vision to make a case for his own research enterprise and the new discipline it

embodied. Having explained its scientific character, detailed its immediate usefulness, and justified its social importance, Serebrovskii emphasized that anthropogenetics must be developed energetically: "We must very rapidly broaden and
deepen our work, make it maximally concrete, study our gene fund, study and
analyze pedigrees, and proceed to the organization of experiments," so that when
anthropogeneticists are asked for advice, they will be able to "go beyond general
answers and give really scientific" information.[55] Because it formed the scientific
basis of practical eugenics, he concluded, anthropogenetics is a science geared to
"helping us maximize the productive forces of our country."

How had Serebrovskii come on such a daring idea for social action? We must
remember that he was not only a drosophila geneticist, a eugenicist, and a Marxist:
his central occupation was poultry breeding. Since 1918 he had headed experimental
poultry stations and, beginning in 1926, he conducted expeditions to investigate
the "gene fund" of domesticated poultry in various tribal, mountainous regions in
order to produce chickens with agriculturally desirable characteristics. As chairman
of the department of poultry breeding at the Moscow Zootechnical Institute since
1923, Serebrovskii was well acquainted with the latest developments in *zootekhnika*.
In particular, he had been impressed by the world-renowned, pioneering work of
Il'ia Ivanovich Ivanov (1870–1932) on artificial insemination. Ivanov, who had
been Filipchenko's teacher and research collaborator from 1913 to 1920, had been
teaching at the Moscow Zootechnical Institute since the early 1920s. In the period
1927–30, his techniques for the artificial insemination of sheep and cows came into
wide use in the Soviet Union. He had also published on artificial insemination in
poultry, and Serebrovskii was seeking to use his techniques.[56]

In 1926-27, Ivanov headed an expedition to West Africa with the purpose of
attempting to hybridize different species of anthropoid apes by artificially insemi-
nating chimpanzees.[57] Although no results were published, Serebrovskii may have
heard of the work when Ivanov returned to the Moscow Zootechnical Institute in
1928, the same year Serebrovskii moved his research base to that institute. Ivanov's
zootekhnika was almost certainly the inspiration for Serebrovskii's antropotekhnika—a word he used explicitly in connection with his plan. Although H. J. Muller
later published the same proposal and claimed to have thought of it in 1910,[58] there
is good reason to believe that Ivanov indirectly inspired Serebrovskii's plan, and
that Serebrovskii directly inspired Muller's.[59]

But if Serebrovskii's proposal synthesized planning, Bolshevism, and zootekhnika, it also grew out of the logic of the Soviet eugenics movement. Over the
preceding decade, Marxist eugenicists had been seeking a way to be useful. The
first widely touted variant, Volotskoi's sterilization proposal, was the quintessential
form of "negative eugenics." It had met with great resistance in the early 1920s;
by the late 1920s, sterilization, marriage restrictions, immigration control, and other
"negative" measures were seen as the hallmarks of "bourgeois" eugenic policy.
The second widely touted Marxist variant, Lamarckian eugenics, had offered little
in the way of policy that was eugenic or new, and in any case it had been partially
discredited by the Kammerer scandal.[60] Following Muller's discovery, it seemed
possible that favorable genetic traits might eventually be induced, but that time was

a long way off. With no support for negative eugenics, and no prospects for inducing desirable hereditary traits, there remained only one option: positive eugenics. Previously, all such proposals had seemed bourgeois, voluntaristic, and trivial in effect. Now, at last, zootechnology had come up with a technique that made positive eugenics a Bolshevik possibility.[61]

THE "DEMISE" OF SOVIET EUGENICS

Within months, the Cultural Revolution was under way and Serebrovskii's scheme had become a major embarrassment. In mid-1930 Serebrovskii published a letter lamenting the fact that some of his comrades had failed to understand his argument. He apologized for his criticism of the Five-Year Plan, agreeing with his critics that the development of oil, gas, minerals, and other natural resources was much more important for the immediate future of the Soviet state than the tabulation of the population's genes.[62] If there was a single event that signaled the demise of eugenics, it was the publication in the June 4, 1930, issue of *Izvestiia* of a stinging poem entitled "Evgenika" by the notorious popular satirist Demian Bednyi (a pseudonym). Bednyi began by noting the similarity between the Russian nobility's love of pedigree horse breeding and their preoccupation with their own genealogy. Then, quoting passages from Serebrovskii's 1929 article, he followed them with his own reductions to absurdity—for example, a future Moscow clogged by 10,000 carbon copies of the director of Serebrovskii's publisher, Gosizdat. Near the end of the poem, his tone becomes indignant: "Our ancestors were all illiterate. They forgot to leave us a note on their pedigrees. . . . They were all mutilated by the old regime, injured by unbearable work, sent to the front—in short, it ruthlessly spoiled our gene fund. Thus contaminated, we finally started the struggle. . . . But our Eugenics is class eugenics—proletarian—and it comes from the masses, not from an armchair in a stuffy room."

Of course, Soviet eugenics was not done in by Bednyi's poem: larger forces were at work. The period of the First Five-Year Plan (1929-33) witnessed, in Stalin's words, a *velikii perelom*—a "Great Break" as Western historians have branded it.[63] The period saw the first show trials, the move to heavy industrialization, the collectivization of agriculture, the imposition of an ideological "Party line" in many new areas, widespread institutional harassment and reorganization, and crackdowns on bourgeois experts. Two of those experts were Kol'tsov and Filipchenko. In 1930, Kol'tsov was relieved of his teaching responsibilities at Moscow University, his Department of Experimental Biology was split apart, and the remarkable collection of young animal geneticists who worked at his institute was dispersed. Filipchenko was relieved of his teaching responsibilities at Leningrad University as of January 1930, and his Department of Experimental Zoology was disbanded.[64] He died suddenly from meningitis in May 1930.

These attacks on bourgeois experts also had a strongly antitechnocratic thrust. As Kendall Bailes has convincingly demonstrated, the "Shakhty" and "Industrial Party Affair" trials singled out those who had been active in Russia's technocracy movement.[65] As is less often noted, however, technocracy was not limited to en-

gineering or industry: there was also agricultural "tekhnika" and "zootekhnika."
During the collectivization of agriculture and the liquidation of the kulaks, technical
agricultural specialists were especially vulnerable: Ivanov was arrested in December
1930 and died in 1932.[66] And there was "antropotekhnika": eugenics itself can be
seen as a form of technocracy.[67]

The "Great Break" also involved the ideological proscription of any attempt
at theoretical links from the biological to the social. During the period, a new
pejorative word entered the Russian language, *biologizirovat'*—literally "to biolo-
gize"—which was understood as one of the several sins collectively referred to
during the period as "Menshevizing idealism." For example, at a March 1931
meeting of the Society of Materialist Biologists of the Communist Academy,
B. Tokin alluded to "the perfectly clear attempts of Comrade Serebrovskii to biolo-
gize social phenomena" and noted with chagrin that "the exposure of the biolo-
gization of social phenomena" had been the work not of Party biologists, but of
the poet Demian Bednyi.[68] As a result of the Great Break, the new biosocial fields
that had developed with such vigor in the previous decade were broken apart,
dissolved, or renamed—for example, "plant sociology" became "phytocoenol-
ogy." As far as I can determine, no field that linked the biological and the social
survived the Great Break intact.

As a field run by bourgeois experts, premised on a biosocial link, and imbued
with technocratic values, eugenics was doomed. The Russian Eugenics Society was
disbanded shortly after the last issue of its journal appeared in 1930, and the eugenics
section of Kol'tsov's institute was abolished. Any lingering doubts about the status
of the field were set to rest in 1931 with the appearance of the article on *evgenika*
in the *Great Soviet Encyclopedia*. It defined eugenics as the "bourgeois doctrine
of the biological improvement of the human race" and declared categorically that
Filipchenko's eugenic ideas were "bourgeois," Kol'tsov's were "fascist," and
Serebrovskii's constituted "Menshevizing idealism."[69]

In retrospect, the demise of Soviet eugenics during the Cultural Revolution may
well seem overdetermined. Eugenics was a utopian biosocial science, founded by
bourgeois liberals, funded by the public health minister, a kind of antropotekhnika
that would have given eugenic experts control over social policy. As such, it could
not survive a period that was characterized by the proscription of the "biosocial,"
attacks on bourgeois experts, the dismissal of its chief patron, and widespread
antitechnocracy campaigns. However malleable, Soviet eugenics could not change
in six months the fundamental nature of what it had become over the course of
more than a decade.

Nonetheless, the sudden end of Soviet eugenics raises troubling comparative
questions. In every one of the more than thirty countries where eugenics developed
during the period 1900-40, it was perforce domesticated. Everywhere, it represented, at least potentially, a federation of differing institutional, professional, the-
matic, and ideological clusters. Far from weakening it, such a structure made it
more adaptable: not only was it able to exist in a variety of political, cultural, social,
and economic circumstances, but it was also able to accommodate itself to rapid

changes in those circumstances. The point is well illustrated by the example of German eugenics, which arose under the Kaiser, flowered during Weimar, and prospered under the Nazis.

If, as I have suggested, the diverse composition of a discipline helps it survive and adapt to rapidly changing political circumstances, why did some part of Soviet eugenics not survive the *velikii perelom*? The simple answer is that some part of Soviet eugenics *did* survive—but not as "eugenics." By 1934, a number of ex-eugenicists had reassembled under Narkomzdrav at Levit's institute to pursue a newly christened specialty: "medical genetics."[70] And when that enterprise, in turn, was dissolved in 1937, some of those former eugenicists continued to pursue their research under the rubrics of anthropology, neurology, physiology, psychology, and medicine. Their efforts persisted through the purges, the world war, and Lysenkoism. Finally, in the 1960s, when Lysenko's hegemony came to an end, students and colleagues of Filipchenko, Kol'tsov, and Serebrovskii were able to resurrect genetics, medical genetics, and even eugenics.

Of course, these events are part of a much larger story that is beyond the scope of the present discussion.[71] Suffice it to say that the networks associated with Soviet eugenics in the 1920s, and the links they forged with Soviet public health, have proved remarkably enduring.

NOTES

Research for this paper has been supported by the History and Philosophy of Science Division of the National Science Foundation; by the Science, Technology, and Society Program of the National Endowment for the Humanities; and by the Department of the History and Sociology of Science of the University of Pennsylvania.

1. For an international comparison of eugenics movements, see Mark B. Adams, ed., *The Wellborn Science: Eugenics in Germany, France, Brazil, and Russia* (Oxford, 1989).

2. For a comparison of British and American eugenics and the sources of their funding, see Daniel J. Kevles, *In the Name of Eugenics* (New York, 1985).

3. Garland E. Allen, "The Eugenics Record Office at Cold Spring Harbor, 1910–1940," *Osiris*, 2d ser., vol. 2 (1986), pp. 225–64.

4. Sheila Faith Weiss, "Wilhelm Schallmayer and the Logic of German Eugenics," *Isis*, 77, no. 286 (March 1986), pp. 33–46, and *Race Hygiene and National Efficiency: The Eugenics of Wilhelm Schallmayer* (Berkeley: University of California Press, 1987). On German eugenics and race hygiene, see also Benno Müller-Hill, *Murderous Science* (Oxford, 1988); Robert N. Proctor, *Racial Hygiene* (Cambridge, Mass., 1988); Peter Weingart, Jürgen Kroll, and Kurt Bayertz, *Rasse, Blut und Gene* (Frankfurt am Main, 1988); and Paul Weindling, *Health, Race, and German Politics between National Unification and Nazism, 1870–1945* (Cambridge: Cambridge University Press, 1989).

5. William Schneider, "Toward the Improvement of the Human Race: The History of Eugenics in France," *Journal of Modern History*, 54 (1982), pp. 268–91.

6. For a suggestive comparison of the German and Russian movements in the 1920s, see Loren Graham, *Between Science and Values* (New York, 1981), pp. 217–56.

7. F. Galton, *Nasledstvennost' talanta, ee zakony i posledstviia* (St. Petersburg, 1875).

8. See Alfred J. Rieber, *Merchants and Entrepreneurs in Imperial Russia* (Chapel Hill, N.C., 1982).

9. On Filipchenko, see Mark B. Adams, "Iurii Aleksandrovich Filipchenko," *Dictionary of Scientific Biography*, supplement 2 (1990), s.v.

10. Iu. A. Filipchenko, "Evgenika," *Russkaia mysl'*, nos. 3–4 (1918), pp. 69–95.

11. N. K. Kol'tsov, "Uluchshenie chelovecheskoi porody," *Russkii evgenicheskii zhurnal*, 1, no. 1 (1922), p. 27; delivered at a meeting of the Russian Eugenics Society, October 28, 1921.

12. Iu. A. Filipchenko, *Chto takoe evgenika* (Petrograd, 1921); *Kak nasleduiutsia razlichnye osobennosti cheloveka* (Petrograd, 1921); *Puti uluchsheniia chelovecheskogo roda (Evgenika)* (Petrograd, 1924); and *Frensis Gal'ton i Gregor Mendel'* (Moscow, 1925).

13. N. N. Medvedev, *Iurii Aleksandrovich Filipchenko* (Moscow, 1978), p. 43.

14. Ibid., p. 44.

15. Iu. A. Filipchenko, "Biuro po Evgenike," *Izvestiia Biuro po Evgenike*, no. 1 (1922), pp. 1–4.

16. See Mark B. Adams, "Science, Ideology, and Structure: The Kol'tsov Institute, 1900–1970," in L. Lubrano and S. G. Solomon, eds., *The Social Context of Soviet Science* (Boulder, Colo., 1980), pp. 173–204; and "Chetverikov, the Kol'tsov Institute, and the Evolutionary Synthesis," in Ernst Mayr and William Provine, eds., *The Evolutionary Synthesis* (Cambridge, Mass., 1980), pp. 242–78.

17. V. V. Sakharov, "Razbor muzykal'nykh genealogii, sobrannykh na evgenicheskom seminare professora N. K. Kol'tsova," *Russkii evgenicheskii zhurnal*, 2, no. 2/3 (1924), pp. 17–25; and A. S. Serebrovskii and V. V. Sakharov, "Novye mutatsii Drosophila melanogaster," *Zhurnal eksperimental'noi biologii*, ser. A, 1, no. 1/2 (1925), pp. 75–91.

18. Charles Rosenberg, "Toward an Ecology of Knowledge," in A. Oleson and J. Voss, eds., *The Organization of Knowledge in Modern America, 1860–1920* (Baltimore, 1979), pp. 440–55.

19. V. V. Bunak, "O deiatel'nosti Russkogo Evgenicheskogo Obshchestva," *Russkii evgenicheskii zhurnal*, 1, no. 1 (1922), pp. 99–101. In addition to N. K. Kol'tsov, that commission included Bogoiavlenskii, Dauge, Iudin, Martsynovskii, Mol'kov, Prokhorov, Sysin, Shifman, Viktorov, and Zakharov.

20. V. V. Bunak, "Iz otcheta o deiatel'nosti Russkogo Evgenicheskogo Obshchestva za 1922 g.," *Russkii evgenicheskii zhurnal*, 2, no. 1 (1924), pp. 66–67.

21. *Eugenical News*, 9, no. 2 (1924), pp. 17–20.

22. M. P. Kutanin, "Otchet o rabote Saratovskogo otdeleniia Russkogo Evgenicheskogo Obshchestva," *Russkii evgenicheskii zhurnal*, 5, no. 2 (1927), pp. 93–96.

23. *Eugenical News*, 10, no. 5 (1925), p. 57.

24. S. N. Davidenkov, "Geneticheskoe biuro pri M. O. N. i P.," *Russkii evgenicheskii zhurnal*, 6, no. 1 (1928), pp. 55–56.

25. Marie-Hélène Mandrillon, "Eugénisme et hygiénisme en URSS: La 'Revue russe d'eugénique' 1920–1929," presented at the Colloque international d'Histoire de la Génétique, May 19–22, 1987, Paris.

26. F. Florinskii, *Usovershenstvovanie i vyrozhdenie chelovecheskago roda* (St. Petersburg, 1866).

27. M. V. Volotskoi, "K istorii evgenicheskogo dvizheniia," *Russkii evgenicheskii zhurnal*, 2, no. 1 (1924), pp. 50–55.

28. V. M. Florinskii, *Usovershenstvovanie i vyrozhdenie chelovecheskago roda* (Vologda, 1926).

29. See, for example, P. I. Liublinskii, "Sovremennoe sostoianie evgenicheskogo dvizheniia," *Russkii evgenicheskii zhurnal*, 4, no. 2 (1926), pp. 63–75.

30. T. I. Iudin, *Evgenika* (Moscow, 1925), p. 6. Iudin's book was published by the Sabashnikov brothers.

31. Bunak, "O deiatel'nosti," p. 101.

32. M. V. Volotskoi, "O polovoi sterilizatsii nasledstvenno defektivnykh," *Russkii ev-*

genicheskii zhurnal, 1, no. 2 (1923), pp. 201–22; and *Podniatie zhiznennykh sil rasy (Novyi put')* (Moscow, 1923).

33. Filipchenko, *Puti*, pp. 156, 162, 186.

34. See, for example, Diane Paul, "Eugenics and the Left," *Journal of the History of Ideas* (October 1984), pp. 567–90.

35. A. V. Gorbunov, "Vliianie mirovoi voiny na dvizhenie naseleniia Evropy," *Russkii evgenicheskii zhurnal*, 1, no. 1 (1922), pp. 39–63.

36. See note 22, and also M. P. Kutanin, "Otchet o deiatel'nosti Saratovskogo otdeleniia Russkogo Evgenicheskogo Obshchestva za 1927 god," *Russkii evgenicheskii zhurnal*, 6, no. 1 (1928), pp. 54–55.

37. See A. E. Gaissinovitch, "The Origins of Soviet Genetics and the Struggle with Lamarckism, 1922–1929," trans. Mark B. Adams, *Journal of the History of Biology*, 13, no. 1 (1980), pp. 1–51.

38. Paul Kammerer, *The Inheritance of Acquired Characteristics* (New York, 1924).

39. M. V. Volotskoi, *Klassovye interesy i sovremennaia evgenika* (Moscow, 1925). For an example of another Lamarckian who advocated sterilization, see Peter J. Bowler, "E. W. MacBride's Lamarckian Eugenics and Its Implications for the Social Construction of Scientific Knowledge," *Annals of Science*, 41 (1984), pp. 245–60.

40. T. H. Morgan and Iu. A. Filipchenko, *Nasledstvenny li priobretennye priznaki?* (Leningrad, 1925).

41. See Gaissinovitch, "Origins of Soviet Genetics."

42. See Mark B. Adams, "Solomon Gregor'evich Levit," *Dictionary of Scientific Biography*, supplement 2 (1990), s.v. He served as scientific secretary from February 1, 1926, through April 16, 1930.

43. S. G. Levit, "Evoliutsionnye teorii v biologii i marksizm," *Vestnik sovremennoi meditsiny*, no. 9 (1925), as reprinted in *Problema konstitutsii v meditsine i dialekticheskii materializm* (Moscow, 1927), pp. 21, 32; from Gaissinovitch, "Origins of Soviet Genetics."

44. See Mark B. Adams, "Aleksandr Sergeevich Serebrovsky," *Dictionary of Scientific Biography*, supplement 2, s.v.

45. A. S. Serebrovskii, "Teoriia nasledstvennosti Morgana i Mendelia i marksisty," *Pod znamenem marksizma*, no. 3 (1926), pp. 98–117; quotation from page 113.

46. M. V. Volotskoi, "Spornye voprosy evgeniki," *Vestnik Kommunisticheskoi Akademii*, no. 20 (1927), pp. 240–41. Serebrovskii had first proposed the term *antropogenetika* in 1923, but at that time he did not distinguish it from eugenics.

47. A. S. Serebrovskii, "Chetyre stranitsy, kotorye vzvolnovali uchenyi mir," *Pravda*, September 11, 1927.

48. The group also included I. I. Agol, N. P. Dubinin, A. E. Gaissinovitch, V. N. Slepkov, N. I. Shapiro, and B. N. Sidorov.

49. On the so-called theory of two sciences, see Dominique Lecourt, *Lyssenko: Histoire réelle d'une "science prolétarienne"* (Paris, 1976).

50. According to Gaissinovitch, who has inspected the records of the meeting, Serebrovskii's position was heavily criticized for his claim that genetics is "an entirely objective field, and as such independent of class . . . it cannot be revolutionary or unrevolutionary"—a phrase omitted from the published version. As a result, Serebrovskii's paper was published not in the journal of the Communist Academy, as was customary, but rather as an article for discussion in *Under the Banner of Marxism*. See Gaissinovitch, "Origins of Soviet Genetics."

51. *Trudy kabineta nasledstvennosti i konstitutsii cheloveka pri mediko-biologicheskom institute*, vol. 1, edited by S. G. Levit and A. S. Serebrovskii (Moscow, 1929), pp. 115–16.

52. A. S. Serebrovskii, "Antropogenetika i evgenika v sotsialisticheskom obshchestve," ibid., pp. 3–19.

53. Ibid., pp. 7, 12.

54. Ibid., p. 18.

55. Ibid., p. 19.

56. For a brief biography of Ivanov by P. N. Skatkin, a list of his publications, and a sample of his works, see *I. I. Ivanov: Izbrannye trudy* (Moscow, 1970).

57. Ibid., p. 16.

58. See the final chapter, entitled "Birth and Rebirth," in H. J. Muller, *Out of the Night: A Biologist's View of the Future* (New York, 1935), pp. 103–127.

59. Mark B. Adams, "Soviet Medical Genetics in the 1930s," *Acts of the XVIIIth International Congress of History of Science* (Berkeley, Calif., 1985), vol. 2, p. 03.4, and "Eugenics in Russia, 1900–1940," in Adams, ed., *The Wellborn Science,* esp. pp. 192–200.

60. See Gaissinovitch, "Origins of Soviet Genetics." In an exemplary toad whose coloration, claimed Kammerer, proved the inheritance of acquired characteristics, the herpetologist G. K. Noble had discovered India ink injected under the skin. See Arthur Koestler, *The Case of the Midwife Toad* (London, 1971).

61. See Mark B. Adams, "From 'Gene Fund' to 'Gene Pool,' " in William Coleman and Camille Limoges, eds., *Studies in the History of Biology,* vol. 3 (Baltimore, 1979), pp. 241–85.

62. A. S. Serebrovskii, "Pis'mo v Redaktsiiu," *Mediko-biologicheskii zhurnal,* nos. 4–5 (1930), pp. 447–48.

63. Stalin used the term *velikii perelom* to refer to the year 1929/30 of the First Five-Year Plan and, more specifically, to the collectivization of agriculture.

64. See the letters from Filipchenko to Theodosius Dobzhansky, Dobzhansky Papers, Library of the American Philosophical Society, Philadelphia.

65. Kendall E. Bailes, *Technology and Society under Lenin and Stalin* (Princeton, N.J., 1978).

66. He was released to internal exile in June 1931, and died in Alma-Ata.

67. Weiss, "Wilhelm Schallmayer."

68. P. P. Bondarenko et al., eds., *Protiv mekhanisticheskogo materializma i men'shevistvuiushchego idealizma v biologii* (Moscow and Leningrad, 1931), p. 20.

69. G. Batkis, "Evgenika," *Bol'shaia Sovetskaia Entsiklopediia,* vol. 23 (1931), pp. 812–19.

70. *Konferentsiia po meditsinskoi genetike: Doklady i preniia,* supplement to *Sovetskaia klinika,* 20, no. 7/8 (1934). The following year, the institute was renamed the Maxim Gorky Scientific Research Institute of Medical Genetics, Narkomzdrav.

71. I have given a fuller account of the development of eugenics and medical genetics in the USSR in "Eugenics in Russia, 1900–1940," in Adams, ed., *The Wellborn Science,* pp. 153–216. I have discussed developments in the 1930s in "The Politics of Human Heredity in the USSR," *Genome,* 31, no. 2 (1989). I treat more recent events in "The Soviet Nature-Nurture Debate," in Loren R. Graham, ed., *Science and the Soviet Social Order* (Cambridge, Mass., 1990).

LEWIS H. SIEGELBAUM

Okhrana Truda

Industrial Hygiene, Psychotechnics, and Industrialization in the USSR

Work-related injury and death predate the industrial age. But the concentration of workers in factories and the concomitant mechanization of production processes—developments characteristic of the nineteenth-century industrial revolutions of Western Europe and North America—were accompanied by carnage on a scale hitherto unknown except in battle. The greater the capacity and speed of operation of machines, the more threatening to limb and life. The more that piece rates and other material incentives were used by employers to urge workers on to a more intense pace, the more fatigued and careless a worker could become. The ever-increasing specialization of labor itself could induce monotony, fatigue, and ultimately accidents.

Industrial accidents and disabilities soon became a major social issue in industrialized and industrializing countries. As a response to the appalling toll that work took on those who perfomed it, trade unions and socialist movements typically demanded improved working conditions, shorter working hours, gender- and age-related restrictions, and compensation paid by employers. Notwithstanding advances in these directions and the passage of legislation to standardize building codes, introduce factory inspection, and otherwise promote safety consciousness, progress in reducing accidents was slow.[1] Many employers continued to circumvent safety regulations where these existed; at the same time, increased mechanization, the introduction of assembly-line production, and the rapid growth of clerical occupations exacerbated problems of monotony and mental fatigue.[2]

It was at this juncture that "science," in the form of applied chemistry, physics, physiology, and, above all, psychology, intervened. The first two decades of the twentieth century saw a veritable explosion of research in Europe and North America on the causes of work-related disabilities and accidents and the concomitant emergence of two new professions—industrial hygiene and industrial psychology or psychotechnics.[3] Spawned by the technocratic approach to curing the ills of industrial society, these professions soon became an integral part of the industrial scene. In this period it was widely believed that the efforts of industrial hygienists and psychotechnicians to understand the causes of accidents and develop strategies for preventing them would reduce their incidence and rates of severity. Yet the historical record is far from clear in this respect.

The purpose of this essay is to trace the early development of these professions in the one country where, putatively at least, the working class was in power, the Soviet Union. On the face of it, a society that had broken with the logic of capitalism and had placed the welfare of its workers among its highest priorities should have conferred considerable power and authority on those seeking to prevent the squandering of workers' blood, flesh, nerves, and brains. Was this the case? Were these specialists able to overcome the deleterious effects of economic and cultural backwardness, the frenzied pace of Soviet industrialization, and the ideologically charged suspiciousness of their expertise? Was there a distinctly Soviet approach to accident and disability prevention, and is it possible to judge the degree of its success? In addressing these issues, special attention will be devoted to the demands placed on hygienists and psychotechnicians, the struggles within the professions, and their relationship to broader socio-political developments.

THE TSARIST LEGACY

The record of the tsarist regime with respect to industrial relations and accident prevention was not exemplary. A factory inspectorate was established in 1882, originally to enforce laws protecting juveniles and women. Following the first serious outbreak of strikes in 1884–85, the jurisdiction of the inspectorate was expanded to include peaceful mediation of labor disputes, supervision of labor contracts, provision of workers' medical assistance, and protection of their lives, morals, and health. But the size of the inspectorate, inadequate from the beginning, did not keep pace with the broadening of its responsibilities. In the words of one historian, "The factory inspector's work, like a housewife's, was never done."[4]

There were other problems as well. Like their contemporaries in the zemstvo administrations, many inspectors were highly educated and intrepid social reformers who sought to expose and thereby alleviate the abuses they witnessed. Others, however, succumbed to pressure from the Ministry of Finance and individual industrialists and refrained from filing grievances on behalf of workers. All the while, as a consequence of desperate conditions on the land and massive foreign capital investment in industry, the number of industrial workers swelled. Precisely because of its relative lateness and intensity, industrialization in tsarist Russia produced conditions highly conducive to industrial accidents and disabilities. The combination of large-scale factories employing advanced technology with a working class that was scarcely removed from the village was sufficient in itself to cause extensive carnage.[5] Moreover, working hours for adult males were not regulated until 1897, and until 1906 workers were deprived of any legal opportunities to improve working conditions.

Neither the creation of the State Duma nor the other concessions wrested from the authorities during the 1905 revolution significantly altered the situation. The only piece of legislation concerning industrial accidents—the Workers' Insurance

Laws of 1912—took nearly five years to draft. Although they provided for elected representatives of workers to administer funds jointly with employers, they failed to address the matter of accident and disability prevention; in any case their provisions did not extend to state-owned or small-scale enterprises.[6]

Whatever progress was made in these respects by 1914 was undone by the First World War. The recruitment of many skilled workers into the army, the running down of capital stock, and the resort to intensification and overtime by employers eager to fulfill war orders took their toll on workers. At the Putilov Works, Petrograd's (and the empire's) largest industrial plant, there were 211 cases of mutilation in 1914, and 305 in 1915. For every 1,000 workers in Ekaterinoslav's factories in 1915, 322 sustained injuries; in Perm's armaments factories, the rate was nearly 300 per 1,000 workers in 1916.[7] The actual rates were undoubtedly higher, for monetary inflation convinced many workers that they could not afford to seek compensation or disability pensions.

INDUSTRIAL COLLAPSE AND PROFESSIONAL GROWTH

Early Soviet legislation on industrial safety reflected the impact of workers' control as it had evolved in the course of 1917–18.[8] On May 18, 1918, the prerevolutionary system of factory inspection was abolished and replaced by one that called for inspectors to be nominated by the factory committee of each industrial establishment and appointed by respective trade unions and social insurance organs. In addition, the new law enjoined each factory committee to form a special subcommittee on labor protection which was to contain from three to seven members, depending on the size of the work force. The administration of this and other laws pertaining to safety was placed in the hands of the Commissariat of Labor (Narkomtrud), which created a Bureau for the Protection of Labor especially for that purpose.[9] By 1920, similar provisions had been made for the appointment of technical and health inspectors.[10]

As promising as these initiatives may have appeared, their immediate impact was severely circumscribed by the circumstances of the Civil War years. With industrial production at a fraction of its prewar level, and the industrial proletariat dispersed throughout the countryside, mobilized for the Red Army, or barely surviving in the cities on whatever could be pilfered from the idle plants and bartered on the black markets, the regulations governing industrial safety had little more than a paper reality.[11] Even after the introduction of the New Economic Policy (NEP) in 1921, the system of labor inspection remained rudimentary, the collection of statistics on occupational diseases and industrial accidents was haphazard at best, and any analysis of the causes of accidents was, perforce, speculative.[12]

This situation began to change in 1923. That year saw the founding of both the Central Museum for the Protection of Labor and Social Insurance and the Obukh Institute for the Study of Occupational Diseases. The former was devoted to the display of protective devices and methods of accident prevention; the latter employed both a research and clinical staff and issued periodic bulletins on dangerous substances used in industry and on instances of occupational disability.[13] Two years later, in 1925, the State Institute for the Protection of Labor was established in Moscow under the auspices of Narkomtrud, the Commissariat of Public Health of the RSFSR, and the USSR Supreme Council of the National Economy. Its director was S. I. Kaplun, a twenty-eight-year-old professor at the Moscow Medical Institute and a party member since 1917.[14]

In the meantime, the first monographs, collections of articles, conference proceedings, and journals dealing with industrial hygiene in the USSR were beginning to appear. Without doubt, the most important of the journals was *Gigiena truda* (Labor Hygiene), a monthly published by the Central Council of Trade Unions under the editorship of Kaplun. *Gigiena truda* reported on the work of labor, technical, and health inspectors, provided space for the discussion of appropriate terminology, reprinted decrees of Narkomtrud and other Soviet organs on labor protection, and summarized international developments in industrial hygiene and related fields. So impressive was the scope of activity in the USSR that Alice Hamilton, the pioneering American industrial toxicologist, could write of her visit to that country in 1924 that ''Indeed, it seemed to me that there was more industrial hygiene in Russia than industry.''[15]

Nor did industrial hygiene exhaust professional concern with the stresses and strains of industrial work. There was also industrial psychology, or psychotechnics, a term coined in 1903 by a German, William Stern, and thereafter used widely throughout continental Europe. Whereas industrial hygienists studied primarily ''objective'' or material conditons such as temperature, ventilation, lighting, the condition of equipment, and the plant in general, psychotechnicians attempted to measure the effects of various kinds and intensities of work on workers' attentiveness, muscular reflexes, pulse rates, and other psycho-physiological functions. Whereas the former experimented with and refined all manner of safety devices (goggles, masks, ear plugs, gloves, boots, safety switches, and locks), the latter developed methods, apparatuses, and test strategies for measuring discrete characteristics and capacities of individuals.

Nevertheless, the two professions shared much common ground and indeed reinforced one another's development in the USSR. First, both emerged as counterweights to the Soviet version of Taylorism, which was being promoted by the Central Institute of Labor and articulated by the institute's visionary director A. K. Gastev. As early as 1921, at the first conference on the Scientific Organization of Labor (NOT—*nauchnaia organizatsiia truda*), psychotechnicians joined forces with trade unionists and hygienists to contest Gastev's narrow approach to vocational training, which emphasized the acquisition of a few basic skills. Typical of their objections was the statement by V. M. Bekhterev, dean of Russian reflexologists, that ''In a socialist society, the rationalization and scientific organization of labor must be based on the fundamental principle that the maximum of productive work can only be procured by fully protecting the health of workers and by guaranteeing the complete development of their personalities.''[16] Adhering to this principle, members of both professions continued to oppose Gastev's definition of the ultimate purpose of NOT—namely, the transformation of human labor into something akin to the movements of machines.[17]

But psychotechnicians and hygienists made common cause not only because they confronted a common enemy. The members of the two professions also shared the same philosophical outlook, influenced by both the Western origins of their professions and factors specific to their circumstances in a "backward" country. Like the statisticians and other professional people who had staffed the zemstvos and other semigovernmental institutions before the revolution, they had a profound sympathy for the long-suffering masses (narod) and an even more profound faith in the uplifting powers of science. Presented with an opportunity to be of assistance to the proletariat, they—and the considerably more numerous doctors and inspectors on whom they relied for diagnoses and data—believed that they were serving both scientific rationality and the building of socialism. If getting the attention of party officials meant packaging their scientism in Marxist terms, they were prepared to do so.

Finally, to a significant degree the two professions crossed institutional boundaries. I. N. Shpilrein, who would eventually become the leading Soviet psychotechnician, began his career in Gastev's institute but moved to the State Institute for the Protection of Labor shortly after its creation. Until 1928, Shpilrein served as a member of the editorial board of Gigiena truda and frequently contributed articles to it. Other prominent psychotechnicians such as S. G. Gellershtein, V. M. Kogan, V. Efremov, and Kh. S. Rivlina continued to write articles and reviews for Gigiena truda even after the Psychotechnical Society began to publish its own journal. And, as we shall see, some of the most penetrating and thorough work on fatigue was conducted by these two groups of specialists in tandem, treating the phenomenon from both psycho-physiological and environmental perspectives.

DISABILITY RESEARCH AND INDUSTRIAL POLICY

One of the critical tasks of the professions concerned with industrial safety was to interpret the statistics on accidents and disabilities collected and compiled by the social insurance offices of the Commissariat of Public Health (see appendix). The quality of the data left much to be desired. Underreporting of accidents in the Soviet Union owing to incomplete information provided by the social insurance offices was estimated at between 10 and 15 percent for these years.[18] This estimate does not include cases in which workers, fearful of losing their jobs, failed to report to the enterprise medical station. Moreover, the standard unit of measure—"accidents per 1,000 insured workers"—included managerial-technical personnel whose chances of incurring accidents were considerably less than manual workers.[19]

Given the limitations of these measurements, how did Soviet specialists approach their research on industrial accidents and disabilities? Among the vast number of studies produced in the latter half of the 1920s, three research strategies can be discerned. The first was to locate as precisely as possible those workers who suffered accidents and to pinpoint when those accidents had occurred; the second was to study the impact of changes in the labor process on fatigue and accidents; and the third was to investigate both the nature and the degree of severity of occupational diseases and disabilities.

Not surprisingly, Soviet investigators found that accident rates differed markedly from one occupation and age group to another and that other factors were involved as well. The studies by Shkliar, Trakhtenberg, and Krol' of accidents at the Petrovskii metallurgical factory in Dnepropetrovsk revealed that accidents occurred most frequently during the second of three shifts and in the "hot" shops, especially the foundry section, that the rate was three times as high among 19- to 23-year-olds as among those who were 18 and under, and that those with one to two years' production experience (*stazh*) had a considerably higher rate than those with less than one year or workers with more than two years' *stazh*. Finally, the accident rate among the enterprise's female workers was negligible, a fact that was explained by the relatively safe, if menial, tasks performed by women.[20]

In their follow-up study, the researchers noted not only the continuing rise in the number of accidents per worker—0.96 in 1926, 1.08 in 1927, and 1.18 in 1928—but also the decline in the proportion of accidents resulting in either temporary or permanent disability. Two other trends, related to the work regimen, were discussed. The rise in the rate of accidents toward the end of each shift was related to the early meal break followed by as much as six hours of continuous work. And, whereas in 1926 and 1927 the frequency of accidents was greatest on Fridays and Saturdays, the introduction in 1928 of a system of staggered days off appeared to have eliminated end-of-the-week fatigue.[21] Other studies of individual metallurgical enterprises, shipyards, machine tool factories, and coal mines tended to replicate the methodology and findings of Shkliar and his colleagues. In some cases, though, a downward trend in the frequency of accidents per worker was recorded.[22]

Industrial hygienists were not content, however, merely to record differential rates of accidents. They sought both to refine their analyses and to generalize about the causes of accidents, with a view to discovering their implications for policy. Such refinement involved breaking down specific occupations into constituent tasks and body movements. For this, hygienists relied on the research of psychotechnicians who reconstructed the work day using time and motion study and minutely detailed occupational schemas, known as *professiogrammy*.[23]

In generalizing about causality, hygienists isolated several factors unrelated to work. Poor living conditions, alcoholism, and family problems—the latter often a result of the first two—were frequently cited. But, overwhelmingly, it was conditions in the factories that bore the brunt of criticism. Inadequate lighting, excessive temperature, humidity, and dust levels, antiquated equipment, excessive crowding of machinery and workers, insufficient rest periods, and other violations of safety codes and factory rules figured prominently in reports of technical and health inspectors.[24] There was also criticism of the tendency of management to staff enterprise safety bureaus with poorly educated and low-ranking technical personnel and to burden them with an excessive range of duties.[25]

As industrial hygienists focused more on the correlates of accidents, they sometimes found that culpability rested with the economic system itself. For example,

in one article, Sinel and Engel, two of Kaplun's assistants at the State Institute for
the Protection of Labor, went so far as to assert that "Under the influence of the
sharp demand for its products, our industry has had to raise its productivity without
at the same time being able to renew or improve its equipment. This circumstance
in connection with the application of unlimited piece rates could not but have
negative repercussions on the dynamics of accidents."[26] This assertion, or at least
part of it, was supported by another article which demonstrated a positive correlation
between increased labor productivity and the rate of accidents at the Petrovskii
metallurgical factory.[27]

The relationship between policy and research was nowhere more complex than
with respect to the question of raising productivity without risking the health of
workers. Labor productivity was, in fact, a highly controversial issue in the late
1920s. Much of the controversy centered on changes in the labor process—in
particular, the intensification of production. One of the earliest and most exhaustive
studies devoted to this question was conducted in 1925 by V. V. Isakov and Iu.
N. Khalturina.[28] The study investigated the effects of increasing from two to three
the number of weaving machines that were operated by female weavers at two
textile mills. Isakov's and Khalturina's conclusions neither condemned nor endorsed
the change; rather, they pointed to the importance of ancillary factors in determining
different rates of productivity and levels of fatigue. Among these, hygienic conditions and the socioeconomic condition of those who had volunteered to work on
three machines were given special emphasis.

Although the study was carried out before the state had launched its economy
and rationalization drives, those campaigns were in full swing by the time the study
was published. Their most concrete manifestations were the seven-hour workday
and the three-shift system, first introduced in the textile industry in January 1928.[29]
Hailed by party leaders as a great socialist innovation, these changes inevitably led
to a more intense pace of production and raised to a matter of urgency the question
of fatigue. In this context, the cautionary notes sounded by Isakov and Khalturina
take on added significance. It was asserted, for example, that "to raise productivity
by means of increasing the weaver's intensity of effort is possible only if in addition
to commercial considerations, the . . . physical expenditure of the vital energy of
the worker is taken into account."[30]

Other researchers noted that the shift to three machines could only be considered
"rational" if proper atmospheric and other environmental conditions prevailed and
if rest periods were properly observed. Yet the reported rise in 1928 of absenteeism
and illnesses among Moscow textile workers was attributed precisely to "unsatisfactory sanitary-hygienic conditions and increase in fatigue as a result of the lack
of normal breaks for food and rest, and the greater intensification of work consequent
upon the consolidation (*uplotnenie*) of the work day."[31]

On a broader, theoretical level, O. A. Ermanskii, a former Menshevik whose
oeuvre defies categorization as either industrial psychology or hygiene, questioned
the correlation between the intensity and the productivity of labor. In his view,
human progress could be measured not by the increase in the quantity of human
energy expended in the transformation of nature (intensity of labor) but, rather, the

reverse, that is, by its reduction per unit output. Mechanized and, in particular, assembly-line production could thus contribute enormously to human progress, but only if certain physiologically based norms or optima of energy expenditure were maintained.[32] In this respect Ermanskii considered the early Soviet experience with conveyor production "dangerous." Writing in March 1927, he noted "the excessive intensification of labor as the first consequence of introducing the conveyor."[33]

But this begged the question of the optimum of energy expenditure or, to put it another way, the speed at which conveyors should be operated and the length of time workers should be on the line without a break. A detailed comparative analysis of manual and assembly-line production of harrows at the Hammer and Sickle Factory in Khar'kov found that there was a "significant economization of energy expenditure" among workers on the assembly line, but that this did not necessarily mean a reduction of fatigue. On the contrary, the investigators concluded that "Workers on the conveyor, although conscious of expending less energy and approving of the collective nature of the work, nonetheless raise an arsenal of complaints ranging from leg and back aches to emotional disorders and protests against the compulsory, elementary and fatiguing monotony (*odnoobraziia*) of work."[34]

In short, mental fatigue or the "subjective element" would have to be taken into account in assessing fatigue and regulating assembly-line production. So, too, would different levels of tolerance among individuals. Soviet psychotechnicians did think about these questions but could not reach any consensus about how to integrate them with physiological considerations. The First All-Union Conference on the Psychophysiology of Labor and Occupational Selection, which met in May-June 1927, merely concluded that there were "certain theoretical problems" that still needed to be worked out and that no single approach to the study of fatigue could be endorsed unequivocally.[35] This remained the situation for several years to come.

Meanwhile, on the practical level, psychotechnicians sought to determine proper rest intervals for a number of occupational groups through a variety of measures. These included the Bourdon cancellation and other attention tests, tremometer readings of hand- and arm-steadiness, metabolic rates, and the so-called work method, whereby investigators perfomed all the tasks associated with a given occupation.[36] The advantages of physical exercise during rest periods were also emphasized; indeed, organized calisthenics in the Soviet workplace apparently date from this period.

Aside from the specification of high-risk occupations and working conditions and the study of work fatigue, Soviet investigators also studied occupational disabilities and diseases. Much of their research dealt with the toxicity of chemical substances used in industrial production and the incidence and nature of diseases such as silicosis, lung cancer, and other respiratory and pulmonary disorders. Cases of mass poisoning, documented by technical inspectors, also received close attention. Perhaps the most interesting research, however, concerned eye and ear disorders. Analyzing the data on eye injuries incurred by workers at the Red Sormovo metalworks factory, S. Ia. Glezerov noted the inverse relationship between age and accident rates and attributed this in part to the fact that older workers tended to wear spectacles. "Out of the enormous and ever-growing number of varieties of protective glasses," he remarked, "not one can be worn by metal workers. . . . All have defects. Either they are too heavy, too large, or restrict the range of vision."[37]

Consequently, the number of eye injuries, particularly in the metal works industry, was staggering. At the Khar'kov Electromechanical Factory, 22 percent of all workers in 1925 were victims, mostly of flying splinters but also of burns. At the Stalingrad Metallurgical Works, the figure was 30 percent. Over the course of two and a half years, there were 1,512 cases of injury at the factory, including 20 that resulted in complete blindness. Not all occupational groups were at equal risk. Among three Leningrad factories, eye injuries affected, respectively, 18, 20.6, and 55 percent of all workers in 1928. But for polishers the range was 263–700 percent and for turret lathe operators, the average was 350 percent, or 3.5 eye injuries per worker.[38]

Hearing defects were found to result not so much from accidents as from the cumulatively debilitating effects of noise. Among workers employed for ten or more years in the flyer-frame division of several large textile mills, 24.8 to 42 percent were found to have had partially or completely damaged cochleae. Studies of railway workers and telephonists revealed that "reduced hearing ability" was widespread.[39]

By the end of the NEP period, Soviet psychotechnics and industrial hygiene could boast of an impressive record of scientific investigation and a sound institutional basis for future research. In addition to those already mentioned, institutes for the study of occupational diseases and labor hygiene existed in Leningrad, Kazan', Kiev, Khar'kov, Stalino, and Tbilisi. In 1927, an All-Russian (later, All-Union) Psychotechnical Society was established with Shpilrein as its chairman. The society's journal began to appear the following year. By 1930, according to one estimate, there were some five hundred psychotechnicians in the Soviet Union, and in just three years, the total number of books and articles in the field had reached more than four hundred.[40]

If, despite this overall impressive growth, the rate of accidents and injuries remained intolerably high, the extent of the problem was far better known and analysis of its causes far more advanced than in the early or even mid-1920s. While the introduction of new technology and revisions to the organization of labor had exacerbated the problem of fatigue, the absence of any artificially imposed consensus about how to deal with the problem meant that lively and fruitful debate could continue. Moreover, there were grounds for optimism in the draft figures for expenditure on technical safety during the First Five-Year Plan. The amount to be allocated in 1932/33 was to be nearly two-thirds more than what was spent in 1927/ 28.[41]

In this respect, as in so many others, the correspondence between plan and reality once again proved to be illusory. It was one thing to apportion funds among industrial enterprises but quite another for them to be applied for the intended purpose. On more than one occasion in 1929, Narkomtrud called attention to the failure of managers to utilize funds for occupational safety, characterizing such inaction as "negligent."[42] By 1932, N. Shvernik, chairman of the Central Council of Trade Unions, used stronger language, referring to the "criminally slipshod relation on the part of management to technical safety and the protection of labor."[43]

This problem, however, paled in comparison with that of absorbing and safe-guarding the new labor recruits who poured into the cities and industrial construction sites from the surrounding countryside during the First Five-Year Plan. Ill-nourished and poorly clothed, crowded into barracks and dormitories, frequently working overtime and even two successive shifts, these largely unskilled peasant-workers injured themselves and their workmates in unprecedented numbers (see appendix).

After 1929, there was, unfortunately, no discussion of the increased rate of accidents in the main journal devoted to industrial hygiene and safety. Observing that no two factories or shops possessed identical conditions, one statistician concluded in 1931 that "the summaries of accidents for all branches of industry in the existing system of statistics represents a typical example of the divorce of statistics as a method from the material reality toward which it is applied."[44] Since material reality was ever-changing, even within a single factory, such an argument could be used to justify the dismissal if not the suppression of statistical series over time. In any case, after 1933, no aggregate figures for industrial accidents or occupational disabilities were published.

It was as though a fog had descended over these questions, a fog that became thicker still by the mid-1930s.[45] When an elaborate statistical compendium appeared on the health of Soviet citizens and the state of health services in 1936, there was but one table on temporary disabilities as a result of industrial accidents. The table compared 1930 with 1934 for four branches of industry, but expressed the comparison in terms of the almost meaningless percentage decline.[46] Statements in the periodical and monographic literature to the effect that there were "13.3 percent fewer accidents among Union of Machine-Instrument Workers in 1937 than in 1936" and that industrial accidents declined in 1938 compared to 1937 by 10 to 20 percent in the major branches of industry should be regarded with a large dose of skepticism, if only because of the political context within which the statistics were reported.[47]

None of this is to deny that the rate of industrial accidents may have declined during the 1930s as the growth in the size of the industrial workforce tapered off, the proportion of skilled workers increased, and industrial equipment was modernized. Yet, in the absence of any concrete data, it is impossible to be precise about the extent of the decline or any other aspect of occupational disability and accidents. On the other hand, the fate of the two professions that were devoted to the investigation of these phenomena is at least partially documented and can be discerned in its broad outlines.

THE PROFESSIONS UNDER FIRE

Like other professions, industrial hygiene and psychotechnics experienced profound upheaval during the period that has been characterized as the Cultural Revolution. A volume devoted to this subject portrays the Cultural Revolution in the professions as arising out of, and interacting with, existing disputes among different schools of thought, disputes which sometimes reflected different political orientations and philosophies. Its agents were usually young communist intellectuals who, in the words of Sheila Fitzpatrick, "were often extremely aggressive, but at the same time unsure of their credentials. They tended to question their own value to society, suggest that factory workers could do their jobs better, and . . . [engaged in] what one observer called 'the disease of self-flagellation in a collective of intellectuals.' "[48] The human behavioral sciences were not immune to this disease, though in their case there was the added factor that "political leaders and scholarly professionals claim(ed) privileged understanding of the same subject matter: people."[49]

These two factors were combined with particular force in the case of psychotechnics and industrial hygiene. First, these fields dealt not only with people, but with people in the process of production, a subject that was particularly dear to the hearts of party leaders.[50] Second, being of recent provenance and having lower status than the "pure" sciences from which they were derived, they did not generate an intense degree of confidence, nor did their practitioners enjoy much professional autonomy. These two circumstances by themselves, not to speak of the traumatic impact of the First Five-Year Plan on Soviet workers, ensured that the Cultural Revolution would reverberate among industrial hygienists and psychologists with particular force.

Those reverberations began during 1930. Shpilrein, in his review of the activities of the All-Russian Society of Psychotechnologists covering the period from its founding to February 1930, noted that the society had failed to popularize its work among the masses and also that one of its members had been excluded as an "anti-Soviet element."[51] But in comparison with what was to come, this criticism was pallid. There was neither a hint of self-criticism nor an invocation of *partiinost'* (party-mindedness). Kaplun, writing in April 1930, was no more provocative with respect to "The Burning Questions of Scientific Work in the Areas of Labor Hygiene and Pathology."[52] He did not take the opportunity to condemn any particular school but, rather, focused on organizational questions such as the lack of coordination among research institutes and the dangers of artificially dividing research on hygiene and pathology. And even as late as August of that year, Kaplun's journal could carry a review of a book on "psychic fatigue" which did not go beyond complaining about the disproportionate emphasis on empirical as opposed to theoretical material.[53]

Roughly at this point a shrill polemic against Shpilrein's approach to psychotechnics appeared in the journal *Psikhologiia*. The polemic, published posthumously, was written by N. F. Kurmanov, a former student of Shpilrein. The essence of Kurmanov's attack was that Shpilrein had never lost his earlier admiration for the idealism of William Stern and had failed to learn anything from Feuerbach, Marx, Engels, Plekhanov, and Lenin. At best, he had adopted a "neutralist empiricist position," but this was only a cover for retaining his idealist perspective.[54] In his reply, printed in the same issue, Shpilrein was indulgent toward Kurmanov, but insisted that Kurmanov had misinterpreted his former teacher's approach.[55]

No doubt aware of similar attacks against analogous authorities such as Deborin, Shpilrein nevertheless tried to distance himself from his past and from the "objectivist" and biological orientation of the field over which he had presided. In September 1930, he delivered a report entitled "What Is Fatigue" to a joint session of the Psychotechnical Society and the newly formed Society of Materialist Psychoneurologists. The report repudiated the decision of the psychophysiological congress in 1927 to accommodate different approaches to this complex subject. Shpilrein explicitly denounced the "purely biological method of studying social processes, whereby the human organism was treated in mechanistic terms." He also condemned the concept of the optimum because of its marginalization of "the social factor." "In reality," he remarked, "the optimum moves (*sdvigaetsia*). The optimum for a worker engaged in socialist construction will be different from the worker of a capitalist factory and significantly higher than for the worker under serfdom. But however great is this optimum (defined as the socially acceptable coefficient of the expenditure of an organism's resources), its biological limit is the energetic maximum."[56]

Still, Shpilrein refrained from characterizing these approaches as anti-Marxist or associating them with any individual except Ermanskii, who in any case had been something of a maverick in the profession for a number of years. Shpilrein may have gone a long way toward applying the lessons of struggles in related fields, but, at least for some of his listeners, he had not gone far enough. Why, it was asked, had he avoided any mention of what workers were doing now, of socialist competition and shock work, "since sometimes one hears . . . discussion about the overwork of workers and a whole series of other purely technical objections leveled against shock work?"[57] Since it was precisely at this time that the Council on Technical Norms was redefining the basis for output norms to be the performance of "workers demonstrating an intense tempo, that is, shock workers," this was a pertinent question.[58]

Kaplun was subjected to the same sort of criticism. His definition of the "burning questions" of labor hygiene was found to be inadequate by several practitioners. In the era of socialist construction, it was now argued, industrial hygiene had to abandon its passive, defensive nature and instead assist in speeding up the tempo of construction—"of course not at the expense of the physical and spiritual powers of the proletariat, but on the contrary, by developing them."[59] Or again, "From the point of view of improving the health of the proletariat, it is much more important to study and establish the most advanced regimen of labor and forms of labor cooperation, than to take multitudinous measurements of energy expenditure."[60] By 1931, these forays had become more generalized and, judging by their sheer repetitiveness, ritualized as well. Under attack by the advocates of "the Marxist-Leninist revolutionary theory of knowledge and practice" were Menshevik idealism and rotten liberalism (read the notion of protecting labor), neutralism (read objectivity), eclecticism (read employing methods devised by Western researchers), empiricism (read paying attention to data), and so forth. Virtually none of the leading lights in psychotechnics and labor hygiene emerged unscathed, although some were attacked more vigorously than others. Two examples will suffice. One was Professor N. A. Vigdorchik of the Leningrad Institute of Occupational Diseases. He had the courage, or stupidity, to suggest as a subject for investigation in December 1930 (!) "The Role of Socialist Competition and Shockwork in Increasing Morbidity." For this, he was rewarded by being denounced in the resolutions of several conferences and journal articles. The other was K. Kh. Kekcheev, whose *Labor Physiology* appeared in a second edition in 1930. Aside from retaining enough of a biomechanical approach to be accused of several of the above-mentioned heresies, the book also contained the statement that "from the productive point of view, man must be exploited as judiciously as the machine."[61]

Kaplun had devoted eight pages of his journal to withering criticism of Kekcheev's book, but what Vigdorchik and Kekcheev had asserted, he only doubted. He, therefore, also came under fire, finding himself the target of a *Pravda* article signed by six militants. Kaplun responded by confessing his "mechanistic and Menshevik idealist views" and admitting that among his friends were several Deborinites, that is, disciples of the recently discredited philosopher of science, A. M. Deborin. More self-criticism followed.[62]

In the meantime, industrial psychologists were undergoing their own process of "socialist reconstruction." The All-Union Psychotechnical Congress, meeting in Leningrad in May 1931, was an occasion for much self-criticism and mutual recrimination. As if to underscore the necessity for a radical reorientation of the profession, the opening speech was delivered by M. B. Mitin, who was then leading the assault against the Deborinites and would soon assume the mantle of authority within the field of philosophy.[63] The conference was noteworthy in another respect. For the first time, "conciliarism, the establishment of a philosophical line by resolutions of conferences," was employed, and *partiinost'*, the right of the Communist party to define truth, was formally invoked.[64]

Thus armed with the insights of Marxist-Leninist teaching, Soviet psychotechnologists were ready to confront their Western counterparts at the Seventh International Psychotechnical Conference, held in Moscow in September 1931. "The position of the Soviet delegation," we are told, "can be characterized as the active, militant contraposition of Soviet psychotechnics and psychophysiology of labor to bourgeois psychotechnical science." This strategy, according to the same account, was a great success. "Soviet psychologists emerged as passionate propagandists of Marxist ideology," contributing to the growing division among the representatives of science in capitalist countries between idealists and mechanists on the one hand and Marxists on the other.[65]

But the unity within the Soviet camp was superficial.[66] As soon as the conference was over, the denunciations were renewed. Now it was the turn of the specialists in occupational selection and industrial accidents to be pilloried. It was discovered that here too "biologism" had crept into Soviet research in the form of the concept of accident proneness, which was associated with the German psychotechnologist Karl Marbe. The concept had never been well received in the USSR, but its fatalistic implications were even more anathema once the transformatory zeal of the Cultural Revolution took hold of the profession. One zealot went so far as to assert that not only "proneness" but "accident" (*neschastnyi sluchai*) ought to be purged from the vocabulary of Soviet psychotechnics, since each mishap could be explained by the socio-material conditions where it occurred.[67] The notion, put forward by Iu. O. Shpigel', that psycho-physiological conditions should also be taken into account, was regarded by Gellershtein as "very closely connected to the views of Marbe."[68]

In this manner, the fundamental premises on which industrial hygienists and psychologists had operated—that workers needed protection from harmful substances, dangerous conditions, and overwork and that statistical analysis and psychological testing could lead to a better understanding of what changes were necessary and which workers were suited to which jobs—were condemned as ideologically incompatible with the tasks of socialist reconstruction. Thus, it would appear that both labor hygiene and psychotechnics were casualties of that process. But if only to avoid sanctimoniousness with respect to fields that in the West saw their fair share of "distortions" and charlatanism, several points need to be made.

First, although the struggles within these professions owed a great deal to the initiative and encouragement of the political authorities, their outcome cannot be considered to have been predetermined. As David Joravsky has pointed out, the insistence by Stalin (among others) that theory be subordinated to practice still left open the question of exactly what practice meant and how it was to inform theory.[69] That this dogma was interpreted in the way it was must be attributed to the apocalyptic nature of the times as well as to the intelligentsia's instincts for survival. The predictions by Communist intellectuals that the contradictions between town and countryside were about to be resolved, that the distinction between mental and manual labor was withering away, and other equally utopian notions were not just flights of fancy but can be seen as "a kind of running commentary on contemporary processes of institutional disintegration and social flux" under the impact of vast and largely uncontrolled socioeconomic changes.[70]

Second, as simplistic and overschematized as the denunciations of "bourgeois psychotechnics and labor physiology" were, subsequent developments within these fields have demonstrated the justice of some of the accusations. The culture-bound nature of many psychological tests, class-based assumptions implicit in the search for psychically maladjusted workers and psychopathic personality types among those who do not "stand up" to stress, and the lack of corroborating evidence that accident proneness is a fixed personality trait have been widely if not universally recognized by industrial psychologists.[71] Put another way, on present evidence, the "reconstructionists" were right to stress the "social factor" and the malleability of individual personalities. Nor should their antipathy to laboratory methods be dismissed as mere abolitionism or anti-intellectualism. For they were only repeating the criticism leveled by worker-delegates against the Moscow Institute of Labor Protection for its failure to study fatigue as experienced in every day assembly-line work.[72]

The problem was that the reconstructionists' impulses were taken to the extreme and transformed into axioms. Emphasizing the social factor did not have to mean eliminating the personal or physiological; invoking practice should not have precluded laboratory experimentation or restricted investigators to the study of the performance of shock workers. Yet those who reminded their colleagues of these points were rebuked because their positions were said to be "objectively" consistent with bourgeois pseudo-science.

IN THE WAKE OF THE CULTURAL REVOLUTION

Nevertheless, neither industrial hygiene nor psychotechnics disappeared entirely. Indeed, by 1932, as the storm whipped up by the Cultural Revolution began to subside, many of those who had been its chief victims resumed their scientific work, occasionally finding that their earlier positions had been vindicated. The case of D. I. Reitynbarg, who wrote extensively on safety propaganda, illustrates well this ironic, if temporary, turnabout. An advocate of socialist competition to reduce accidents in production, Reitynbarg had also urged the adoption of techniques pioneered in the United States. These included brief orations during the intermissions of theatrical performances, the inclusion of a "lucky number" among tickets distributed to workers before meetings, and street theater performances.[73] In his writings on safety posters, he pointed out that, in contrast to the positive and often humorous content of their Western counterparts, Soviet posters tended to depict blood, severed limbs, and other negatively emotive themes.[74] At the height of the upheavals within the profession, Reitynbarg came under attack and duly engaged in self-criticism. Indiscriminately borrowing from American experience, he had failed to relate his work to Soviet circumstances. This was largely because he had not worked out any theoretical approach but, rather, had unconsciously relied on utilitarian and empiricist instincts.[75] Yet within a year the effectiveness of "before" and "after" signs hung in the lavatories of workers' clubs and the buffet of a workers' theater in Moscow could be measured in precise percentages "naturalistic" posters in the factories were being condemned for frightening newly recruited workers, and the "theory" that was being advanced seemed decidedly utilitarian.[76]

This is not to suggest that industrial hygiene and psychotechnics had returned to the status quo ante. The scope of what could be published and, presumably, researched had been considerably narrowed, and public debate about the merits or weaknesses of different approaches had ceased. Nonetheless, something of a modus vivendi had been achieved. As long as they invoked (if only in preamble form) the classics of Marxism-Leninism—appropriately digested by the now chastened authorities within the field—specialists were able to pursue their work. Psychological testing and vocational training methods and the rationalization of technical processes now came back into vogue.

But this arrangement did not last. As in the past, official faith in technics eventually gave way to a violent swing in the direction of voluntarism and intolerance of the technical experts. The termination of the journal *Sovetskaia psikhotekhnika* in 1934 and the closure of the Psychotechnical Society the following year marked the beginning of a new onslaught on the professions that was more devastating and long-lasting than the Cultural Revolution. This time, the challenge came not from zealots within the professions, but from outstanding workers, known as Stakhanovites, whose production feats appeared to confirm political authorities' suspicions of the experts.

Stakhanovism, which emerged in the autumn of 1935, was to have immense significance for industrial hygienists and psychologists. It served to discredit all the old calculations about the productive capacity of workers and their machines, dubbed the "theory of limits," and hence all those theorists associated with their formulation. Not only did Stakhanovites "smash" the old technical and output norms, but after doing so they testified to being less tired than previously.[77]

Separating fact from fiction in the accounts of Stakhanovites' records is not easy. It would appear that in many cases their achievements were not the result of the speed-up of production processes or "sweating" but, rather, an increased division of labor or a more rational use of tools. Despite pressure from above, management proved unable to replicate the special circumstances in which they set their records. The resulting gross disparities in output and wages between Stakhanovite and non-Stakhanovite workers and the herky-jerky pace of production exacerbated tensions throughout the industrial system which fed into the Great Terror of 1937–38.

Some industrial hygienists and psychologists salvaged their careers (if not their self-esteem) by attesting that Stakhanovites had fewer accidents, produced a smaller proportion of defective goods, and suffered less from fatigue than other workers.[78] Given that Stakhanovites generally were better equipped and serviced and had a higher standard of living, these claims could well have been true. But the empirical evidence provided was so slim as to preclude a definitive judgment. In any case, as both Kravchenko and Scott point out, the overstraining of machines and workers during periods of intense activity (so-called Stakhanovite days, five- and ten-day periods) was a major cause of breakdowns, fatigue, and accidents.[79] Soviet officials had another explanation, namely, sabotage. With rare exception, the only industrial accidents reported in the Soviet press from 1936 to 1938 were in connection with accusations against hapless engineers and managers, many of whom received the ultimate sentence or long prison terms.

The politicization of industrial accidents, coinciding with the virtual cessation of research into this and related phenomena and the closure of the institutes that had sustained such research, constitutes a terminal landmark for this essay. In 1940, the Commissariat of Public Health published a large and well-illustrated textbook by Kaplun which it recommended for use in the medical institutes of the USSR. The book was remarkable in a number of respects, not the least of which was its failure even to mention psychotechnics. Typical of its approach to topics which had been "burning questions" a decade earlier was the following statement:

> In rare cases, fatigue among individual workers is still possible, but as a whole, the problem of fatigue as a mass, typical phenomenon in the contemporary stage of the construction of communism has already unquestionably been removed, since all possibilities for the maximal prevention of reduced work capacity and the breach of both urban and rural workers' health have been created.[80]

Public acknowledgment that fatigue and other phenomena associated with accidents and disabilities had not disappeared would have to await the post-Stalin era.

The fates of those who had been active in the fields of industrial hygiene and psychology were varied. Shpilrein was arrested sometime in the late 1930s and died not long thereafter, but his close associates, Gellershtein and Shpigel', were able to preside over a revival in the late 1950s and early 1960s of the field they had helped pioneer. Kaplun continued to write propagandistic literature on Soviet achievements in occupational safety until his death in 1943. Meanwhile, Ermanskii, the ostracized ex-Menshevik, continued to lead a charmed existence. In 1940, not without difficulty, he managed to publish a study of Stakhanovism that was critical of the many distortions and excesses inspired by that movement. The book remains to this day the most interesting one on the subject.[81]

CONCLUSION

The evolution of the professions of industrial hygiene and psychotechnics illustrates the ways in which science and politics were inextricably connected during the formative decades of Soviet power. Research agendas and even the conclusions drawn from empirical investigation were determined not only by official policy, but also by politics within the professions.

During the NEP years, industrial hygienists and psychotechnicians developed a wide range of methodologies to analyze the causes and prevention of industrial accidents. But the failure of such techniques to stem the growth of accidents and disability heightened the impatience of younger, more party-minded members of the institutes. Whether inspired by the new tasks of socialist construction or eager to make a name for themselves, they went on the attack against the relatively narrow professionalism of their elders. In response to these attacks, industrial hygienists and psychotechnicians immersed themselves in criticism and self-criticism. Meanwhile, reality had its own logic. Although it is entirely possible that the rate of accidents fell in the 1930s, the fact that the industrial labor force more than doubled meant that the number of disabled workers swelled. The extent of that increase cannot be known, for in the late 1930s the professions dedicated to studying the phenomenon were all but obliterated.

Viewed in comparative terms, the USSR appears to have avoided the pressures of market competitiveness and corporate profitability which have been and remain major underlying causes of industrial accidents in both underdeveloped and advanced capitalist societies. Yet, the forced pace of industrialization itself and the suppression of experimentation and statistical inquiry into the effects of that process meant that Soviet workers were no less at risk of being maimed, blinded, deafened, or otherwise disabled than their Western counterparts, and perhaps even more so.

NOTES

1. For general histories of industrial hygiene, see Bernhard J. Stern, *Medicine in Industry* (New York, 1946); Ludwig Teleky, *History of Factory and Mine Hygiene* (New York, 1948); and Irma Rittenhouse, "Industrial Hygiene: Legislation and Reform," in *Encyclopaedia of the Social Sciences* (New York, 1932), 7: 112–27.

2. For discussions of these developments and their relationship to fatigue, see A. Mosso, *Fatigue* (New York, 1904); F. B. Gilbreth and L. M. Gilbreth, *Fatigue Study* (New York, 1916); and Morris S. Viteles, *Industrial Psychology* (New York, 1932), pp. 438ff.

3. Industrial hygiene was and remains a branch of occupational hygiene; psychotechnics is synonymous with applied psychology. Industrial work is only one of many spheres in which psychotechnical research has been conducted.

APPENDIX

Rates of Industrial Accidents, 1926–33

Branch of Industry	Accidents per 1,000 Insured Workers							
	1926*	1927*	1928*	1929	1930	1931	1932	1933
Coal mining	283.3	471.3	469.8	509.3	477.0	359.0	269.6	291.6
Oil extraction	251.2	338.8	298.3	†	†	†	†	†
Ore mining		215.7	197.7	314.4	327.8	379.2	239.5	192.1
Metallurgy	259.5	269.4	256.4	337.6	315.6	267.7	211.0	198.1
Machine building	281.8	276.6	286.1	298.6	307.6	297.6	192.1	168.5
Chemicals	221.9	164.3	157.8	230.1	215.4	227.9	170.5	NA
Woodworking	318.2	336.6	384.2	281.5	268.1	252.7	186.3	173.9
Hides and leather	†	†	†	239.9	219.8	204.6	137.2	111.3
Textiles	72.2	76.1	72.8	67.8	76.9	72.6	76.6	48.0

Sources: For 1926, N. I. Sinev and I. F. Engel', "Promyshlennyi travmatizm v SSSR," *Gigiena, bezopasnost' i patologiia truda* [hereafter *GBPT*], no. 3 (1929), pp. 69–70. For 1927 and 1928, I. Engel', "Metody ucheta neschastnykh sluchaev i promyshlennyi travmatizm v SSSR," *GBPT*, no. 11 (1929), p. 71. For 1929 and 1930, *Sotsialisticheskoe stroitel'stvo SSSR, Statisticheskii ezhegodnik* (Moscow, 1934), p. 424. For 1931 and 1932, *Gigiena i bezopasnost' truda*, no. 1 (1933), p. 4. For 1933, ILO, *Industrial Safety Survey*, 12, no. 2 (1936), pp. 52–53.

Note: The Soviet method of computation was the same as (and probably derived from) that of Germany. In Germany the overall rate of industrial accidents was 77.3 in 1927, 82.2 in 1928, and 80.7 in 1929, according to F. Ritzmann, "German Accident Statistics, 1928–1930," *Industrial Safety Survey* (ILO), 8, no. 6 (1932), p. 151.

* RSFSR only

† Statistics not available

4. Theodor von Laue, "Factory Inspection under the 'Witte System', 1892–1903," *American Slavonic and East European Review,* 19 (1960), p. 356. See also Frederick C. Griffin, "The 'First Russian Labor Code': The Law of June 3, 1886," *Russian History/ Histoire russe,* 2, pt. 2 (1975), pp. 83–100. The classic Russian study is A. A. Milukin, *Fabrichnaia inspektsiia v Rossii, 1882–1906* (Kiev, 1906). In 1894, there were a mere 143 inspectors. For a vivid personal account by the first chief inspector in Moscow, see I. Ianzhul, *Iz vospominanii i perepiski fabrichnogo inspektora* (St. Petersburg, 1907).

5. Indeed, many workers were seasonal and therefore sought overtime as a means of supporting their families back in the village. See Robert Eugene Johnson, *Peasant and Proletarian: The Working Class of Moscow in the Late Nineteenth Century* (New Brunswick, N.J., 1979), pp. 29–30, 35–40, 43–50.

6. Compare V. Ia. Laverychev, *Tsarizm i rabochii vopros (1861–1917 gg.)* (Moscow, 1972), pp. 236–43, and Ruth Amende Roosa, "Workers' Insurance Legislation and the Role of Industrialists in the Period of the Third Duma," *Russian Review,* 34, no. 4 (1975), pp. 410–52.

7. L. S. Gaponenko, *Rabochii klass Rossii v 1917 godu* (Moscow, 1970), p. 202.

8. Blair A. Ruble, *Soviet Trade Unions: Their Development in the 1970s* (Cambridge, Mass., 1981), pp. 11–15.

9. "O deiatel'nosti otdela okhrany truda v Moskovskoi oblasti," *Vestnik Narodnogo Komissariata truda,* nos. 2–3 (1918), pp. 335–40; *Sobranie uzakoneniia i rasporiadeniia rabochikh i krestianskikh pravitel'stva* (1918), cols. 36–474.

10. Margaret Dewar, *Labour Policy in the USSR* (London, 1956), pp. 180, 187, 188; George M. Price, *Labor Protection in Soviet Russia* (New York, 1928), pp. 86–93.

11. By 1920, there were an estimated 1.2 million industrial workers as compared with 2.6 million in 1917. Large-scale industrial production in 1921 was one-fifth of what it had been in 1913. See Alec Nove, *An Economic History of the USSR* (London, 1969), pp. 66–68.

12. As late as 1924, the Ukraine had only forty-one health inspectors. A. E. Pasternak, "Deiatel'nost' sanitarnoi inspektsii Ukrainy v 1923g.," *Gigiena truda,* no. 1 (1924), p. 86.

13. The latter was named after B. A. Obukh who had been a Bolshevik since 1902, served as one of Lenin's physicians after the Revolution, and was the founder and director of the institute that bore his name. See *Bol'shaia Sovetskaia entsiklopediia* [hereafter *BSE*], 3d ed. (Moscow, 1970–78), 18:1 233–34.

14. *BSE,* 11: 361.

15. Alice Hamilton, *Exploring the Dangerous Trades: The Autobiography of Alice Hamilton, M.D.* (Boston, 1943), p. 332.

16. Quoted in Richard Schultz and Ross A. McFarland, "Industrial Psychology in the Soviet Union," *Journal of Applied Psychology,* 19 (1935), p. 266.

17. For these early controversies, see especially S. Leiberstein, "Technology, Work, and Sociology in the USSR: The NOT Movement," *Technology and Culture,* 16, no. 1 (1975), pp. 48–55; Zenovia A. Sochor, "Soviet Taylorism Revisited," *Soviet Studies,* 33, no. 2 (1981), pp. 246–64; Steven Smith, "Taylorism Rules OK? Bolshevism, Taylorism and the Technical Intelligentsia in the Soviet Union, 1917–41," *Radical Science Journal,* no. 13 (1983), pp. 3–27. For the now-classic discussion of the many guises that Taylorism assumed in interwar Europe, see Charles S. Maier, "Between Taylorism and Technocracy: European Ideologies and the Vision of Industrial Productivity in the 1920s," *Journal of Contemporary History,* 5, no. 2 (1970), pp. 27–61.

18. I. F. Engel', "Metody ucheta neschastnykh sluchaev i promyshlennyi travmatizm v SSSR," *Gigiena, bezopasnost' i patologiia truda* [hereafter, *GBPT*], no. 11 (1929), p. 69.

19. See V. A. Beleliubskii, "Znachenie orientirovochnoi statistiki pri izuchenii professional'nogo travmatizma," *GBPT,* no. 10 (1929), p. 90, where mention is made of this fact with respect to statistics derived from social insurance offices.

20. B. M. Shkliar, M. S. Trakhtenberg, and N. D. Krol', "Dinamika razvitiia na metallurgicheskom zavode im. Petrovskogo v Dnepropetrovske za 1927," *Gigiena truda,* no.

8 (1928), pp. 68–79. The same reason might apply to workers with less than one year's *stazh*.

21. B. M. Shkliar, M. S. Trakhtenberg, and N. D. Krol', "Dinamika travmatizma na metallurgicheskom zavode im. Petrovskogo za 1926–1928 gg.," *GBPT*, no. 12 (1929), pp. 96–107.

22. V. N. Popovitskii, "Dinamika travmatizma na metallurgicheskom zavode 'Krasnyi Oktiabr,' " *GBPT*, no. 9 (1929), pp. 83–90; V. S. Ikriannikov, "Travmatizm na pogruzochno-razgruzochnykh rabotakh vo Vladivostoke," *Gigiena truda*, no. 12 (1928), pp. 79–87; A. V. Bronevskii, "Dinamika travmatizma na Taganrogskom instrumental'no-mekhanicheskom zavode IuMTa i metody bor'by s nim," *GBPT*, no. 4 (1929), pp. 87–96; A. Plotnikov, "K voprosu ob izuchenii travmatizma v kamennougol'noi promyshlennosti," *Gigiena truda*, no. 8 (1928), pp. 87–90.

23. See extracts from S. G. Gellershtein, "Psikhotekhnika" (1926), in *Informatsionnyi Biulleten'*, no. 2 (17), seriia: iz istorii sovetskoi sotsiologii, Psikhologiia truda, chap. 1 (Moscow, 1969), pp. 45–62; S. G. Gellershtein, "K voprosu o professional'noi tipologii," in *Istoriia sovetskoi psikhologii truda, teksti (20–30 gody XX veka)* (Moscow, 1983), pp. 118–27; I. N. Shpilrein, "Osnovye teoreticheskie problemy psikhotekhniki," pp. 64–68; and A. A. Gaivorovskii, "Sravnitel'naia otsenka metodov psikhotekhicheskoi kharakteristiki professiia," pp. 69–74, in *Vsesoiuznaia konferentsiia po psikhofiziologii truda i professional'nomu podboru. Tezisy dokladov* (Moscow, 1927).

24. See, for example, S. Ia. Glezerov, "Professional'nyi travmatizm glaz na zavode 'Krasnoe Sormovo,' " *Gigiena truda*, no. 2 (1928), pp. 47–49; D. R. Balianskii, "K voprosu o bezopasnosti raboty na pressakh," *Gigiena truda*, no. 2 (1928), pp. 70–75; S. M. Stakhorskii, "Travmatizm v metalloprommyshlennosti Ukrainy," *Gigiena truda*, no. 6 (1928), p. 82.

25. V. A. Krukovskii, "Ob organizatsii tekhniki bezopasnosti v promyshlennosti predpriiatiiakh," *Gigiena truda*, no. 9 (1928), pp. 78–82.

26. N. I. Sinev and I. F. Engel', "Promyshlennyi travmatizm v SSSR," *GBPT*, no. 3 (1929), p. 65.

27. B. M. Shkliar, "Promyshlennyi travmatizm i ego sviaz' s proizvoditel'nostiu truda i sverkhurochnymi rabotami," *GPBT*, no. 8 (1929), pp. 58–61. Kaplun dissociated the journal from the article's findings by claiming in an editorial note that "the author's data do not provide a basis for serious methodological or practical conclusions."

28. V. V. Isakov and Iu. N. Khalturina, *Izuchenie proizvoditel'nosti i utomliaemosti pri perekhode na tkatskikh fabrikakh s 2-kh na 3 stanka* (Ivanovo-Voznesensk, 1928).

29. See E. H. Carr and R. W. Davies, *Foundations of a Planned Economy*, 3 vols. (Harmondsworth, England, 1974–77), 1: 516–53, and for a Soviet view, A. P. Finarov, "Perevod promyshlennykh predpriiatii na 7-chasovoi rabochii den' v 1928–1932 gg.," *Istoriia SSSR*, no. 6 (1959), pp. 107–14.

30. Isakov and Khalturina, *Izuchenie proizvoditel'nosti*, p. 29. The statement appears in the section by Isakov.

31. N. Rozenbaum, Kh. Rivlina, E. Belorets, L. Seletskaia, "Vliianiia intensifikatsii truda na utomliaemost' tkachei," *Gigiena truda*, no. 8 (1928), p. 15; N. E. Akim, "Okhrana truda na tekstil'nykh fabrikakh Moskovskoi gubernii s semichasovym rabochim dnem," *GBPT*, no. 5 (1929), p. 98; and the circular dated May 9, 1929, reprinted in *GBPT*, no. 9 (1929), p. 117.

32. O. A. Ermanskii, *Teoriia i praktika ratsionalizatsii*, 5th rev. ed. (Moscow-Lenigrad, 1933), pp. 117–18. Earlier editions were not available to me, but see the review of the first edition in *GBPT*, no. 1 (1929), pp. 141–43.

33. O. A. Ermanskii, "Opasnost'," *Komsomol'skaia prvada*, March 17, 1927.

34. E. M. Kogan, et al., "Opyt sravnitel'nogo izucheniia ruchnoi i konveirernoi raboty," *Gigiena truda*, no. 8 (1928), pp. 17, 22.

35. *Psikhofiziologiia truda i psikhotekhnika*, 1 (1928), p. 67.

36. Schultz and MacFarland, "Industrial Psychology," pp. 284–95; I. N. Shpilrein, "O

trudovom metode v professiografii," *Gigiena truda*, no. 10 (1927), pp. 68–71; and extracts from Shpilrein, "Chto takoe 'Trudovoi metod'?" in *Informatsionnyi Biulleten'*, pp. 63–72.

37. Glezerov, "Professional'nyi travmatizm glaz," p. 47.

38. "Obzor russkoi literatury po voprosam travmatizma i gigieny glaza," *GBPT*, no. 6 (1930), p. 115, and nos. 10–11 (1931), p. 161.

39. "Obzor russkoi literatury po professional'nym zabolevaniiam ukha, nosa i gorla," *GBPT*, no. 2 (1929), pp. 128–29.

40. A. V. Petrovskii, *Istoriia sovetskoi psikhologii, Formirovanie osnov psikhologicheskoi nauki* (Moscow, 1967), p. 269.

41. B. L. Markus, "Piatiletnyi plan ozdorovleniia uslovii truda v RSFSR," *Gigiena truda*, no. 11 (1928), p. 97.

42. "Zakonodatel'stvo," *GBPT*, no. 1 (1930), p. 104; "Zakonodatel'stvo," *GBPT*, no. 2 (1930), p. 119.

43. XVII Konferentsiia VKP(b), Stenograficheskii otchet (Moscow, 1932), p. 113.

44. G. I. Lifshits, "Statistika proftravmatizma na sovremennom etape (v poriadke sa- mokritiki)," *GBPT*, no. 12 (1931), p. 22.

45. This metaphor is borrowed from Carr's "Preface" to Carr and Davies, *Foundations*, p. vi.

46. Tsentral'noe upravlenie narodnogo khoziaistvennogo ucheta, *Zdorov'e i zravookh- ranenie trudiaschikhsia SSSR, Statisticheskii sbornik*, ed. by I. A. Kraval' (Moscow, 1936), p. 25.

47. *Profsoiuzy SSSR*, no. 7 (1938), p. 59; V. I. Prokhorov, "Profsoiuzy i voprosy truda," in G. A. Prudenskii, ed., *Voprosy truda v SSSR* (Moscow, 1958), p. 151.

48. Sheila Fitzpatrick, "Cultural Revolution as Class War," in Sheila Fitzpatrick, ed., *Cultural Revolution in Russia, 1928–1931* (Bloomington, Ind., 1978), p. 28.

49. David Joravsky, "The Stalinist Mentality and the Higher Learning," *Slavic Review*, 42, no. 4 (1983), p. 586.

50. The reader is reminded that just as industrial hygiene is a subspecialty within the field of social hygiene, so industrial psychology is merely one of many applications of psychology.

51. *Psikhotekhnika i psikhofiziologiia truda* [hereafter, *PPT*], no. 1 (1931), pp. 66–67.

52. S. I. Kaplun, "Bol'nye voprosy nauchnoi raboty v oblasti gigieny i patologii truda," *GBPT*, no. 4 (1930), pp. 3–25.

53. The review is in *GBPT*, no. 7 (1930), p. 127. This is worth highlighting, for labor physiology and, in particular, fatigue study were soon to bear the brunt of attacks from within and outside the profession. The review was by Gellershtein.

54. N. F. Kurmanov, "Idealizm v psikhotekhnike rekonstruktsionnogo perioda i otsutstvie rekonstruktsii v psikhotekhnike," *Psikhologiia*, 3, no. 3 (1930), pp. 385–408. Shpilrein indeed had been an early champion of Stern's "personalist" approach.

55. I. N. Shpilrein, "Mekhanicheskaia bor'ba za rekonstruktsiiu psikhotekhniki," *Psi- khologiia*, 3, no. 3 (1930), pp. 409–19.

56. I. N. Shpilrein, "Chto takoe utomlenie," *PPT*, no. 1 (1931), pp. 67–75.

57. "Voprosy po dokladu," ibid., pp. 75–76.

58. See L. H. Siegelbaum, "Soviet Norm Determination in Theory and Practice, 1917– 1941," *Soviet Studies*, 36, no. 1 (1984), p. 54.

59. S. R. Dikhter, "Ob organizatsii nauchno-issledovatel'skoi raboty v oblasti organizatsii i ozdorovleniia truda v period sotsialisticheskoi rekonstruktsii," *GBPT*, no. 11 (1930), p. 49.

60. V. Stroganov, "K voprosam organizatsii nauchnoi raboty v oblasti gigieny i patologii truda," *GBPT*, no. 11 (1930), p. 52.

61. Both were attacked (along with Kaplun) in "Za partiinost' v nauke po gigiene i fiziologii truda," *Pravda*, June 16, 1931. For Kaplun's review, see *GBPT*, nos. 4–5 (1931), pp. 147–53.

62. *Pravda*, June 20, 1931; S. I. Kaplun, "Za razoblachenie sobstvennykh oshibok v poriadke samokritiki," *GBPT*, nos. 8–9 (1931), pp. 3–22; and his "Reorganizatsiia IOT

kak realizatsiia itogov diskusii na fronte gigieny i fiziologii truda," *GBPT,* no. 12 (1931), pp. 3–18.

63. On the struggle between the "Bolshevizers" led by Mitin and the Deborinite "dialecticians," see David Joravsky, *Soviet Marxism and Natural Science, 1917–1932* (New York, 1961), pp. 250–71.

64. Ibid., p. 261. For the resolutions, see *PPT,* nos. 4–6 (1931), pp. 374–80.

65. Petrovskii, *Istoriia sovetskoi psikhologii,* p. 273. See also T. L. Kogan, "K VII mezhdunarodnoi psikhotekhnicheskoi konferentsii," *Psikhologiia,* 5, no. 5 (1931), pp. 161–69.

66. See the comment by Iu. O. Shpigel' that "in connection with the political tasks which stood before us at the conference, we sought to criticize bourgeois authorities rather than engaging in self-criticism." *Sovetskaia psikhotekhnika,* nos. 5–6 (1932), p. 47.

67. K. Pauker, "Obezopasit' put' avto i peshekhoda," *Pravda,* December 13, 1931.

68. "Doklad Iu. O. Shpigelia na plenume moskovskogo otdeleniia Vsesoiuznogo obshchestva psikhotekhnika, 31 ianvaria 1932 g. (sokrashchennaia stenogramma)," *Sovetskaia-psikhotekhnika,* nos. 5–6 (1932), pp. 420–28.

69. Joravsky, "Stalinist Mentality," pp. 591–92.

70. Fitzpatrick, "Cultural Revolution as Class War," pp. 31–32.

71. See, for example, Morris S. Schulzinger, *The Accident Syndrome* (Springfield, Ill., 1956); W. Ryan, *Blaming the Victim* (New York, 1971); and D. Berman, "Why Work Kills," in Vincent Navarro and Daniel Berman, eds., *Health and Work under Capitalism: An International Perspective* (Farmingdale, N.Y., 1983), pp. 168–92.

72. *Rabochie o nepreryvnom potoke: vtoraia Moskovskaia konferentsiia rabochikh s predpriiatii vvedshikh nepreryvnyi potok* (Moscow, 1931), pp. 34–35, 49–51.

73. D. I. Reitynbarg, *Sotsialisticheskoe sorevnovanie na snizhenie neschastnykh sluchev v proizvodstve* (Moscow, 1930).

74. D. I. Reitynbarg, *Plakat po bezopasnosti truda v SSSR i za granitsei* (Moscow, 1931).

75. E. A. Rakhmel', "K itogam I Vsesoiuznogo s"ezda psikhotekhniki i psikhofiziologii truda," *Psikhologiia,* 5, no. 2 (1931), p. 175; Reitynbarg, "Plakat pobezopasnosti truda na novom etape," *Sovetskaia psikhotekhnika,* no. 4 (1932), pp. 269–78.

76. M. D. Karnaukhov, "K voprosu ob izuchenii effektivnosti plakata," *Sovetskaia psikhotekhnika,* no. 4 (1932), pp. 289–300; V. V. Reutov, "Ob ustrashaiushchikh plakatakh i novykh kadrakh-rabochikh," *Sovetskaia psikhotekhnika,* nos. 5–6 (1932), pp. 397–98.

77. See *Labour in the Land of Socialism, Stakhanovites in Conference* (Moscow, 1936), pp. 147, 222–23; and B. L. Markus, "The Stakhanov Movement and the Increased Productivity of Labour in the USSR," *International Labour Review,* 34, no. 1 (1936), pp. 23–25.

78. S. I. Kaplun, "Zdorovyi i zhizneradostnyi trud," *Pravda,* December 19, 1935; S. S. Val'iazhnikov and A. A. Alekseev, "Sistema propagandy bezopasnosti (opyt raboty na I GPZ im. L. M. Kaganovicha)," p. 34; and V. M. Davidovich, K. M. Karaul'nik, Kh. O. Rivlina, and Iu. O. Shpigel', "Psikhotekhnika v dele perenosa stakhanovskogo opyta," pp. 108–113, in VTsSPS, *Vsesoiuznyi nauchno-issledovatel'skii institut okhrana truda, Tezisy dokladov nauchnoi sessii, 14–19 aprelia 1936 g.* (Moscow, 1936).

79. Viktor Kravchenko, *I Chose Freedom* (New York, 1946), pp. 187–91, 193–94; John Scott, *Behind the Urals* (Bloomington, Ind., 1973, reprint of 1942 ed.), pp. 163–68.

80. S. I. Kaplun, *Obshchaia gigiena truda* (Moscow-Leningrad, 1940), p. 75. See also page 45.

81. O. A. Ermanskii, *Stakhanovskoe dvizhenie i stakhanovskie metody* (Moscow, 1940). See especially the note from the publisher and the introduction.

Afterword

Was the tsarist regime the real, or merely the perceived, obstacle to health reform in Russia? Prerevolutionary reformers were convinced that it was their enemy, and hence many of them turned their backs on St. Petersburg and looked to local governments to lead the way to a better future. Yet as some began to realize even before 1917, this tactic was bound to fail: the needs of the country were so great that only an enormous effort mounted and sponsored by the central government could begin to address them. But the tsarist regime passed from the scene without any resolution of the conflict over the role of the state and of medical professionals in planning and executing health reforms. Meanwhile, Russia's problems were only increased by the consequences of war and the breakdown of both central and local government.

If the ideology of Russian community medicine was to be believed the Revolution ought to have brought the dawning of a new era. With the monarchy gone, the old estate structure destroyed, and the influence of the church severely curtailed, the way was open—at least in theory—for bold new policies designed by medical professionals and implemented by a regime that proclaimed its dedication to reason and science. Yet, paradoxically, Bolshevik health reformers, like their tsarist predecessors, found that ideology limited their choices about the future. Once in power, the party had to decide not only what goals the new state was to pursue, but what was to be the role of experts—in this case medical professionals—in reaching those goals. It also had to confront the agonizing question of whether the proletariat was to constitute a new privileged class, and, if it was, what its privileges would mean in the field of health care. Finally, like their tsarist predecessors, the Bolsheviks had to grapple with the problem of providing health care to the peasants whose suspicion of modern medicine almost equaled their ignorance of its fundamental principles.

The essays in this volume draw attention to a number of important continuities and discontinuities between prerevolutionary and Soviet public health. Even as they answer some questions, these essays reveal, as any pioneering effort must, how much ground remains to be plowed.

A balanced assessment of Soviet public health requires an understanding of the goals of its architects. A number of the essays refer to the important role played by Nikolai Semashko as commissar of public health. Did Semashko have an original conception of the aims and methods of the new Soviet medicine? Or, as Lenin's comrade-in-arms, was his task merely to set the system on track? Scholars engaged in writing the history of both Russian and Soviet public health would profit enormously from a political biography of Semashko. No less would we benefit from a biography of his deputy Z. P. Soloviev, nicknamed "the enforcer," the tough administrative genius who translated Semashko's conceptions into practice. Another figure worthy of close attention is A. N. Sysin, who played a crucial role in the rapprochement between the Bolsheviks and the Pirogov Society.

What of the organizations that were constructed by these leaders? As some of the essays suggest, the architects of Narkomzdrav were determined to avoid the jurisdictional nightmare that had inhibited health reform prior to 1917 and insisted from the outset on the organic unity of Soviet health administration under the aegis of one commissariat. Nevertheless, there was a great deal of administrative overlap and bureaucratic infighting. To what extent were these features inevitable given the division of powers between Narkomzdrav and other commissariats? To what extent were they the result of the continuity in administrative personnel from the tsarist period? To address these questions, we need an institutional history of the development of Narkomzdrav in the 1920s and early 1930s, with particular attention to the way in which Narkomzdrav hammered out its relations with the *oblast* health departments and with the republican commissariats of health. An institutional history of relations between the center and periphery would be enormously enriched by studies of the health departments of the local soviets, both urban and rural. Close reading of the records of those departments might reveal a good deal about the relations between physicians, workers, and party officials in the cities and might shed some light on the vexing question of the extent to which folk medicine survived, perhaps even flourished, in the Soviet countryside.

What of the physician in all this? In Russia, as in many other settings, physicians were among the earliest groups to come to an accommodation with the new regime. A reading of the contributions to this volume suggests that the timetable of that accommodation varied from one medical specialty to the next. What did the different groups of specialists (for example, psychiatrists, industrial hygienists) expect from the government in making their accommodation? What, for its part, did the new government anticipate from its "experts"? How much and what type of medical professionalization would be tolerated? A related subject, much in need of further investigation, is the rapid feminization of the medical profession in the late 1920s. Was this development a deliberate goal or an unintended consequence of state policy, and what were its consequences for health care delivery?

One of the major conduits in the relationship between the state and the physicians was the physicians' unions. The relationship between the unions and the state is a fascinating but unexplored topic. As some of the contributors remind us, questions of medical organization were very much part of the work of Narkomtrud. Those interested in Soviet labor history would find a rewarding subject in the prolonged and, at times, heated battle between the rival medical unions VSPOV and Vsemediksantrud.

To be sure, not all physicians were state employees. After 1917, as indeed before it, there was in the Soviet Union a substantial private medical practice. Under the tsarist regime, private practice (which constituted about one-third of the profession) was excoriated as a manifestation of the Western entrepreneurial spirit. How was it that private practice, so antithetical to the Bolshevik ideology, was tolerated after 1917? In part the answer to this question lies in the overburdened Soviet medical system which, as several of the contributors point out, was woefully inadequate to handle the medical problems of a nation that had endured war, civil war, and revolution in the space of less than a decade. In part the answer lies in the attitude of the medical practitioners themselves. What did the ordinary physician, both Russian and Soviet, think? The records of the enormous numbers of local medical societies that sprang up in 1917 and were soon incorporated into VSPOV should provide some insight into the response of private practitioners to the Revolution.

Closely related to the questions of professional behavior is the question of professional training. The Revolution of 1917 triggered renewed interest in the reform of medical education, an issue which had been on the agenda of the Pirogov society well before the Revolution. Scholars would benefit significantly from an analysis of the projects for educational reform proposed during the 1920s. What were the views of those in the Commissariat of Enlightenment who had jurisdiction over the medical schools from 1922 to 1930? What positions on the requirements for medical training were taken by the leading figures in Narkomzdrav? As the commissariat responsible for the work done by physicians after they graduated, Narkomzdrav championed the inclusion of a variety of new disciplines in the curriculum of the medical schools. In this connection, one of the intriguing questions that remains to be addressed is how a single commissariat could serve as the patron of disciplines as divergent as social hygiene, with its strong nurturist philosophy, and eugenics, with its heavily naturist emphasis.

Finally, there are the citizens, the clients as it were of the medical system. The Bolsheviks had made a commitment to providing quality medical care for all Soviet citizens, but soon after the Revolution they had to confront the painful question of whether the workers were to have privileged access to health care. And what about workers' families? A fierce debate arose over whether the catchment areas for medical care should be tied to place of work or place of residence. An analysis of these debates promises to reveal a great deal both about the regime's priorities and about the categories of citizens which were ill-served or, in many cases, not served at all by the medical system.

The task of bringing medicine to the countryside was every bit as difficult as that of providing health care to the swelling cities. Programs to improve rural health care were crippled by the reluctance of physicians to work in outlying areas. Fearing that as members of the rural intelligentsia they would find themselves even more isolated than in tsarist times, they clung to the cities: their reluctance to practice in rural areas forced the new regime to abandon, however unwillingly, its original intention to eliminate the feldshers. The few physicians who did brave the countryside often found that, despite the pronouncements of Narkomzdrav, their day-to-day problems were much the same as those encountered by community physicians decades earlier: nowhere to live, no horse to ride, and a populace whose hostility to modern medicine and its spokesmen was profound.

How scholars evaluate Soviet medicine will depend to a great extent on the yardstick they use to measure its successes and failures. Is Soviet public health in the first decade and a half after the Revolution best compared to public health in the late tsarist period? Or ought we judge Soviet public health against its own oft-declared aspirations to change? Or, yet again, is the Soviet system best understood by comparing it to the German or French models which its spokesmen frankly acknowledged as the source of inspiration for many of their ideas? Whatever yardstick is used, the essays presented here attest to the rich potential of the material on social medicine for the large questions of interest to historians of Russia and the Soviet Union.

Contributors

MARK ADAMS is Associate Professor in the Department of History and Sociology of Science, University of Pennsylvania. His most recent publication is *The Wellborn Science: Eugenics in Germany, France, Brazil, and Russia* (Oxford, 1989). He is the head of the Soviet-American Project on the great emigre biologist Theodosius Dobzhansky.

LAURIE BERNSTEIN is Visiting Assistant Professor in the Department of History, Swarthmore College. She is currently revising for publication her dissertation on prostitution, and is planning a work on the cult of domesticity in the USSR in the 1930s.

JULIE BROWN is Associate Professor in the Department of History, University of North Carolina at Greensboro. Her articles have appeared in *Russian Review, Social Problems,* and *Social Research.* She is currently working on a monograph on the history of the Russian psychiatric profession.

CHRISTOPHER M. DAVIS is Lecturer in Soviet Studies at the Centre for Russian and East European Studies, University of Birmingham. He is the author of numerous articles on the Soviet health sector, co-editor of *Models of Disequilibrium and Shortage in Centrally Planned Economies* (London, 1979), and is now engaged in research on the economics of Soviet defense.

SALLY EWING is a Fellow of the Russian and East European Studies Center, University of Illinois at Urbana-Champaign. Her research interests are the sociology of law and cultural studies. She is currently preparing a study of the impact of the social sciences on the development of cultural forms after the Russian revolution.

JOHN HUTCHINSON is Associate Professor in the Department of History, Simon Fraser University, and the author of *The Cleansing Hurricane: Politics and Public Health in Revolutionary Russia, 1900–1918* (Johns Hopkins University Press, 1990). He is now working on a history of the Red Cross.

SAMUEL RAMER is Associate Professor in the Department of History, Tulane University. His research interests lie in the area of Russian social and cultural history from 1861 to 1941.

LEWIS H. SIEGELBAUM is Professor in the Department of History, Michigan State University. He is the author of *Stakhanovism and the Politics of Productivity in the USSR* (Cambridge, England, 1988), and is currently writing a book on the Soviet state and society in the 1920s.

SUSAN GROSS SOLOMON is Associate Professor in the Department of Political Science, University of Toronto. She is the author of *The Soviet Agrarian Debate: A Controversy in Social Science, 1923–1929* (Westview Press, 1977) and the editor of *Pluralism in the Soviet Union* (Macmillan, 1983). She is currently writing a history of Soviet social hygiene between 1921 and 1936.

NEIL WEISSMAN is Associate Professor in the Department of History, Dickinson College. He is the author of *Reform in Tsarist Russia: The State Bureaucracy and Local Government, 1900–1914* (New Brunswick, N.J., 1981). He is currently writing a book on police and deviance in early Soviet Russia.

Index

Agriculture: public health, 147, 154, 160; eugenics, 205

Alcoholism: constraints on health reform, xiii; social hygiene research, 185–89; postrevolutionary increase, 197n; restriction of liquor, 198n

All-Russian Medical-Sanitary Workers Union. *See* Vsemedikosantrud

Anthropogenetics: eugenics and public policy, 215–18

Anthropology: Russian eugenics, 208

Army, Red: physicians and Civil War, 106; sanitation and Civil War, 107; feldshers, 123–24, 126, 130

Asylums: origins of psychiatry, 27–29; cost and zemstvos, 29–30; 1905 Revolution and political prisoners, 32–33; police and control of, 33; decentralization of psychiatric care, 34–38; early twentieth century, 38–41; World War I, 42

Bacteriology: community physicians and health reform, ix–x; populist ideology and zemstvo medicine, 10, 12; general hygiene, 176

Bolsheviks: health reform, xi, 246; destruction of zemstvo medicine, 3–4; from workers' insurance to unified Soviet medicine, 73–76; medical policy before October Revolution, 99; centralization of medical administration, 100–102; urbanism and political base, 121; eugenics and public health, 200

Brothels: government regulation, 45, 58–61. *See* Prostitution

Centralization: Lenin and Bolshevik Revolution, 19; tsarist regime and health administration, 98–99; establishment of Narkomzdrav, 101; Narkomzdrav and New Economic Policy, 115–16

Cholera: medical centralization and tsarist regime, 99

Civil War: working-class politics and insurance movement, 74; accounting and control of workers' insurance, 84; jurisdictional struggle between Narkomtrud and Narkomsobes, 93n; Narkomzdrav and health administration, 102–107; *rotnye* feldshers, 130; industrial safety, 226

Class: early psychiatry, 29; police and regulation of prostitution, 49; proletariat and Soviet medicine, 69–70, 76–83, 154–55; politics and Soviet medicine, 78; workers' insurance medicine, 82, 90–91; Bolsheviks and Soviet medical administration, 106; expertise and health administration, 127

Collectivization: rural feldshers, 138; public health in 1930s, 160

Commissariat of Labor. *See* Narkomtrud

Commissariat of Public Health. *See* Narkomzdrav

Commissariat of Social Welfare. *See* Narkomsobes

Community medicine: general hygiene, 176; social hygiene, 180

Criminals: psychiatrists and control of asylums, 33–34

Cultural Revolution: workers and social insurance, 94n; social hygiene, 192; eugenics, 218–20; industrial revolution, 233–37

Economics: constraints on health reform, xii; tsarist regime and asylums, 29; zemstvos and asylums, 35, 43n; Narkomtrud and Medical Experts Commission, 88–89; Medical Commissions and Narkomzdrav, 95n; New Economic Policy and funding of medical facilities, 108; funding of Narkomzdrav and New Economic Policy, 111–12; transfer of public health to local budgets, 132–33; Narkomzdrav and five-year plans, 146–47, 151–52, 156–57, 163, 166–67; medical system in 1927–28, 147–50; medical system in 1929, 152, 154–56; medical system in 1930–32, 160–63; industrial safety, 229–30

Education, medical: constraints on health reform, xiii; feldshers, 123, 124–25, 128–29, 129–32, 134–35, 139; physicians and Narkomzdrav, 127–28, 248; physicians in 1930s, 161–62; social hygiene, 181–85, 190, 191

England: health reform and zemstvo ideology, 14

Ermanskii, O. A.: industrial hygiene, 230–31, 239–40

Eugenics: Bolsheviks and public health, 200; origins and definition, 201–202; origins of Russian, 202–203; postrevolutionary Russia, 203–205, 208–10; organizations, 205–206; discipline-building, 206; Russian Eugenics Society, 207–208, 219; public policy, 210–18; Cultural Revolution, 218–20

Europe: prostitution regulation and venereal disease, 61; physicians and social insurance system, 95n; Soviet health care during 1920s, 110

Factories: workers and medical care, 83; medical care in early twentieth century, 91n–92n; tsarist regime and working conditions, 225; working conditions and accidents in 1920s, 229

Faingold, B. I.: workers' insurance, 76–82

Feldshers: Narkomzdrav and Soviet health care in 1920s, 116; prerevolutionary Russia, 121–24; professionalization prior to 1917, 124–25; professional movement and revolutions of 1917, 125–27; Soviet regime, 127–29; education and rural health care, 129–32; transfer of public health to local budgets, 132–33; elimination and